Made Whole

More Than 145 Anti-Inflammatory Keto-Paleo Recipes
to Nourish You from the Inside Out

CRISTINA CURP

from *The Castaway Kitchen*

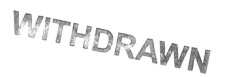

VICTORY BELT PUBLISHING INC.

Las Vegas

First Published in 2018 by Victory Belt Publishing Inc.

Copyright © 2018 Cristina Curp

ISBN-13: 978-1-628602-94-4

Cover Design by Charisse Reyes and Justin-Aaron Velasco
Interior Design by Yordan Terziev and Boryana Yordanova

Printed in Canada
TC 0318

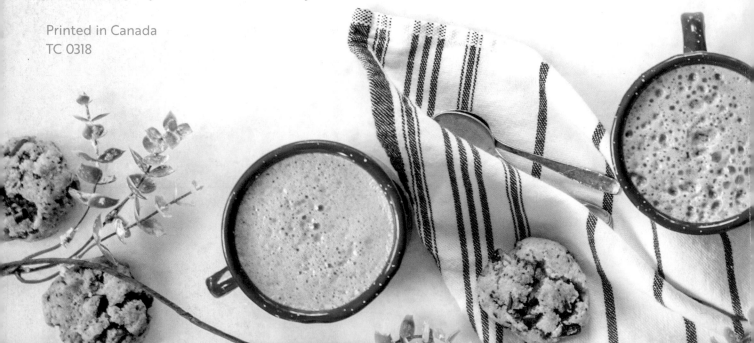

I dedicate this book to my mother, my greatest teacher and best friend.

And to all of you who have been overlooked and cast aside by doctors and society, left to live with chronic pain, fatigue, and mystery symptoms, told that there is no cure for what ails you and that you just have to deal with it. All of you who have ever felt "less than," I see you. This book is for those who look beyond, the Google doctors and self-taught researchers, those who refuse to give up and who know that they deserve more. You are pioneers, and this book is for you, your health, and your vitality!

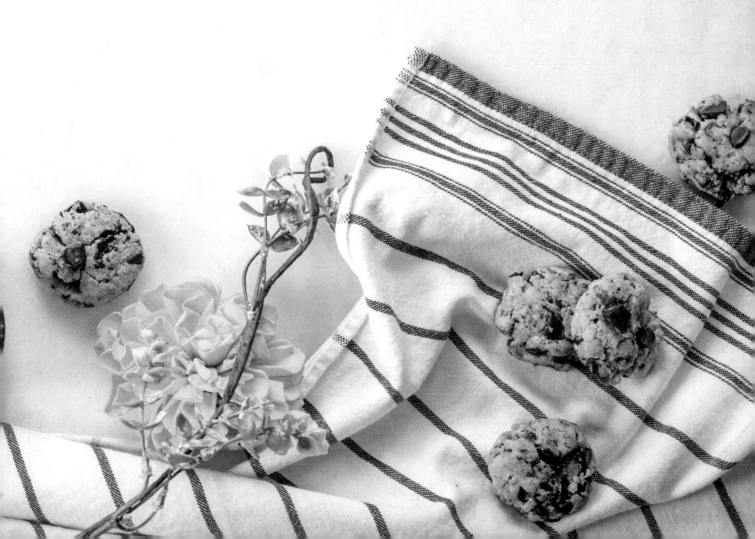

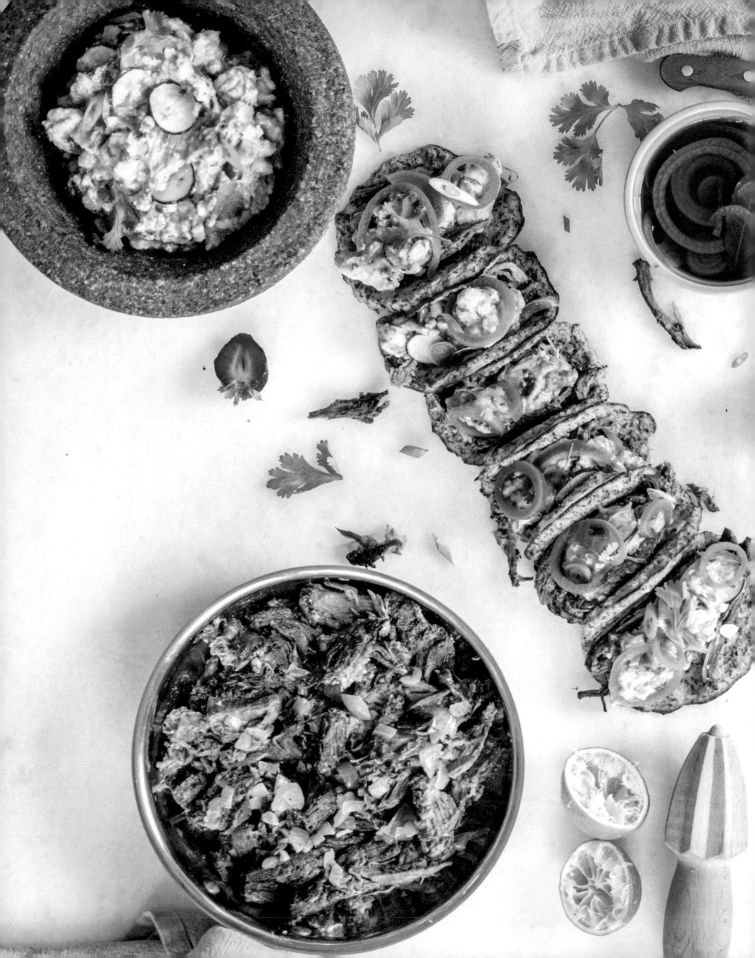

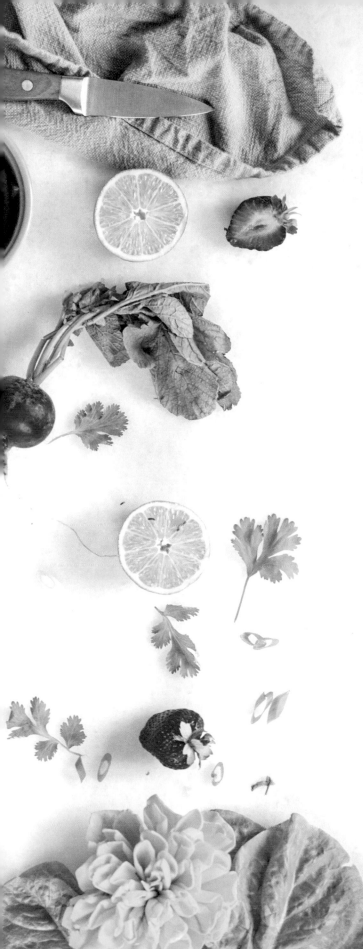

contents

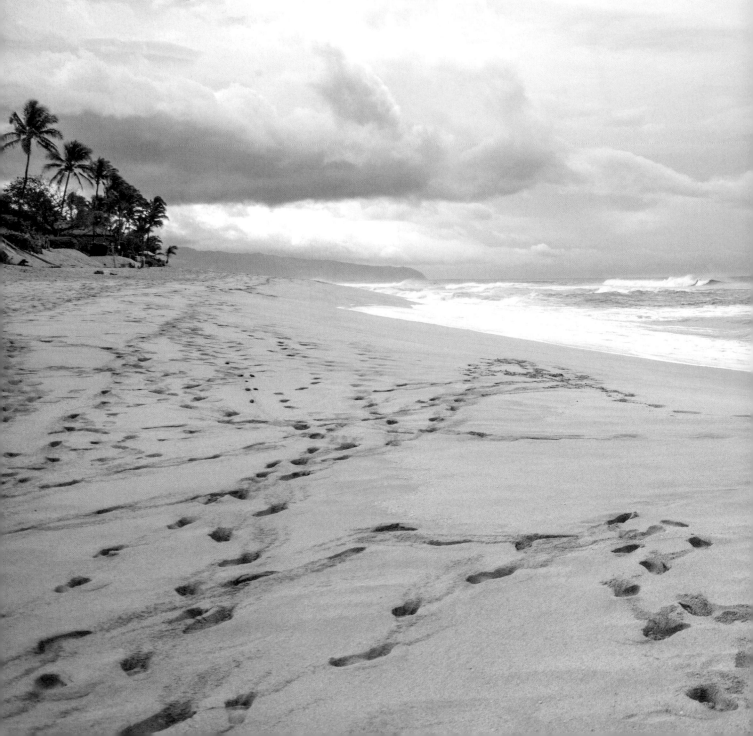

Make Whole (VERB):

To restore to a sound, healthy,
or favorable condition.
To repair. To heal.

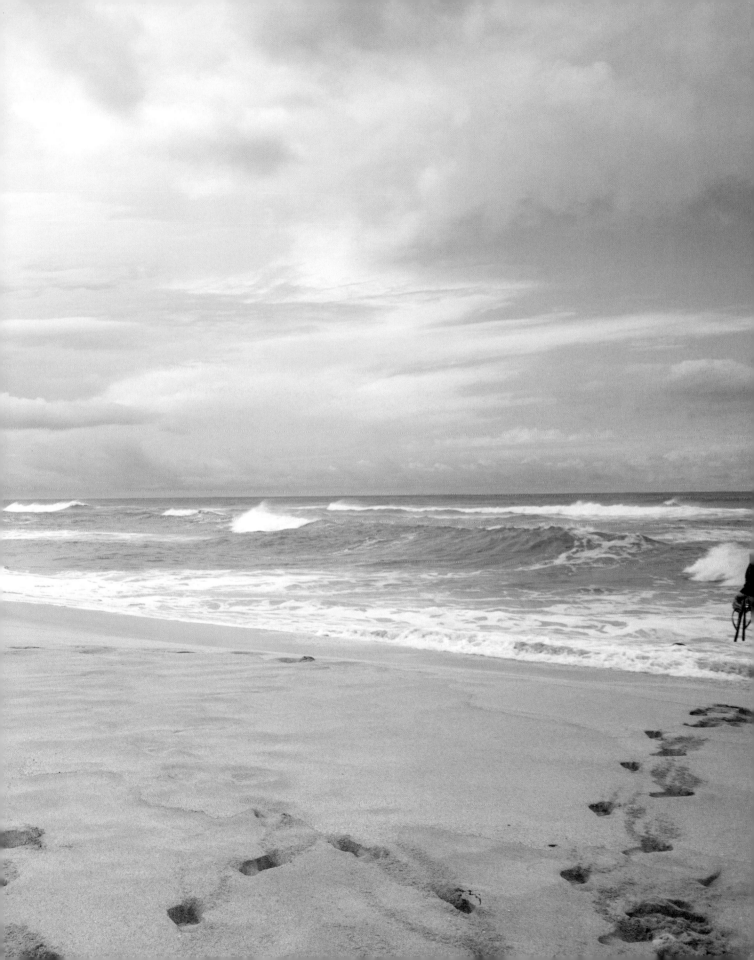

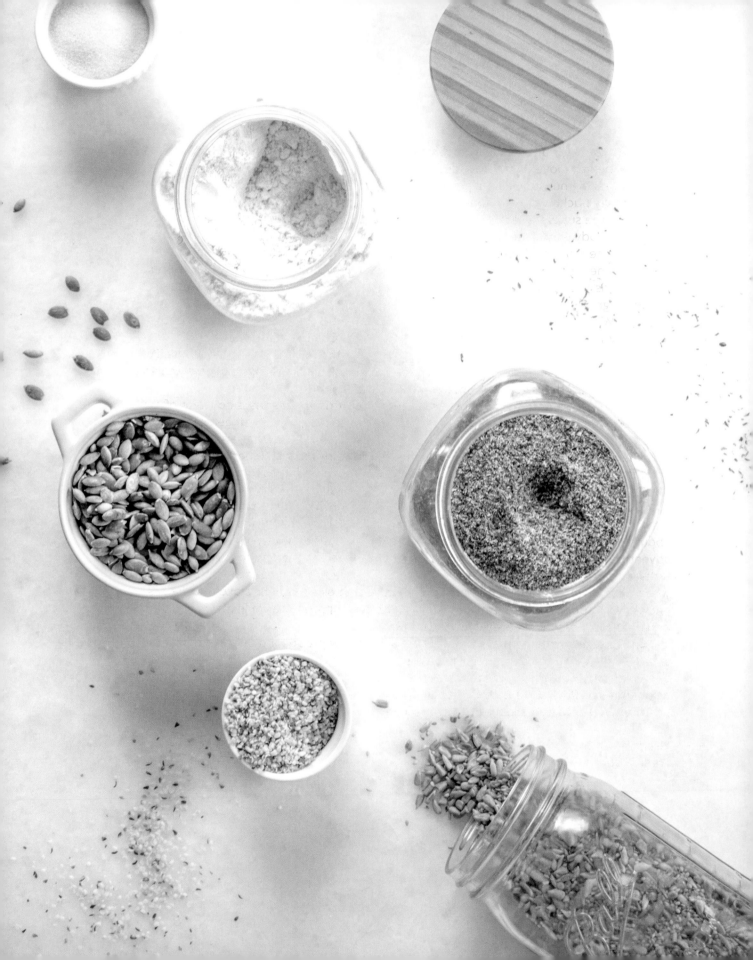

foreword

Over the past three and a half years, Cristina Curp has embodied the rise of the ancestral health movement. Grounded in her commitments to appreciating quality food, embracing nutrition as the greatest wellness weapon at our disposal, and unabashedly bucking conventional wisdom, her rapid ascension from a little-known blogger to the superstar behind *The Castaway Kitchen* is as inspiring as it is unsurprising to me. Anybody who's interacted with Cristina has felt the authenticity and unapologetic optimism she radiates. These are just a few of the attributes that shine through in her mission to help others reach their greatest heights. This relentlessly vivacious spirit has become Cristina's calling card—and is the common thread that runs throughout this book, her greatest creation yet.

Made Whole is an absolute knockout. Crafted masterfully in a manner that's both informative and entertaining, this book is packed with Cristina's unmistakable wit, culinary genius, and unapologetic belief in embracing the best life has to offer. Just like its author, it's approachable, easy to relate to, and prioritizes what matters most: making damn good food that's good for you. In the end, that's what it's all about.

Fueled by her contagious enthusiasm for quality nutrition, Cristina is now one of the top resources for every culinary offering in the Paleo, low-carb, and ketogenic realms. As a result, every recipe in *Made Whole* is made with only whole, natural, and unprocessed ingredients. They're also free of gluten, grains, sugar, dairy, nuts, starches, nightshades, and alcohol, making it perfect cookbook for anybody who adheres to the keto, Paleo, AIP, or allergen-free diets. It's like a primal Swiss Army knife.

If you're new to the ancestral health world or are cooking for the whole family, fear not: *Made Whole* is neither militaristic nor rigid in its approach. Instead, it's all about accessibility and making pushing your culinary boundaries what it should be: an adventure. Paired with beautiful photography, every recipe is easy to follow and created to take the intimidation out of cooking. Whether you're a food fanatic or somebody who wants to get in and out of the kitchen, you've come to the right place. This baby's packed with tools and tips to minimize your effort and prep time while making nutrient-dense, easy-to-make meals everyone will love.

I can't say enough about this must-read book or how proud I am of Cristina. This user-friendly guide to eating well will help you discover your inner gourmet chef while enjoying every last bite of the healthiest meals you've ever made. In truth, this isn't just a cookbook: it's the ultimate trail map to ditching diets and discovering a path to health and happiness created especially for you. Enjoy every step of the journey, my friends.

Yours in health,
Mark Sisson

You've entered the
realm of real food in
search of something.
Let me help you
navigate your way
through this realm and
teach you what I have
learned in my own
journey. As the proverb
goes, I won't give you
a fish—I will teach you
how to fish.

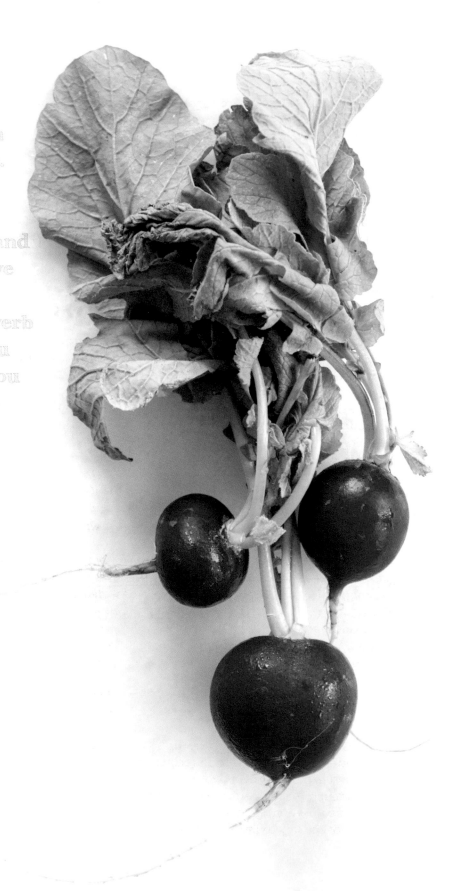

Introduction

Food and I have been through a lot together. We've loved each other for as long as I can remember, but food hasn't always been a friend to me. Sometimes I couldn't get enough of it. It would comfort me, delight me. I could lose myself in food. Sometimes food was the cause of illness; often it was a source of guilt. As with all relationships, we had to change, evolve—mature. I'm proud to say that since I've reexamined what's important, we're stronger than ever. We make each other better.

I'm not a nutritionist, a professional athlete, or a hundred-pound-weight-loss success story. I am a chef, a mother, and a food lover who wanted to remedy my relationship with food. I wanted to enjoy it without feeling sick and tired all the time. I was that person who would complain of health issues, weight issues, and mood issues and immediately follow those complaints with, "But I eat healthy enough."

Was I eating healthy enough? Maybe for someone else, but as it turned out, not for me, even though I have always loved vegetables and have always cooked from scratch. Eventually, when I became serious about optimizing my diet, I went gluten-free, which led me to the Whole30, which converted me to Paleo, and finally I did the autoimmune protocol (AIP). I went through more than two years of elimination diets and self-experimentation—healing, moving, reading. Through research, trial and error, and troubleshooting, I found my way to keto.

It hasn't been easy learning the causes of inflammation in my body. Changing from overeater couch potato to health advocate, active go-getter, and self-employed mom. Finally learning the cause of my hidradenitis suppurativa and regaining control of my health. I had to fight tooth and nail for every inch of success.

The good part: I made progress! I committed for the long haul. I put my autoimmune disease in remission, and, yes, I lost some weight along the way. For someone who has struggled with being overweight most of her life, it was a big win. My biggest triumph, though, has been the lasting changes in my life. Eating whole foods is no longer a chore, a fad, a means to an end. It's a forever way of eating.

This diet is different for everyone; my keto might not look like your keto, and that is okay. The way you eat is a very personal, biological, and emotional choice. That's where this book comes in. Here, I share my favorite recipes—delicious, I-can't-wait-to-make-it kinds of meals—with options for customizing them for your needs.

Focusing on an anti-inflammatory approach to keto, this book goes the distance. You'll notice a few ingredients "missing" in a lot of these recipes, from nuts and dairy to sugar and gluten. I wanted to show the world that no matter what your food triggers are, no matter what ails you, you can eat well.

This book is an "I cook for my family every damn day" book. It's for those who are still figuring out how they will eat like this forever, and for those who want to eat better, feel better, and be better but don't know where to start or feel stuck in their journey.

This book is for you. Since you picked up a cookbook with the title *Made Whole*, you're surely interested in whole-food recipes. Maybe you're a foodie who loves cooking from scratch and exploring new flavor profiles—or maybe you're not completely at home in the kitchen. Maybe you've tried a lot of diets, yo-yoing for years, always let down by ultrarestrictive programs that yielded subpar results. I bet a lot of you are like me, searching for the key to lifelong vitality!

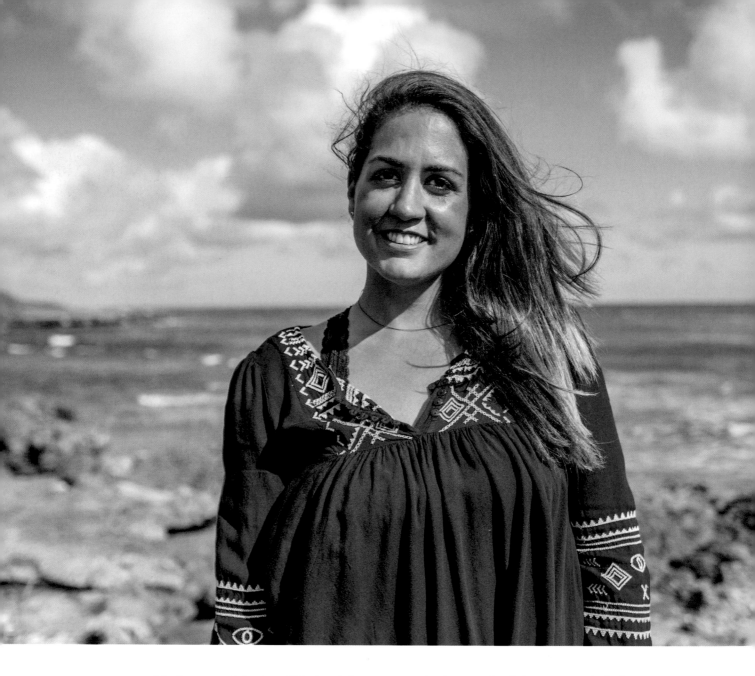

Maybe you picked up this book because you're in search of the missing link. I'm not talking about the lizard man; I'm talking about recipes that consistently make you feel your best without spending loads of time in the kitchen or sacrificing flavor.

Maybe you are a Paleo, AIP, or Whole30 veteran and are interested in trying keto. Perhaps you have been keto for a while but like the sound of a squeaky-clean anti-inflammatory approach. Maybe you just love pretty pictures of delicious food.

I take all kinds. Welcome, all of you. Whatever it is you're here for, I know two things for sure: there are no negative side effects to eating well, and eat well we will!

In these pages, you will find more than 145 recipes that will nourish your body, tantalize your taste buds, and expand your dietary horizons. Warning: We're going to do some pretty crazy stuff with cauliflower.

I want you to love the food that loves you back!

my story

I'm Cristina, a thirtysomething mother and wife. I've been overweight my whole life. I have suffered from a pretty ugly skin condition since I was a tween (did I just use that word?). I always felt a little lost, a little foggy—distracted. There was this overwhelming sensation of *I can't* that rippled throughout my life.

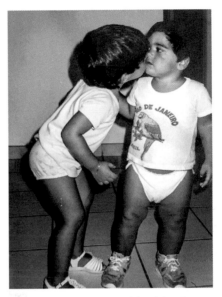

My sister Laura, age 3, and me, age 2

Obviously, that changed, because you're reading this book. And let me tell you, "can't" isn't going to get a book written—or a life changed, or a diet cleaned up, or a body healed.

I was born in Miami to Cuban immigrants. My parents' lives have been difficult; they suffered more than most before they were even teenagers. It often seems as if their past—living in a communist country, being persecuted, fleeing in boats, starting over with nothing—happened to other people. My parents are the most loving, hardworking, and honest humans I have ever met. My childhood was one of dreams and fairy tales. So much love, amazing family adventures—and an abundance of good food. Really good food.

My family is full of avid cooks and maternal figures who dote on their loved ones by feeding them. Cooking is in my blood. My father owns a butcher shop, and my mother owns a farm-to-table café. As schoolchildren, my sister and I were those kids who took giant thermoses of picadillo and rice for lunch. My mother, famous for her delicious meals, was—and still is—unwavering in her commitment to nourish her family…and everyone else. Our house was always brimming with guests relishing large, vibrant salads and grilled meats. This was where my love of food was born, where I first learned to cook: an eat-in kitchen with a red ceramic sink and a table full of friends and family.

Perhaps my love of food growing up was too big, or perhaps I had metabolic damage and leaky gut at a young age, or maybe it was just because of the unhealthy food reward system I had going on, but I don't have memories where I wasn't overweight. Pair that with my autoimmune skin condition, hidradenitis suppurativa, which showed up during puberty, and my insecurities spiraled; I suffered through my school years and beyond.

After graduating from college and spending a few sordid years exploring the Miami nightlife, burnt out from my marketing job and going nowhere, I went to work for my mother. I know what you're thinking, but it was actually really fun (most of the time). She's a tough boss. That lady expects nothing but the best. At Green Gables Café, her successful restaurant in the heart of Coral Gables, I fine-tuned my natural ability to cook into professional chef skills. I learned from a host of multicultural chefs who came through that kitchen. I also washed dishes, bussed tables, made deliveries. When it's a family business, you have to do it all.

One fine day, or should I say night, I met a sailor at a bar. We fell in love and moved to San Diego. Justin and I loved being in San Diego—the weather, the farms, the food! I worked on a biodiesel food truck that served up farm-fresh food. Newly wed and living in a beautiful city, we adopted our handsome schnauzer, Bruce, and sometime around Justin's first deployment, we got some news. Jack came about nine months later, two weeks late and weighing almost 11 pounds. Our lives and hearts would never be the same.

When we PCSed (a military term for moving, again) to Hawaii, Jack was nearly two and my inflammation and body fat were at an all-time high. I was riddled with hidradenitis suppurativa (that skin condition I mentioned). I had postpartum depression. I didn't know anyone in Hawaii, and without a support system, feeling completely lost, overwhelmed, and unhappy, I hit rock-bottom. This is coming from a Miami nightlife veteran, so I know rock-bottom, and surprisingly, it wasn't in the bathroom of a seedy bar. It was in me. It came from years of abusing my body, my hormones, and my metabolism. My system had been mistreated and put under enormous amounts of stress. Taking care of a toddler was the straw that broke the camel's back. I'm fairly certain I temporarily lost my mind, going through the days like a mindless robot, so unhappy I couldn't stand my own company. Dramatic much? You betcha!

I felt so awful that I needed a change. When life seems crazy and out of your control, the one thing you can *always* control is what you eat. No one will ever tie you down and shove food in your mouth. So I took control of what I could, and I did a Whole30, an amazing, totally free, community-oriented thirty-day program. Thirty days of whole foods, with no grains, no dairy, no sweets, no booze—just plants, animals, nuts, and seeds. It's a reset diet, and it works. (You can learn more about the program at Whole30.com.) That first Whole30 kicked off what became the most transformative years of my life.

Since then, I've put my skin condition in remission (life-changing!), shed quite a bit of body fat, gained muscle and confidence, and, most of all, reclaimed my sense of self-worth. I never thought I would love, worship, and care for myself the way I do now. Even writing that feels weird.

In this society of ours, we're conditioned to be more comfortable with hating ourselves than loving ourselves. Time to cut that out. Self-love is back, baby. Self-love is the key: eating well is a way of respecting yourself, and working out is a celebration of what your body is capable of. I spent my whole life on a diet, punishing myself at the gym for the food I had binged on the night before in a vicious cycle of guilt and punishment. Now I've found a way of eating that isn't about dieting, and when I talk about working out or movement, I mean moving your body in a way that feels good for you. That shift in focus, from thinking of food and exercise as punishment to thinking of them as forms of self-love, was just as revolutionary as the changes I made in what I put on my plate and in my body. It's about shifting your perspective from *I can't* to *I choose*, from *restriction* to *celebration*. That, folks, is the key to making lasting positive change.

My one superpower, other than making a beautiful child and having a super-cheesy sense of humor, is my uncanny ability to create a delicious meal from anything, and I mean *anything*. Got some beef jerky, a can of olives, and one egg? I can make it work— I'm part MacGyver, part Julia Child. In college, I could scrounge up whatever scraps and leftovers were left in the fridge and create a hangover brunch that resembled a royal feast. I attribute this skill to being raised by Cuban immigrants, and it has come in handy as I have navigated the many roads to health. I created tons of new recipes during my three years of Paleo, six rounds of Whole30, six months of the autoimmune protocol, and more than a year of keto. What you will find in these pages is the final destination of my search for a way of eating that heals my body while nourishing and supporting my (newly) active lifestyle.

When we moved to Hawaii, I found solace in cooking and sharing my meals online. This has evolved into my full-time work, and it is truly my dream job—creating recipes, providing resources, and spreading inspiration to those who need it. *The Castaway Kitchen* is my website, a tool, a collection of recipes and entries chronicling my own healing journey. More than just a blog, *The Castaway Kitchen* has become an amazing online community; on Instagram and Facebook, thousands share and support each other in their quest for health and wellness. Creating recipes is my favorite thing to do, bested only by the amazing feeling of helping others. Through *The Castaway Kitchen,* I get to do both, and it is truly magical.

You know the saying, "When Mama's happy, everyone is happy"? The change in me has truly changed our family for the best. We're thriving and healthy, positive and stronger together. Hawaii will always be special to us. It's where it all happened: starting *The Castaway Kitchen* out of a hotel room, coming in somewhere over 250 pounds, feeling pretty miserable about myself, yet finally seeing the light at the end of my postpartum depression. Hawaii is the place where we healed as individuals and as a family, inside and out. Now Jack, Justin, Bruce, and I are headed to Washington, DC. We're excited to be closer to our family back east and are embracing this new chapter in our lives.

As I write this in Kailua, Hawaii, I truly hope the love and energy poured into this book transcend these pages and give you some semblance of the inspiration I have felt creating it for you.

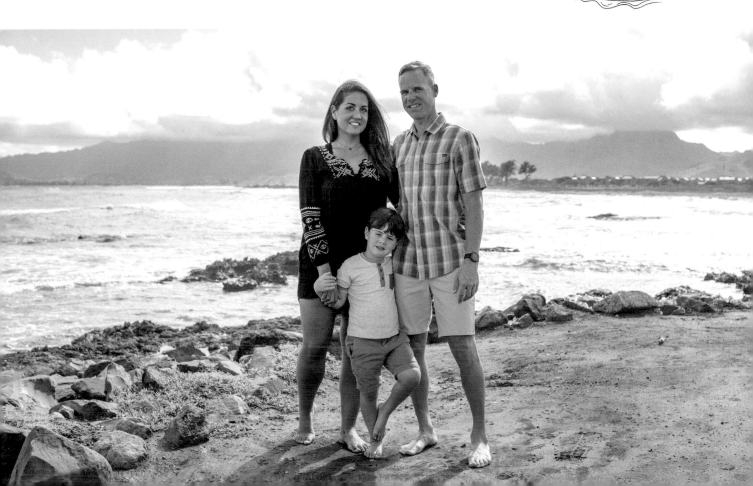

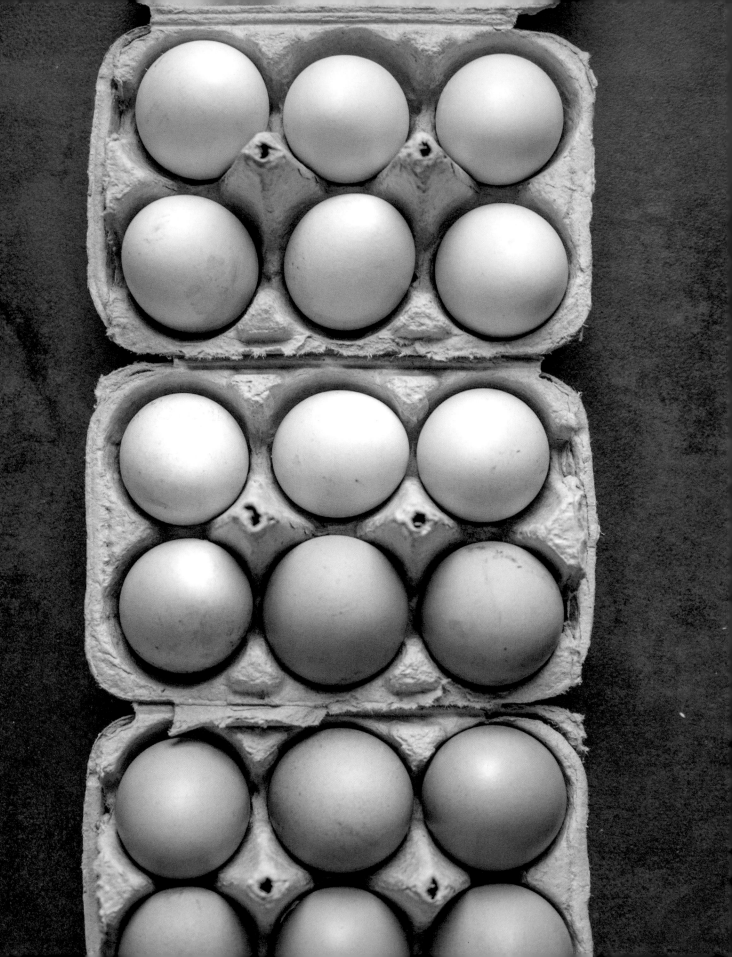

Knowledge Is Power

This book combines a few popular gut-healing, fat-burning, inflammation-crushing approaches to food: Paleo, the autoimmune protocol, and keto. They're all well-known, proven diets that can change and heal your body.

But before we get into the details of Paleo, AIP, and keto, let's talk about why so many of us need a healing diet in the first place. And for that, we need to talk about what's going on under the hood—and how what you're using to fuel your body might affect more than just your gut.

connecting the dots...or symptoms

It's amazing how much what we eat is connected to how good we feel. And I'm not just talking about feeling sluggish after a carb-heavy meal or sick after gorging on candy. What we eat directly affects how the body's systems function, and it's linked to three problems that are common in Americans today: leaky gut, liver dysfunction, and insulin resistance.

leaky gut

Gut health—*not weight*—is the key to good health. Skinny does not equal healthy, and the scale and your waistline need to take a back seat to gut health, which affects not only physical but also emotional health and therefore determines your quality of life. One of the biggest threats to gut health is leaky gut.

"Leaky gut" has become a buzz term in recent years, the mysterious source of so many chronic illnesses. It's exactly what it sounds like: with leaky gut, proteins and bacteria escape through tiny gaps between the cells lining the intestines and hitch a ride in the lymphatic system or bloodstream. This sounds the alarm for the immune system, which releases cytokines, little messengers that get our white blood cells to attack foreign bodies—exactly as they're supposed to. Unfortunately, the immune system can get overzealous and begin to attack not just foreign bodies but also our own healthy cells, causing inflammation. When this happens, your body is literally attacking itself.

There are many possible symptoms of leaky gut, ranging from digestive discomfort (bloating, burping, constipation, diarrhea) to skin conditions (acne, rashes, psoriasis, itchy skin), neurological symptoms (brain fog, fatigue, headaches, depression), and general aches, pains, and malnutrition.

Sometimes the immune system has no specific target and any part of the body is open to attack. Other times, when autoimmune disease is present, the immune system attacks specific parts of the body. In folks with rheumatoid arthritis, the joints are attacked. In people with multiple sclerosis, it's the nerves. With Hashimoto's, it's the thyroid. And so it goes.

Well, that sounds scary as hell, Cristina. How do you get leaky gut in the first place? Excellent question. Food definitely plays a role, which I'll talk about in a minute, but not everyone has the same reactions to the same foods. Some people have very healthy guts and can eat anything under the sun with little to no reactions at all (like my husband, insert grumble here). Unfortunately, those of us who suffer from leaky gut likely got it because we have a predisposition to autoimmune disease (family history), we abused our systems with too much medicine (medical history), or it was triggered by severe stress (prolonged or in one event). Again, though, some people could have all of these risk factors and still not have leaky gut. Food plays a role, too, and to understand that, we need to understand what antinutrients are.

Antinutrients are plants' natural defense system. They're mild toxins or irritants that make the plant hard to digest—basically, something that keeps the plant from being eaten. They also can impair the absorption of healthy nutrients, causing nutrient deficiency. Most importantly, some antinutrients harm the lining of the gut. Remember how, in leaky gut, proteins and bacteria in the gut escape through gaps in the intestinal wall? Antinutrients are one reason those gaps develop. And if you already have leaky gut, consuming antinutrients can cause inflammation.

There are several types of antinutrients:

◦ **Lectins, solanine, saponin:** Found in beans, nuts, wheat, and most vegetables with skin and seeds, these antinutrients survive digestion and can penetrate the gut lining.

◦ **Gluten:** The most difficult to digest protein, extremely irritating to the gut, gluten is found in wheat, barley, and rye. Gluten is also found in a lot of unsuspected products, like soy sauce, supplements, commercially produced soups and broths, and more.

◦ **Tannins:** Found in red wine, these enzyme inhibitors prevent the proper digestion of protein.

◦ **Oxalates:** Found in coffee, sesame seeds, and beans, these can interfere with nutrient absorption. Never take medication or supplements within two hours of drinking coffee.

◦ **Phytic acid:** Found in grains, legumes, nuts, seeds, and coconut, this can interfere with the absorption of minerals and inhibits the digestive enzymes that break down starch and proteins.

Antinutrients are found in all plants; however, many foods, like those allowed on the autoimmune protocol, contain lower levels, and the benefits of eating them greatly outweigh any possible harmful effects of antinutrients. After all, we have to eat something!

The good news is that there are many ways to further reduce the antinutrient content of foods, so even though you may not be able to enjoy nuts or seeds now, perhaps after healing your leaky gut, you can enjoy them sprouted! Look at how our ancestors prepared foods—sprouting, fermenting, and soaking are all preparation methods that make foods much easier to digest.

liver dysfunction

The gut is rarely in jeopardy alone. Because leaky gut often develops as a result of a combination of severe stress, genetics, and medical history, the body as a whole is overburdened—overmedicated, overstressed, suffering from not enough sleep, and exposed to environmental toxins. And all of these factors come together to overwork the liver.

The immune system isn't the only thing that responds to the bacteria and proteins that get into the bloodstream because of leaky gut. The liver filters these toxins out of the bloodstream. But when the liver is overworked because of all the factors that led to leaky gut in the first place, the toxins can run amok. And since part of the liver's job is to filter out hormones, when the liver is overworked, those hormones can become out of balance. It's all tied together.

On top of stress, lack of sleep, medications, and environmental toxins, food itself can burden the liver. Nonalcoholic fatty liver disease is on the rise, and it's directly related to the consumption of carbohydrates. The liver converts excess carbohydrates to fatty acids, which are stored in the liver as well as in fat tissue. Over time, this fat in the liver can build up, leading to fatty liver disease. In addition, insulin resistance (which I'll talk more about in a moment) increases this accumulation of fat in the liver.

This diseased and taxed liver now has trouble doing its many important jobs—including filtering out excess estrogen. Yup, the liver (and the gut) is in charge of filtering out excess sex hormones. With so many estrogenic compounds in today's environment, it's got a big job to do. And it can't do it if it's overworked and diseased.

insulin resistance

Insulin resistance occurs when your body cannot use carbohydrates efficiently. Normally, when carbohydrates are ingested, they're broken down into glucose and shuttled into the bloodstream. Blood sugar rises, and insulin is secreted by the pancreas to move this glucose into cells, which use it for energy. As insulin moves glucose from the bloodstream into cells, blood sugar returns to normal.

But if you're constantly eating a lot of carbs, your pancreas has to pump out more and more insulin to handle all the glucose. In response, your cells, overwhelmed by insulin, stop listening to it and no longer accept the glucose it's trying to move out of the bloodstream. This is insulin resistance: your body has become resistant to insulin's message.

When you're insulin resistant, the pancreas secretes more insulin to get the cells to listen. Eventually, though, the pancreas wears out and can't produce enough insulin to keep blood sugar stable. Then blood sugar is chronically elevated, and when it gets high enough, you're diagnosed with type 2 diabetes.

In addition, insulin resistance can impede weight loss, even when you're doing everything right. What we eat directly affects our insulin, which affects our hormones, which affect our liver—and when it comes to the body, that kind of synergy is the rule, not the exception. While I made a point about your weight not being a primary marker for health, once you have healed leaky gut and hormone imbalance, shedding excess body fat should happen organically with a whole-foods keto lifestyle.

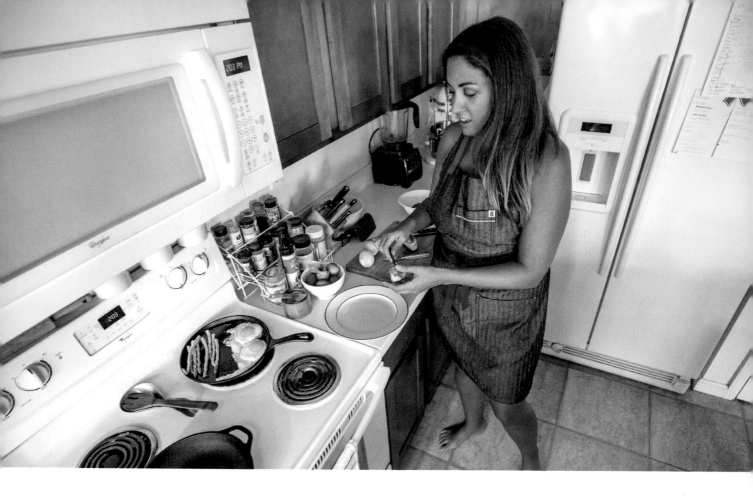

the healing process

Although I've talked about leaky gut, liver dysfunction, and insulin resistance separately above, let's be clear: When healing your body, you can't look at problems in different systems as isolated issues. Rather, you have to look at your body as a whole, as an ecosystem that needs to find balance. And keep in mind, too, that healing is a process, and it's not always an easy one. While going gluten-free and/or dairy-free is enough to help a lot of people resolve their inflammatory issues, some of us—ahem, me (maybe you too)—need to go the extra mile (or ten).

In my case, with a lot of stored fat on my body—body fat that I carried around through years of drug use, smoking, drinking, and eating crap—there were a lot of toxins (which are stored in fat) in my system. I also had insulin resistance and estrogen dominance, which usually go hand in hand. All of this was hard on my liver. I needed to give my liver a break and lower my estrogen levels so my liver could focus on eliminating toxins instead of being overburdened by estrogen.

For me, going keto is what helped. I'll talk a lot more about keto later in this chapter, but for now, the important part is that keto keeps blood sugar stable and gets the body to burn stored body fat. From self-experimentation and research, I deduced that this would alleviate the stress on the liver. No longer taxed with excess insulin, it would metabolize stored body fat and the body would begin to heal and detoxify.

As my body began to metabolize this toxic body fat, free radicals were released into my system. I experienced short bouts of detox symptoms, usually loose stools, fatigue, and acne. During these times, I supported my system by sticking to very simple, clean meals—no processed foods—and lots of water, as well as plenty of sleep. This could happen to you too. Healing isn't linear. Do not despair. Trust the process. Keep moving forward.

After each healing crisis passed I had more energy, less body fat, more muscle. With each passing month, I felt my digestive system and menstrual cycle regulate. I was sleeping better; I didn't need that afternoon coffee. I was able to tolerate foods previously omitted from my diet. When I went from being terrified to eat at restaurants to having the flexibility to have some nuts or dairy occasionally without reaction, I knew my body was healing!

There are numerous reasons why people have setbacks or hit roadblocks on their way to feeling awesome all the time, and I'll help you troubleshoot on pages 37 and 38. But let me be clear, it is possible to feel awesome all the time, and you don't have to settle for less. You don't have to live with chronic pain and inflammation. You deserve to have energy and mobility, and it *is* within your reach!

And remember, it's not *all* about food. Emotional and physical stress are big players, too. Stress is a killer, especially on a system that is already crippled. Knowing how to manage stress with healthy coping mechanisms, prioritizing self-care, and getting good sleep are key in healing. No matter how well you eat, if you are under a lot of stress or overtired, the body will not heal. I know that is hard to hear, because slowing down and making commitments to your health that affect your schedule are difficult—but they're absolutely necessary.

Overwhelmed yet? I know, it's a lot. The great thing is that you don't have to take it all on at once. Make one change at a time and deal with things as they come. Once you make dietary or lifestyle changes, you will see improvement, and then you might find something else that needs work. The body is like an onion—there are layers. As you heal, your body will finally open itself up for healing in areas you didn't even know needed it. Do not let this discourage you! Troubleshoot as you go. Know that eating real food, moving your body, sleeping well, and practicing self-care are never going to harm you.

Eventually you will switch from survival mode to thriving, and the good days will outnumber the bad. Give yourself grace, be patient, stay positive. You can do this.

the healing diets

I've combined three well-known diets to create a clean, whole-foods-focused, anti-inflammatory way of eating. As a basic template, we have the Paleo diet, which strongly focuses on whole foods and unprocessed high-quality ingredients. Then we have the autoimmune protocol, the gold standard in elimination diets, which helps people discover trigger foods that cause symptoms of autoimmune disease, leaky gut, and inflammation. Last, we apply that whole-foods, anti-inflammatory template to a keto approach, which eliminates sugar and reduces carbohydrates to transition the body from using sugar for energy to using fat, both dietary and stored on the body!

These three highly successful, well-tested, and trusted diets have a lot in common, and I've combined them to design a way of eating that's low-carb, that focuses on whole foods and nutrient density, and that reduces inflammation. As a bonus, it comes with finger-licking good recipes.

paleo!

The Paleo diet is widely known as the caveman diet, but it has greatly evolved from just trying to mimic the eating habits of prehistoric men and women. The basis of Paleo is avoiding all grains, dairy, gluten, legumes, refined sugars, and processed foods and focusing on whole foods. Think foods that you could eat without farming—plants that you could forage, animals you could hunt. Yet we live in a modern time, where we make flour from coconuts! So while cavemen certainly didn't have access to ghee or almond meal, these things are allowed on Paleo. Think plants and animals plus a few modern-day comforts like maple syrup and grain-free flour.

Folks on Paleo enjoy plenty of high-quality animal protein, with a big emphasis on sourcing (grass-fed meat in particular); healthy fats like coconut oil, avocado oil, olive oil, and animal fats; all the vegetables, including tubers; fruit, nuts, and seeds; and of course the ever-popular Paleo treats. While it is advised to stick to plants and animals, à la Whole30, most folks enjoy the occasional piece of cake, cookie, stuffed sweet potato, bacon-wrapped date, and other deliciously indulgent Paleo treats.

On the Paleo diet, cane sugar and other forms of processed sugar are not allowed. Most folks severely cut their sugar intake on Paleo and use sweeteners like coconut palm sugar, honey, and maple syrup in *much* smaller amounts.

Paleo is not a low-calorie diet. However, it is naturally lower in carbs than the Standard American Diet (SAD), which includes a lot of processed foods and about 500 grams of carbs per day. Paleo, which is made of ingredients, not packaged foods, naturally has around 150–200 grams of carbs per day. This reduction in carbs, along with the elimination of gluten and dairy (the two most common inflammatory foods), is why folks feel *amazing* when they make the switch to Paleo.

Plus, once you ditch processed foods, thereby eliminating a slew of filler ingredients—from binders, starches, and various forms of sugar to preservatives and artificial coloring and flavors—you can expect to see and feel some great things: clearer skin, better digestion (more regular bowel movements), even better sleep.

All the recipes in this book adhere to the Paleo approach, except in their use of sweeteners—as I'll discuss later, I've found that it works best to avoid sweeteners like honey and maple syrup, which are used without limit on Paleo. The sweeteners I use are borrowed from keto and are technically considered "processed." But I've found that they allow for a necessary reduction in carbs that's truly beneficial—see page 38 for more information.

HIGHLIGHT REEL

The Paleo template is a great starting point, with a focus on whole, grain-free, unprocessed foods and a lot of flexibility. Getting rid of processed foods, focusing on high-quality sources (especially of animal products), and naturally cutting down on carbs goes a long way toward making Paleo anti-inflammatory and healing.

the autoimmune protocol

There are more than eighty autoimmune diseases, they are notoriously difficult to diagnose, and most people with autoimmunity live with their diseases for decades without getting much help from their doctors. Which is why the autoimmune Paleo community is so vast, so active, and so strong. Citizen health activists are taking health care into their own hands. In forums, Facebook groups, meetups, and more, people are sharing what they learn, supporting each other, and helping each other heal.

The autoimmune protocol is one way people with autoimmune diseases and leaky gut can figure out how to heal their bodies. It's designed to uncover an individual's trigger foods—any foods that cause symptoms, from migraines and swollen joints to runny noses. A lot of people are ingesting foods that are causing them harm on a daily basis. Often the symptoms are so mild that people just live with them, but other times, they can be absolutely debilitating.

The autoimmune protocol eliminates specific foods based on their levels of antinutrients and gut permeability. All the excluded foods have the potential to irritate the digestive system, damage the gut, and, when leaky gut is present, even seep through the intestinal wall and trigger inflammation.

Unfortunately, leaky gut and autoimmune disease are the plague of my generation. It seems like more and more people are dealing with chronic pain, digestive issues, hormone imbalance, and other problems directly connected to systemic inflammation. Becoming familiar with the autoimmune protocol and the foods that can be inflammatory is very useful for troubleshooting!

Here's how to do it: Omit all of the foods listed below from your diet. Keep a log of how you sleep, your stress levels, and everything you eat. Take notes on everything. When you begin to feel better, add the excluded foods back in *slowly*. Reintroduce just one food at a time, wait, and brace yourself for a reaction. Take notes again on how you feel. If you feel fine, great! Add the food back to your diet. If you experience symptoms, it might be best to continue to stay away from that food. I did this, and while it didn't solve all my issues, it revealed a huge piece of my health puzzle and was a very informative and empowering experience.

✗ FOODS TO OMIT ON THE AIP ✗

- Coffee (I know, it's brutal)
- Cacao
- All grains
- All legumes (even green beans)
- All nuts
- All seeds
- Spices from seeds, nightshades, and berries (e.g., cumin, peppercorns, paprika)
- Eggs
- All dairy (even ghee and butter)
- All nightshades (peppers, eggplants, tomatoes, potatoes—sweet potatoes are fine)
- Processed sugars (honey and maple syrup are fine)
- Artificial sweeteners (even stevia)
- Processed foods (check labels for preservatives and emulsifiers)

FOODS ACCEPTED ON THE AIP ✓

- All animal proteins
- All vegetables and fruits (except nightshades—see the "omit" list)
- Coconut and coconut products (e.g., coconut milk, coconut flour)
- Non-seed-based spices (turmeric, cinnamon, etc.)
- Rendered animal fats
- Lard
- Bacon
- Avocados
- Olive oil
- Salt
- Herbs

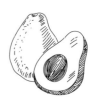

Yup, it's a doozy. But it helps. Now, as you will hear me say a few times in this book, there is no one-size-fits-all diet. Everyone has different trigger foods. No one can do the AIP for you, not even someone with the same autoimmune disease. Your trigger foods are specific to you and only you!

Tapioca and cassava root are used as binders in most AIP recipes, and plantains, sweet potatoes, and other starchy vegetables are used liberally. I ate them all! And while this elimination diet greatly helped me, I noticed that the starchy nature of the diet was causing some distress for me. That's when I began to dabble in low-carb and keto, which I'll talk more about in a few pages. Tweaking. Troubleshooting. Experimenting. It's the only way to really know what works for you. The point is, try everything, don't write anything off, no matter how scary it seems. *How you feel, your symptoms and your reactions, whether or not they show up on a lab test, are real to you. This is your health. You are the captain of your journey.*

That being said, the autoimmune protocol is widely successful. The first medical study on it was conducted last year with patients who had inflammatory bowel disease, and 73 percent saw improvement or remission! Here's what the researchers said: "Clinical remission was achieved by week 6 by 11/15 (73%) of study participants, and all 11 maintained clinical remission during the maintenance phase of the study. [This] rivals . . . most drug therapies for IBD."*

* G. Konijeti et al., "Efficacy of the Autoimmune Protocol Diet for Inflammatory Bowel Disease," *Inflammatory Bowel Diseases* 23, no. 11 (November 2017): 2054–2060.

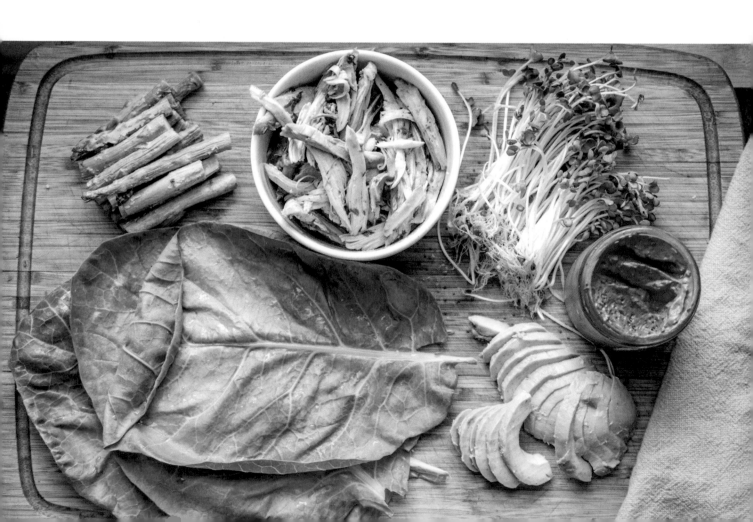

The recipes in this book borrow from the AIP by omitting—in addition to grains and processed foods, which Paleo also omits—nuts, dairy (except butter and ghee), and nightshades. Here is why.

 NIGHTSHADES: These are super sneaky and cause inflammation in a lot of unsuspecting folks. But if someone told you to stop eating them, you would be like, *What?? No way, not possible—how can you make a meal without these?* Well, with these recipes you have 148 ways you can do it. Most nightshade plants are poisonous, as in deadly. The edible ones—tomatoes, eggplants, peppers, and white potatoes—are edible, yes, but they still contain higher-than-normal levels of toxins, their natural defense system, which some folks can deal with just fine. Others, like Tom Brady and myself, not so much. Stiff joints, swelling, digestive distress—no thanks. We prefer to avoid the inflammation. (The internet said that Tom Brady avoids nightshades because it helps him recover faster by preventing inflammation. The internet doesn't lie.)

 NUTS: Nuts are one of those foods that are grossly overconsumed on most grain-free diets. These little delicious nuggets are meant to be eaten sparingly, not by the cup or repeated spoonful. They are also best consumed after soaking or activating (an ancient practice of soaking and drying nuts to make them easier to digest) to reduce their amount of phytic acid, an antinutrient that can interfere with nutrient absorption and disrupt digestion. Also, there are lots of allergies to nuts out in the world—so again, a whole book of delicious, without nuts.

 DAIRY: Milk from any animal is breast milk, and as such it's designed to permeate the gut lining to share the mama's immunity with the baby. Plus, when we drink another mammal's breast milk, we're taking in that animal's antibodies and hormones—and humans have bioidentical hormones to cows', and those hormones are in cow's milk. So when we drink cow's milk, those hormones may interact with our bodies. Thanks, but no thanks. The proteins in milk (lactose and casein) are the parts most likely to trigger reactions, and because their molecular structure is similar to gluten's, people with gluten allergies may have a reaction to them. No cow's milk, heavy cream, or cheese here. Cultured butter and ghee have little to no casein and lactose in them, so I do use them occasionally, but those with severe dairy allergies still need to avoid them. (More on butter and ghee on page 41.) Some people do better with goat's or sheep's milk and milk products, but these are still not AIP-compliant, and since they are also difficult to source, they're not used in this book.

HIGHLIGHT REEL

AIP is an awesome elimination diet that helps heal leaky gut and reverse autoimmune disease by omitting all foods that can permeate, damage, and irritate the gut lining and cause inflammation. For people suffering from chronic illnesses, particularly autoimmune diseases, completing the autoimmune protocol can be very helpful in identifying foods that aggravate their symptoms.

keto

To explain keto and why it works, let's back up a minute and start with how the body is fueled. There are two primary ways that we get energy: we burn sugar (glucose), or we burn fat (both from the diet and what's stored on the body). While in reality everyone burns both, in varying amounts, you're either primarily a sugar-burner or primarily a fat-burner. The body generally prefers to burn glucose when it's available, so when you eat more than a minimal amount of carbs—which are made up of glucose—you're a sugar-burner, and you don't burn a lot of fat.

Here's the kicker: when you consume excess glucose, it's stored as body fat. One too many baked potatoes literally goes straight to your thighs (eye roll). And as long as you're primarily a sugar-burner, it's really hard to burn off that body fat.

The other major problem with being a sugar-burner is that it makes you a slave to the refuel. Right after you eat, your blood sugar spikes. As your body uses that sugar for fuel, your blood sugar falls, triggering hunger (and sometimes other unpleasant symptoms, like low energy, mood swings, lack of focus, and more). That 3 p.m. slump? You betcha! Welcome to the blood sugar roller coaster and the need to snack every few hours.

This is where keto comes in. "Keto" is short for "ketogenic," which means "ketone-creating." Ketones are particles that are created when you metabolize fat, and they're what your body's cells use for fuel. A ketogenic diet is one that leads to the creation of ketones—in other words, it helps your body burn fat as its primary fuel. As you become a fat-burner, the level of ketones in your body rises, and when it reaches a certain level, you're in a state of nutritional ketosis. There are benefits to having high levels of ketones—a ketogenic diet has been used for a hundred years to treat epilepsy, for instance. But there are also great benefits to simply being a fat-burner.

The body stores up to 80,000 calories of fat at any given time, an endless energy source. When you're a fat-burner, you don't need to refuel every few hours—instead, you'll just access some of those calories stored as body fat. There are endurance athletes who thrive on keto, bodybuilders and soccer moms. All folks who constantly have to push the limits of what their minds and bodies can handle. When you are using fat for fuel, you no longer experience those drastic highs and lows in energy and hunger. Your mind is focused, your body satisfied. And because your body is adapted to use fat for fuel, you'll be burning some of that body fat, too.

Right now you're probably thinking, *Well, all that sounds great! So how do you become a fat-burner?* You start by starving the body of glucose by eating a low-carb, high-fat diet. This will cause your body to use up its small amount of stored glucose (glycogen) and begin to use fat for fuel. In the beginning, your body isn't efficient at this. It takes a while to become fully fat adapted—anywhere from a few weeks to a few months. (Keep in mind that fat adaptation and ketosis aren't the same thing. Being fat adapted means that your body prefers to run on fat. Being in ketosis simply means that you have a certain amount of ketones—yes, your body is burning fat to generate those ketones, but it doesn't necessarily *prefer* fat as its main fuel.)

THE NUTS AND BOLTS OF KETO

There are a few ways to get your body to prefer fat as a fuel, and I will warn you, there are very, very dividing and extreme opinions on that matter. When I say *extreme,* I mean there are those who adhere to a zero-carb diet, which is only meat, eggs, and butter. Others eat a lot of dairy and processed foods and focus on their macronutrients (fat, protein, and carbs), with little regard for micronutrients (vitamins and minerals). There are folks who fast for days at a time and those who fast for only sixteen hours a day. Some swear by butter coffee, others scoff at sipping on fat. But most keto folks do eat grain- or gluten-free, focusing on getting plenty of healthy fats, proteins, and veggies, with dairy, nuts, and seeds thrown in the mix. Still, it's a polarized community. I'm like Switzerland. Hanging out over here, sipping on some matcha, saying, "You do you, boo."

The main thing is to omit added sugars from your diet, lower carbohydrates, and incorporate plenty of healthy fats. For most people, it takes a few weeks to a few months of eating less than 50 grams of total carbs a day, with moderate amounts of protein and high amounts of healthy fats, to become fat adapted. What a moderate amount of protein is for you will depend on your activity level, as explained below.

The ketogenic diet is usually described as about 75 percent fat, 20 percent protein, and 5 percent carbs. But the ratio that works best for you may look slightly different. As I'll discuss more on page 35, pay attention to how you feel and tweak those numbers as needed.

The most effective way to calculate your macros is to start by choosing your carb limit. I suggest 50 grams total carbs a day. Second, choose your protein goal. The rule of thumb is 0.6 gram of protein per pound of lean body mass for a sedentary person, 1 to 1.2 grams for active people. For example, I have about 140 pounds of lean body mass and I am active, so I strive for about 140 grams of protein a day. Both carbs and protein have 4 calories per gram, so 50 grams of total carbs comes to 200 calories and 140 grams of protein comes to 560 calories. So far that's 760 calories for one day—definitely not enough to sustain me. The remaining calories will come from fat, which has 9 calories per gram. I add enough to my meals to keep me full and satisfied, roughly 100 to 120 grams per day. That leaves me at 1,840 calories per day. Calories aren't the focus here, but when you're plugging these numbers into an app, like MyFitnessPal, it will ask you for this information.

FAT AS A LEVER

Luis Villasenor of KetoGains.com has coined the phrase "fat as a lever." It's a fantastic way to describe a balanced keto diet once you're fat adapted. (Until then, make sure you're eating high amounts of fat to help your body make the transition.) You set your protein goals, you limit your carbohydrates, and then you use fat as a lever. Add it to your meals until you are full; reduce the amount of dietary fat to lose weight. Remember, once you are fat adapted, your body can use stored body fat for fuel in the absence of dietary fat!

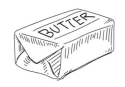

Believe me, you don't need to eat bowls of fat: due to the high-caloric nature of fatty foods, it adds up rather fast. It can take some getting used to the lower carbohydrate intake as well as the higher fat; go ahead, eat the whole avocado!

Tracking your macros can be a short-term solution and tool for getting started on keto, but I have a hate-love relationship with macros and tracking. I do think the information is important and tracking can help someone new to keto get a hang of this way of eating. Even for a Paleo veteran, getting those carbs around 50 grams can be a challenge. However, I have personally experienced the obsession, the feeling of restriction and failure that comes when you don't feel great sticking to preset macros. I have witnessed people asking things like, "I have x amount of fat grams left for the day, but I'm not hungry. Do I just eat a spoonful of coconut oil?" What?? No! If you're not hungry, don't eat. Alternatively, if you *are* hungry, even if your macros are up, EAT! You see what I'm getting at? Tracking can be great, but it's also a slippery slope.

My hope is that you will use macros to get a handle on this whole keto thing and then go on to eat intuitively, making choices that make you feel good. Don't let keto become another diet focused on overrestriction. That, my friends, is not sustainable. This is not a diet, it's a lifestyle, and sustainability is the name of the game.

Fat is not the enemy on keto, but bad fat is. While your body can use any dietary fat to create ketones, hydrogenated vegetable oils and highly processed seed-based oils are very inflammatory (more on fats on page 40). Your body needs clean fuel, like an eco-friendly car. This means unprocessed saturated fats: grass-fed butter or ghee, coconut oil, pastured animal fats, and avocados.

WHY IS KETO SO DAMN POPULAR?

Keto has become more and more popular in recent years. Why? Bottom line: results.

Everything we were ever told about heart health, diabetes, and cholesterol was wrong. A diet high in fat and sodium is supposed to be the worst for health. Could it actually lower cholesterol and reduce the risk of heart disease and diabetes? You betcha! (But let's not forget the real-food part, eh?)

Studies have shown that following a keto diet results in weight loss, lower cholesterol, and lower blood glucose. In one study of eighty-three obese adults who were put on a keto diet, the results were amazing!* In six months, the weight and body mass index of the patients decreased significantly, as did total cholesterol. HDL cholesterol ("good" cholesterol) levels significantly increased. Triglycerides significantly decreased. So did blood glucose. These are all fantastic indicators that overall health improved on the keto diet.

Keto has also been used in clinical settings to treat epilepsy and diabetes. Plus, more and more studies are finding that ketones help with Alzheimer's, ADD, cancer, and more. One study I found really intriguing suggested that a keto diet may reduce inflammation.

* H. M. Dashti et al., "Long-Term Effects of a Ketogenic Diet in Obese Patients," *Experimental and Clinical Cardiology* 9, no. 3 (2004): 200–205.

In a study conducted on rats, the group was fed a ketogenic diet had reduced signs of inflammation and pain than the group fed standard rat chow! Here's what the researchers said:

> Clinically, maintenance on a ketogenic diet has been proven effective in treating pediatric epilepsy and type II diabetes, and recent basic research provides evidence that ketogenic strategies offer promise in reducing brain injury.... The ketolytic metabolism induced by the diet could [also] reduce pain and inflammation. To test the effects of a ketone-based metabolism on pain and inflammation directly, we fed juvenile and adult rats a control diet (standard rodent chow) or ketogenic diet (79% fat) ad libitum [without limit] for 3–4 weeks.... Independent of age, maintenance on a ketogenic diet reduced the peripheral inflammatory response significantly.... These data suggest that applying a ketogenic diet or exploiting cellular mechanisms associated with ketone-based metabolism offers new therapeutic opportunities for controlling pain and peripheral inflammation, and that such a metabolic strategy may offer significant benefits for children and adults.*

On an anecdotal note, many women are using a dairy-free keto approach to manage hormonal issues, from polycystic ovary syndrome to estrogen dominance. In Facebook groups and Reddit forums, folks are researching, troubleshooting, and helping each other figure out how to decipher their health puzzles. It's a beautiful thing.

All the recipes in this book are keto-friendly—low in carbs and high in healthy fats. At the same time, I maintain Paleo's focus on whole foods and quality ingredients.

HIGHLIGHT REEL

The keto diet is all about turning you from a sugar burner into a fat-burner. That means eating high amounts of healthy fats and dropping your carb intake way down. It's an outstanding diet for good health and weight loss.

* D. N. Ruskin, M. Kawamura Jr., and S. Masino, "Reduced Pain and Inflammation in Juvenile and Adult Rats Fed a Ketogenic Diet," *PLOS One* 4, no. 12 (2009): e8349.

finding the sweet spot between paleo, aip, and keto

All the recipes in this book are keto- *and* Paleo-friendly, with the exception of the sweeteners. The reason keto-approved sweeteners are not Paleo is because they technically fall into the category of processed foods. Nor are they AIP-compliant, because they can potentially irritate the gut. Now, on Paleo and AIP, natural sweeteners like honey and maple syrup are used pretty freely, and there's no limit on carbs. Works for a lot of folks. Didn't work for me, might not work for you.

No matter how "clean" I ate on Paleo and AIP, I was hungry all the time, and my sugar cravings were pretty bad too. While Paleo is a nutritious way of eating, when you're slamming sweet potatoes and Paleo sweets on the regular, the pounds will pack on—and eventually the inflammation, too.

After reading Mark Sisson's *The Primal Blueprint* and Robb Wolf's *Wired to Eat*, I began to experiment with testing my blood sugar after eating certain carby foods, and I began to limit fruit and tuber consumption.

I learned a few things about myself. For one, my old food-abuser ways had begun to creep into my Paleo lifestyle. You can still overeat on real food, ya know? I also learned through Robb Wolf's seven-day carb test that I was in fact insulin resistant. After eating 50 grams of effective carbs (or net carbs, the grams of carbohydrates minus the grams of fiber) on an empty stomach, I would immediately feel tired and my blood sugar would stay elevated for quite some time. That means that when I eat carbs (which are, remember, composed of sugar molecules), my body secretes insulin, but my blood sugar stays high because my body doesn't use the insulin effectively. This is a prediabetic state.

Since I am more sensitive to carbs, especially sugar, Paleo treats and tubers were triggers for my sugar/carb addiction and inflammation. Applying the real-food Paleo principles to a low-carb lifestyle was my ticket. This low-carb Paleo looks a lot like keto, but traditional keto was not the path for me. As I searched for recipes and resources online, I found a lot of low-carb keto recipes full of ingredients I didn't eat (especially dairy, nuts, and nightshades), so I made my own recipes.

I settled into a low-carb Paleo diet and kept researching and tweaking it, lowering my carbs further and troubleshooting the infamous keto flu (see page 37). Then one day it happened. I had energy, and the scale began to move again. I wasn't thinking about food (read: sweets) all the time. My inflammation was nonexistent. My finicky ankle wasn't swollen; that hot spot on my knee was gone. My joints didn't hurt, my skin was clear, and I felt amazing. I was fat adapted.

I believe very active people and those who naturally limit their starch and sugar consumption on Paleo are probably fat adapted too, or at least enjoying metabolic flexibility, where they go in and out of ketosis without even noticing it. This, folks, is where it's at! This is where Paleo and keto overlap, and it's a beautiful thing.

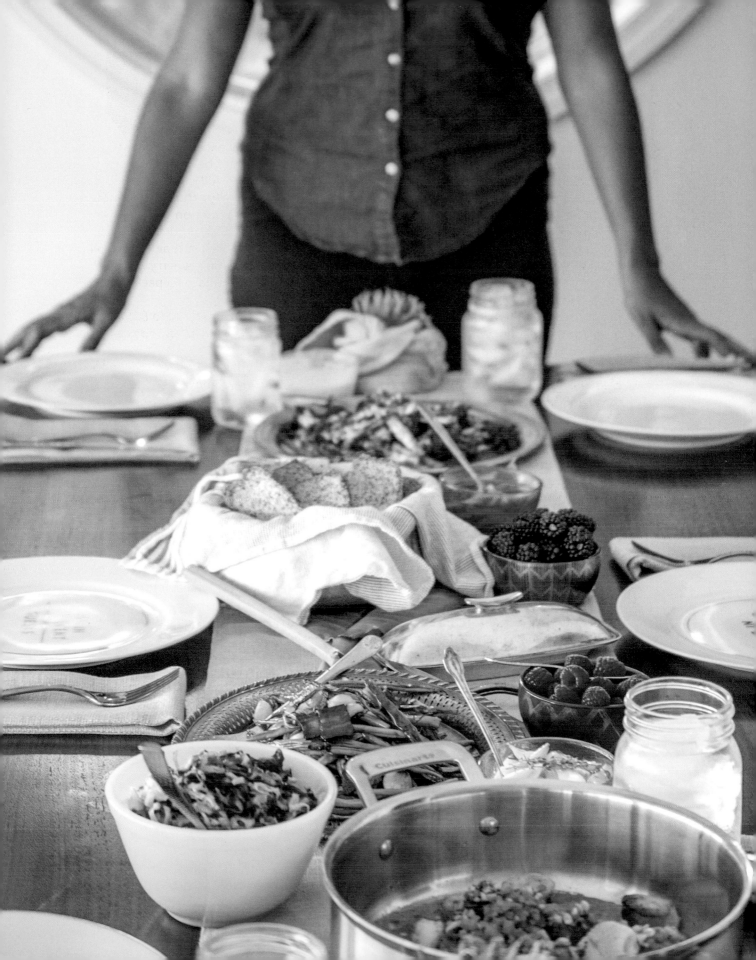

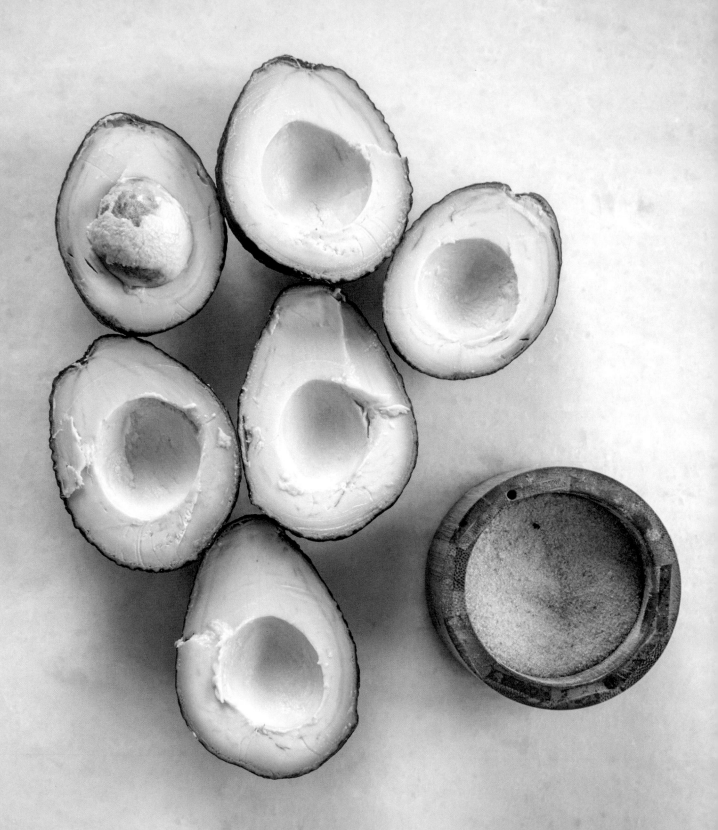

Keto in Practice

A keto lifestyle is life-changing, in the best way. I—and so many others—have found that it's the key to feeling good and staying healthy without feeling restricted. There is freedom in this keto, Made Whole lifestyle! That said, because it really is about using food to change your body, there's a lot to consider and a lot of information to absorb. In this chapter, I'll walk you through the ins and outs of keto and give you my best advice and tips for making it work for *you*.

a day in the keto life

While your meals will be more calorie-dense on keto (remember, fat has more calories than carbs and protein), fat is extremely satiating, so you will quickly notice that you're eating fewer or smaller meals and can easily go hours without eating.

   The easiest way to explain this to you is to tell you what a regular day looks like for me.

 Wake up, drink a tall glass of water with a pinch of pink salt (great for hydration).

 Drink two cups of coffee or tea made delicious and frothy with plenty of good fats. Get a workout in.

 Get some work done.

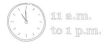 *Have an early lunch of a big salad, like Castaway Chicken Salad (page 164). Take any medication or supplements.*

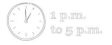 *Get more work done. Run errands. Pick up Jack from school, go to activities. Maybe have an afternoon herbal tea or another tall glass of water with a pinch of salt, which I take with me in my reusable water bottle.*

 Home for dinner: Shrimp + Grits (page 296), a little Spinach Salad (page 348) on the side. Perhaps a sweet treat for dessert.

That's it. I won't eat a meal again until noon the next day.

This is way less than I used to eat, three meals a day plus snacks! What's more, these meals are rich in green vegetables, proteins, and good fats. They're efficient meals that fuel your body. With a focus on whole foods, keto can be extremely nutrient dense!

It's all about eating a healthy balance of colorful plant-based foods and quality animal proteins, all packing lots of essential vitamins and minerals. An easy way to accomplish this is to strive for colorful meals.

the ins and outs of fasting

Fasting is not necessary to be successful on a keto diet, but it often happens naturally. The satiating nature of the diet and the body's ability to use stored body fat for fuel means your body won't signal you to eat (through hunger) just because you have run through the calories obtained at your last meal. It's quite easy to get your fill with just one meal or two each day.

I remember listening to a podcast with the godfathers of Paleo, ancestral health and keto experts Mark Sisson and Robb Wolf, where they spoke about fasting as the time when the magic happens, when your body repairs and replenishes. Eastern medicine and religions all over the world have implemented fasting for centuries. It's not a new idea at all and is quite safe for most people.

However, fasting is not about starving yourself. It's about getting your calories in during a designated window so then you can give your body quiet time outside that window to do other important tasks that don't involve digestion.

For me, fasting came naturally once I was fat adapted. As I write this, it's nearly noon, I have been up since 6 a.m., and I haven't even thought about food today.

The most common fasting practice is to eat in an eight-hour window each day and fast the other sixteen hours. Some folks like to fast one full day (twenty-four hours) a week. Some folks do extended fasts, more than twenty-four hours. While fasting technically means you consume nothing but water, not even black coffee, on keto a lot of people (including myself) "fast" with coffee or even butter coffee. This type of fasting is great for keeping insulin low and energy up. (Butter coffee, or bulletproof coffee, attributed to Dave Asprey, is a blend of coconut oil and/or grass-fed butter or MCT oil mixed into your coffee beverage. Check out my recipe on page 352.)

Let me reiterate that fasting is not necessary, so don't force it. And if you have a thyroid or hormone imbalance, do your research before diving in, as fasting isn't for everyone.

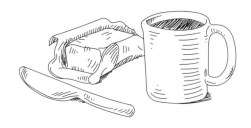

listen to your body, not an app

Eat when you're hungry, and only when you are truly hungry. Stop eating when you are full. Simple, right? Ideally. But when you're transitioning from a Standard American Diet to a healthier one, or when you're healing leaky gut or balancing your hormones, your hunger cues can be a little out of whack. And metabolic damage (or, more accurately, metabolic adaptation), which can result from yo-yo dieting, can really mess with how your body communicates with your brain. Long periods of calorie restriction can cause the metabolism to slow down, reducing the number of calories you use to preserve energy and signaling your body to consume more food. This survival technique came in handy for our ancestors, who often had to go long periods of time without food, but for the modern-day sugar-burner, it means a vicious cycle of binging and restricting.

I think it's a good idea to track your intake of macronutrients (fat, protein, and carbs) for a few weeks or even a few months, until you find a natural rhythm and can recognize when you're really hungry and when you're just bored or anxious. This will also help you learn what a good ratio of macros looks like on keto, and you'll learn what measurements of foods look like. One serving of protein is about the size of your palm. A handful is about a cup. The tip of your thumb is about a tablespoon. As someone who cooks a lot, I can eyeball a lot of measurements, but this takes practice. Tracking your food will help you learn what portions look like and what amounts of food satisfy you.

The standard keto macros look something like 75 percent fat, 20 percent protein, 5 percent carbs. However, this is not a hard-and-fast rule. I feel that 70 percent fat and 10 percent carbs works better for me. This doesn't impede my fat-burning state because most of my carb intake is from green vegetables. Not all carbs are created equal. Green vegetables do not cause the same insulin response as, let's say, a sweet potato. Exactly what macros work for you is something you will have to figure out for yourself. Find a template, apply it to your situation, tweak as needed.

Some people like to count net carbs rather than total carbs. Net carbs are total carbs minus fiber—since fiber is indigestible, many don't count it when tracking their carb intake. I like to count total carbs and keep my carb limit between 30 and 50 grams a day (when I track at all—more on that in a moment). Counting net carbs can be misleading. A lot of packaged foods add fiber to lower the net carb count. If you eat a bagel and then a cup of fiber, does that negate the carbs in the bagel? No.

Yes, I know you might want to omit the carbs for sugar alcohols from the carb count. I get it, we don't absorb them, we pee them out (more on that on page 38). But the next thing you know you're eating a fiber-and-sugar-alcohol cookie that is 0 net carbs, and that kind of food voodoo doesn't sit well with me. It goes against my intuition. If a zero-carb cookie sounds too good to be true, it probably is. The majority of my carbohydrates come from vegetables, coconut foods, and avocados. Tracking total carbs is just easier. Also, it requires less math, and I hate math. I also make better food choices, choosing nutrient-dense foods over foods that just fit into my macros.

But I don't track my macros all the time. I use tracking as a tool to get on course and get an idea of where I am, and then I aim to eat intuitively. I strongly suggest—nay, I *urge* you to stop tracking at some point, even if just for a while. You need to learn to trust your hunger cues and trust yourself with making conscious and intuitive food choices. If you never give yourself the chance, you won't know what you're capable of.

There are no one-size-fits-all ideal macros. Everyone and their mothers will tell you otherwise, but in the real world of unique biological and physiological needs and vastly different lifestyles, you have to figure out what works best for you. Don't be afraid to experiment. What is the worst that can happen? You gain two pounds, but you learn something! So much is at play when it comes to dietary needs—metabolism, activity level, medical history. At the end of the day it's about finding a template you like and applying it to your specific needs.

Remember, the point is to eat nourishing foods, keep your blood sugar stable, keep your energy up, and keep your inflammation down. The rest is just gravy.

the big question: how do I know if I am fat adapted?

You will *feel* it. Sustained energy. Mental clarity that almost feels a little buzzy. You might experience some dry mouth (because you are not retaining water). You might need less sleep. You will be less hungry, and you might notice you go hours without thinking of food. You might feel these things intermittently for a few weeks or months until you are fully fat adapted. There is a transition period and a learning curve when changing your way of eating. Once you're fat adapted, cravings for sugar and carbs are a thing of the past. It's magical.

But Cristina, that all sounds a little woo-woo. Aren't there any more concrete ways to test for fat adaptation? There are ways to test for ketosis, and the two are linked—although being in ketosis and being fat adapted are not the same thing, you have to crawl before you walk, and being in ketosis more often than not will help your body become fat adapted. But I don't think the tests for ketosis are worth it, and here is why.

- **Ketone test strips.** These little strips change color when you pee on them, according to the amount of ketones in your urine. The problem is that they only measure the ketones you are peeing out, and when you're fat adapted, you won't be peeing out ketones—you'll be using them for energy. Don't waste your money.

- **Breath ketone meter.** Just like the test strips, it measures ketones you're *not* using—those exhaled in your breath. It's not very accurate and you will just get confused. Don't waste your money.

- **Blood ketone meter.** Blood testing, while accurate—it measures the ketones circulating in your blood, which you *are* using for energy—can be expensive, and you simply don't need it. I've never tried it.

If you're super curious about your metrics, get a blood glucose meter, which measures your blood sugar levels. It's way cheaper than a ketone meter, and I think knowing how your blood sugar responds to different foods and how stable it is overall throughout the day is more valuable than knowing your ketone level. Low and steady blood sugar levels are always a win.

 Tracking macros and testing ketones or blood sugar can trigger obsessive or compulsive behaviors in some folks. If you are prone to ultrarestriction or binges, don't track—and proceed with caution.

troubleshooting

Due to the highly scientific nature of the keto diet, there is a lot of information out there about numbers, statistics, and macros—a lot of ways to measure your success (or failure) on keto. There are a lot of people out there giving a lot of advice on keto, and quite frankly, I think some of it is dangerous. If something sounds extreme or off to you, it probably is. Always use your best judgment when trying something new, and remember, how you feel will always be a great measure of a program's efficacy.

I get hundreds of messages from people who think they're doing something wrong or feel they have failed because their macros were off. But most of the time all they need to do is tweak something slightly, wait, or change their perspective. Here are few of my simple troubleshooting techniques for common keto issues.

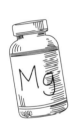

YOU THINK YOU'RE DOING IT WRONG.

Stop comparing yourself to other people. Forget what so-and-so posted on Instagram. Ask yourself how you feel and go from there. If you don't feel well, you might need to tweak your macros, sleep more, or get more sodium.

YOU'RE EXPERIENCING FLU-LIKE SYMPTOMS.

When you feel like death in the early days of the diet, you're experiencing the "keto flu" because your body is weaning off of sugar and detoxing. You will have low energy, headaches, grumpiness. It can suck. Get plenty of sleep, and give it time.

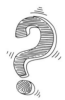

Supplementing with up to 500 mg a day of magnesium can help with keto flu symptoms. I like magnesium glycinate because it's relaxing and doesn't have a laxative effect. Also, make sure you're eating enough potassium-rich foods (hello avocado)!

I also like to supplement with iodine, since I don't use table salt, which has iodine added to it. Iodine is essential in thyroid production, and an iodine deficiency can cause low energy levels. However, if you have a thyroid dysfunction, consult your doctor before using iodine supplements or consuming iodine-rich foods.

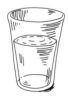

YOU FEEL DEHYDRATED.

For every gram of glycogen (stored glucose), your body stores 3 grams of water. So as you use up your glycogen stores in the early days of keto, you're also losing water. In addition, the drop in insulin has a diuretic effect, so you may get a bit dehydrated as your body adjusts to the new level. Make sure you drink lots of water, and add a pinch of fine Himalayan salt to your drinking water, or sip on bone broth during the day.

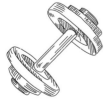

YOU DON'T HAVE ENERGY FOR WORKOUTS.

This is because you're not fat adapted yet. It will get better eventually. In the meantime, scale it back at the gym for a few weeks and try lower-intensity workouts. Focus on really dialing in your eating habits and your new keto lifestyle. Eventually you'll be back full force—and with the awesome muscle-building power of keto.

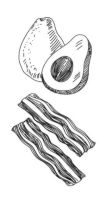

YOU FEEL LIKE YOU CAN'T GET ENOUGH FAT IN YOUR DIET.

This is where tracking goes wrong. If you're not hungry, don't eat. You don't need tons of extra fat in your diet to get into ketosis or become fat adapted. Eating minimal carbs, paired with moderate protein and just enough fat to keep you satiated, is enough to get you into ketosis and, even better, eventually use stored body fat instead of dietary fat for fuel. However, make sure you are eating enough, without snacking. When you're focused on your macros, it's easy to overeat keto snacks because of their high fat content, and next thing you know, your micronutrients are nonexistent. Instead, sit down for satisfying meals with lots of nutrients, so you know you're getting all your vitamins and minerals.

the lowdown on low-carb sweeteners

Low-carb sweeteners are an ever-growing market, with new products coming out every day. I'm always wary of new products with unknown long-term effects. I do, however, love chocolate as much as the next person, and being able to include some sweetness in my life makes this whole way of eating a lot more sustainable. At the same time, I know for sure that natural sweeteners, like honey and maple syrup, just don't work for me. (I talk more about this on page 30.) So I do use low-carb sweeteners, but I use them sparingly.

I prefer granulated erythritol and liquid stevia. Liquid stevia glycerite is my preferred form of stevia. Erythritol, particularly Swerve brand (which combines erythritol with oligosaccharides, chains of sugar molecules), performs really well in baking, and although it's not quite as sweet as sugar, it's close enough to measure cup for cup like sugar. I have also recently tried another non-GMO sweetener by Ketologie, a blend of erythritol and stevia, which I like a lot and also use cup for cup.

Erythritol is a sugar alcohol made by fermenting the sugar in corn (read labels to make sure the corn is non-GMO). When you consume erythritol, most of it is absorbed in the small intestine, but it is not metabolized, so we pee it out. Stevia is also plant-based, and like erythritol, we simply pee it out. This is why both stevia and erythritol are considered zero-calorie and low-carb—and they don't affect blood sugar at all.

Sounds great, right? Yes, but they can also cause gut irritation and/or digestive distress. These sweeteners are not good if you have IBS or candida issues. If you know you have leaky gut or consuming these causes any kind of discomfort, omit them from your diet. You may consider using raw honey in very small amounts instead.

Another reason I only use these sweeteners in the smallest amount possible is that our bodies, our brains, like and expect that sweet taste. It signals that food is coming. When you eat noncaloric sweeteners, there is a disconnect between that signal and what we actually get: the message is not fulfilled and our bodies can often be left feeling hungry. In short, eating too many sugar alcohols can mess up your hunger signals.

carbs on keto

Following keto can often make you feel that carbs are the devil. I get it, I had that reaction too! Yet the keto diet isn't a zero-carb diet. Plenty of healthy foods, from cauliflower to coconuts, have carbs in them. The point of eating a keto diet is to train your body to prefer using fat as fuel, to use ketones for energy, but that's not to say our bodies won't on occasion use glucose.

I like a nondogmatic approach on this front. I believe keto is much more sustainable if you don't feel like starchy vegetables are completely and forever out of your reach. One thing to remember is that you can always change your approach. Here are a few ways people manage carbs on keto.

- **Abstaining:** These people stick to 20 grams of total carbs a day. If you're in this camp, I recommend these 20 grams come from above-ground vegetables. Sticking to this amount of carbs leaves little room for seeds, coconut foods, and the like. But if you're on keto for clinical reasons, staying under 20 grams of total carbs—and eating high amounts of fat—is paramount.

- **Moderating:** This strategy calls for eating 30–50 grams of total carbs a day, with these carbs coming mostly from vegetables, a few seeds, coconut foods, and treats.

- **Counting net carbs:** These folks aim for 20–50 grams of carbs a day and only count the net carbs. Net carbs, remember, are calculated by subtracting the grams of fiber from the grams of carbs in foods. As a rule, when using the net carb approach, I suggest counting total carbs for seeds, sweeteners, and nuts (if you eat them) and only counting net carbs for green vegetables and avocados.

- **Carb cycling:** These folks stick to less than 50 grams of carbs on most days, but on some days they incorporate more carbs (from starchy vegetables or fruit) into meals in the evening, consuming up to 150 grams of carbs in a day. This evening carb cycling is recommended for people with thyroid issues or those who do CrossFit or other high-intensity workouts. These breaks, or refeeds, keep the metabolism on its toes. They refuel the stores of glycogen (stored glucose) temporarily. For those with thyroid issues, they can give energy and keep weight loss moving. For those who do high-intensity workouts, they can help with muscle recovery. The glucose will be burned off quickly and the body will return to a fat-burning state.

- **Allowing a cheat day:** Some people are abstainers (20 grams of carbs a day) or moderators (30–50 grams of carbs a day) six days a week, but one day a week, they allow themselves a free-for-all.

I'm going to flat-out say it, I don't like cheat days, do cheat days, or recommend them. I think even the term *cheat day* implies that the way you eat is not a lifestyle or permanent. However, if you have a special occasion or you're on vacation, and you don't have any food triggers (i.e., you won't feel sick from eating gluten or dairy or other foods), then go forth and make your choices.

I used to carb cycle, and when I first began keto it helped me get through the keto flu. I also lift weights a lot, and I would carb up in the evenings of workout days. Organically and without much thought, I stopped carb cycling, and I don't miss it. However, if one day I want some sweet potato fries with dinner, I will have them and it's not a big deal. It's just not a regular occurrence.

Feel free to play around with your approach. You can even make up your own. Go with what feels good to you, and don't feel married to any one way to manage your carbs. In the spirit of self-experimentation, stay fluid and open to change.

Vegetables are not the enemy. Broccoli isn't going to kick you out of ketosis, and if you're scared of a carrot, you need to check yourself. While animal proteins are some of the most nutrient-dense foods available, I am a huge advocate for vegetables. Coming from the AIP background, I know that what you do eat (vegetables and organ meat) is just as important as what you don't (sugar and gluten), and I firmly believe eating vegetables is essential. Take, for example, Dr. Terry Wahls, who reversed her multiple sclerosis through diet and functional medicine. The Wahls Protocol, a protocol very similar to the AIP elimination diet, recommends consuming 9 cups of fruits and vegetables a day. She went from wheelchair-bound to riding a bicycle, and her story and her book, *The Wahls Protocol,* are amazing.

Food is fuel, and once you're fat adapted, think of yourself as an eco-friendly car. You prefer to run on your battery (ketones), but you can crank the gas (carbs) when needed.

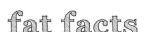 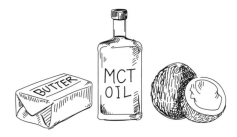

fat facts

If you're new to this way of eating, you might be surprised that canola oil, grapeseed oil, and other vegetable oils are a big no-no, and the fats that have the green light cost a lot more. It can be quite the deterrent. So let's talk vegetable and seed oils really quick. These are extremely bad for the body.

Vegetable and seed oils are high in polyunsaturated fatty acids (PUFAs). PUFAs are highly unstable and prone to oxidation, especially under heat (doh!). During oxidation, free radicals, highly reactive molecules, cause cell damage and essentially make the PUFA carcinogenic. Our system reacts by countering them with antioxidants and—more problematically—inflammation. Oh yeah, vegetable and seed oils are also not natural at all; they're made using chemicals, extreme heat, and whatnot. Garbage. Don't use them.

That's not to say that PUFAs themselves are inherently bad when they come from healthy whole foods and, crucially, not from cooking oils. There are two main kinds of PUFAs: omega-6 fatty acids and omega-3 fatty acids. While we need both, it's important to have the right balance of omega-6 to omega-3. The Standard American Diet is way, way too high in omega-6, which throws off the balance, and too much omega-6 can be inflammatory. Hence the importance of omega-3-rich foods (hello salmon!) to balance it out. But it's just as important to avoid foods high in omega-6, especially those damaging, chemical-laden vegetable oils.

When fueling your body, you want clean, healthy fats that will help reduce inflammation! Enter deliciously natural saturated and monounsaturated fats.

Saturated fats are found in pastured egg yolks, fish, nuts and seeds, coconuts, and pastured animal fats (like butter or ghee). Using cooking fats that are high in saturated fat—like tallow, lard, coconut oil, butter, and ghee—is key. These highly stable fats have high smoke points and won't oxidize when exposed to heat, unlike cooking oils high in PUFAs. Monounsaturated fats, like olive oil, are best used for cold dishes like salad or added after cooking. They're not as stable as saturated fats and could oxidize when used in high-heat cooking.

When sourcing animal fats, it is important to choose grass-fed. Pastured butter, for instance, is high in vitamin D_3, vitamin K, and omega-3 fatty acids. Fats from animals that ate grass is the good stuff—grain-fed animal fat does not have the same benefit.

Medium-chain triglycerides (MCTs) are an easily digestible kind of fat that go straight to the liver to be metabolized into ketones for energy. This specific type of fat is very common on the keto diet because it helps your body achieve or stay in ketosis. Think of MCTs as very efficient fuel. MCTs are most abundant in coconut, but they're also found in butter and ghee in small amounts.

When cooking with a fat, know its smoke point—if the heat you're using is higher than that, the fat will begin to smoke, a sign that it's breaking down and will have a burnt, acrid flavor. Know where your fats come from. Store as directed.

keto in a nutshell

Okay, let's call this what it is: a recap. Because I just talked your face off about a whole lot of stuff.

This book is about the keto diet as I follow it, with a Paleo emphasis on whole, nutrient-dense foods and without some of the foods omitted in AIP. The main goal of keto is to switch your body from burning primarily sugar to burning primarily fat. You do this by starving your body of sugars (carbs), so that your body will metabolize fat for energy, which results in the release of ketones.

Eat plenty of high-quality animal protein, nonstarchy vegetables, and healthy fats. Eat berries, nuts, and seeds in moderation. Eat to satiety. Drink plenty of water. Get plenty of sleep. Move your body. See results.*

I think some folks go a little dairy- and nut butter–happy when they first go keto. In my experience, this doesn't help with reducing inflammation, healing a leaky gut, or losing weight, so I don't include those foods in this book. I want you to cook, eat, and kick ass without having to think too much about it. That is what this book is about. I did the legwork so that you don't have to troubleshoot as much as I did—just cook, eat, and enjoy! Think of the recipes in this book as your own keto-fied elimination diet, a baseline from which you can do your own self-experimentation. Dive in, embrace the changes, and look forward to feeling better than you ever have.

These recipes will get you there.

---

*That doesn't automatically mean "lose weight," people. Reprogram your brain. "Results" are better energy, less pain, greater mobility, improved vitality, and overall wellness.

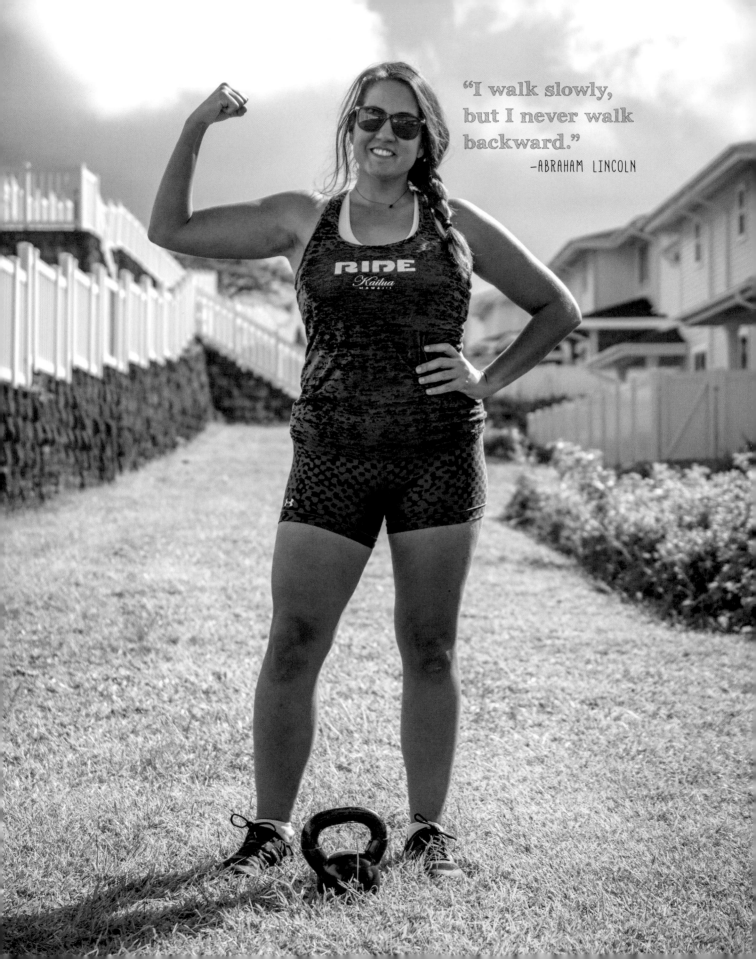

"I walk slowly,
but I never walk
backward."

—ABRAHAM LINCOLN

Creating Your Own Path to Health

For a long time, I thought that I wasn't qualified to give advice on lifestyle or health. After all, I was just like everyone else, trying to figure it all out. Waiting for the day that I felt I had accomplished enough—enough to make me qualified, a "success story."

What I came to learn through experience, exposure, and research is that we're all qualified to share our personal experiences and that no one has all the answers, no matter how well they sell it. I've learned that you can like and respect someone and not agree with everything they say. When it comes to health, nutrition, and especially weight loss, there are a lot of people who are convinced that they have the answer—that their way will work for everyone. As someone who's tried a whole lot of those ways—who has done all the diets and followed all the rules—the one thing I know for certain is that one person, diet, philosophy, or set of rules won't fix all your problems. That might not sell a lot of books, I get that. The promise of results does. You want answers; you want a manual. But guess what? There is no manual. You have to take what you learn from others and make it work for you. You have to apply a combination of dedication, general knowledge, and an understanding of extremely specific details that pertain to your body, life, DNA, history, and so on.

I want you to feel empowered to make a series of choices that all add up to you reaching your goals. I want you to be prepared for setbacks, stalls, and the unknown. These things are inevitable. They are frustrating, and they can make you question your resolve. I know, I have been there, and I am telling you that *you can do it*. You will figure it out. Stay the course.

There are a lot of research studies out there that attest to the effectiveness of keto and Paleo. I know they work—I *live* it. But let me tell you, all the sound science in the world isn't going to help you until you are ready to help yourself. As a reformed overeating, overweight, self-loathing food addict—someone who used food as a form of self-harm—I can tell you that no lifestyle or way of eating will help you lose weight or heal your body until you're ready to love yourself.

Healing, losing weight, gaining strength, and nourishing your body can only come from a place of self-love and self-respect. If you lie to yourself about eating too much or too little, if you are stuck in a cycle of binging and purging, you will not evolve. Honesty is the basis of all healthy relationships—especially the one you have with yourself. Moving forward to a place of freedom when it comes to nutrition takes a lot of self-awareness and commitment. Set your intentions and change for the sake of growth, not from a place of self-loathing. Love begets love.

a new relationship with food

Through a series of dietary resets, reevaluations of what my body needed for nourishment and what healthy food meant to me, and examinations of why I had formed so many negative habits, I learned to communicate with my body. I found that a grain-free, dairy-free keto diet was what my body needed to thrive. Fat and protein satisfy me in a way that carbohydrates never did. I could eat a bowl of pasta and be hungry two hours later. Today my meals sustain me for hours without my needing to snack or graze in between. Every time I eat, I have a purpose: to nourish myself, to satisfy my hunger, and to enjoy the process. The experience of learning to eat healthy transcended the physical: I had abused food for so long that it was intertwined with my emotional health, and the experience of finally choosing healing foods was cathartic.

I want you to experience this, too, and the information, meal plans, shopping lists, and recipes in this book are all aimed at helping you find a better relationship with food—one in which you cook, eat, listen to your body, and focus on choosing foods that nourish and satisfy you physically and emotionally.

For me, eating this way was the key for my hunger cues to finally come from my body, not my mind. But it wasn't diet alone. I worked on self-love; I worked on listening to my body. And over time, I began to notice when I was full—and I would stop eating. Something I never had done before. Instead of overeating and purging, I found a healthy rhythm where, if I felt that my body needed more nourishment, I would eat more without guilt, and if I was full, I simply stopped eating. The lights on my dash were finally blinking, and I was reading them loud and clear.

The single biggest change: I no longer use food to cope with my emotions. If I'm sad or upset, I don't reach for ice cream to make myself feel better. Which is not to say that eating should be void of emotion. Food makes me happy; certain flavors and smells remind me of happy or sad memories. Our traditions and celebrations revolve around food. But Christmas is still Christmas whether I have cookies or not. I enjoy cooking and sharing with my loved ones. I love making delicious, tasty food that my guests devour. The happiness doesn't come from the amount of food I eat but the social aspect of sharing with others, and the pride I take in my work and in my choices.

The people in your life might not support you or understand the changes you are making at first. If you feel attacked by them or feel that those around you threaten your success, shift your focus. Take the power away from their actions by focusing on how you react to them. Remember that it's not about them—the way you eat is about you, and you choose not to let them wear you down.

You never have to eat anything that would harm you or make you feel less than fantastic. Our bodies are incredible machines. They want to work well; they want to thrive. Survival is in your DNA, so listen to your body! You have thousands of years of evolutionary wisdom inside.

Remember that eating healthy is a choice, and choosing your well-being—over quick fixes, over cravings, over peer pressure—is not selfish, it is self-care. Stop waiting for lightning to strike. The road to wellness is built on the mundane and consistent, on series of small, everyday choices. Choose you.

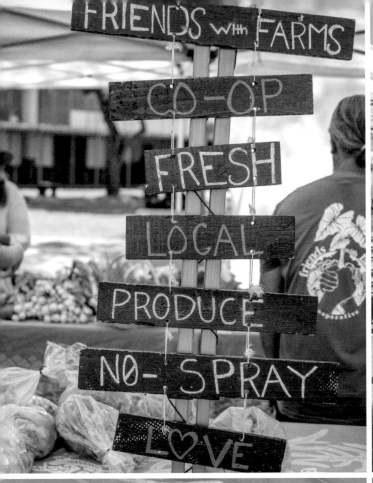

FRIENDS with FARMS
CO-OP
FRESH
LOCAL
PRODUCE
NO-SPRAY
L♡VE

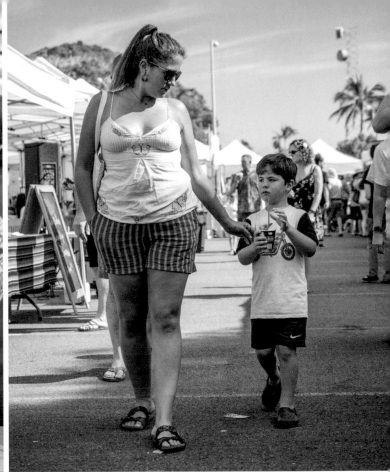

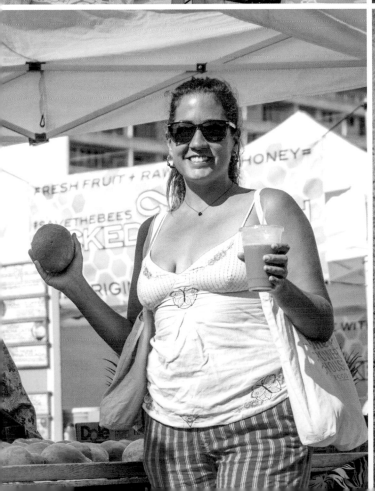

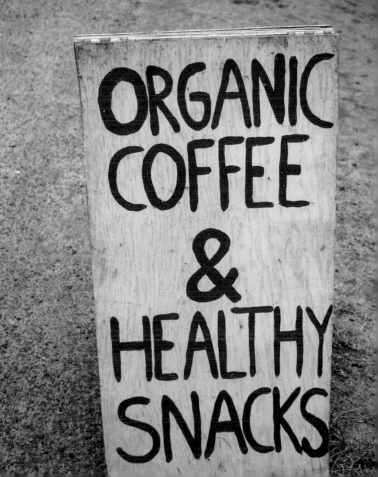

ORGANIC
COFFEE
&
HEALTHY
SNACKS

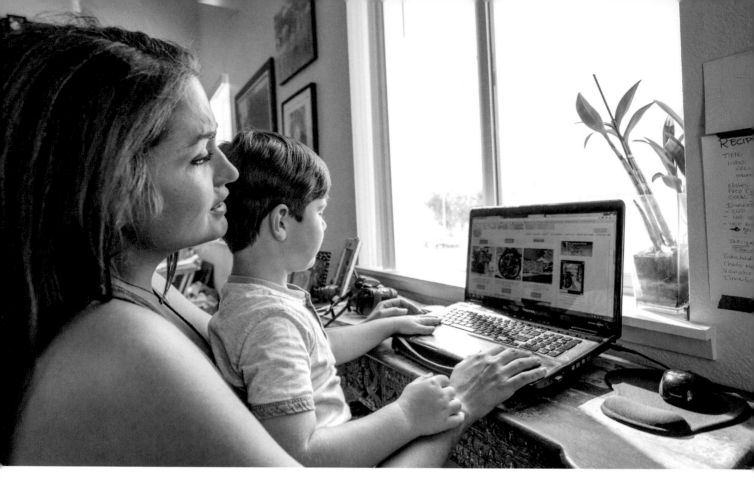

lifestyle factors

While I firmly believe that what you eat will either heal or harm you, I have learned that diet alone doesn't paint the complete picture of health. Lifestyle factors are just as important, if not even more so—I'm looking at you, sleep. That's right, getting your z's isn't a sign of laziness. It's essential for reducing inflammation, balancing hormones, healing leaky gut, and even shedding body fat. Managing stress is up there too!

Here are my tips and tricks for doable lifestyle changes, so you can make sure your dietary changes aren't in vain.

◦ SLEEP: Turn your phone off at night, put it in airplane mode, or just leave it in another room. Get an old-school alarm clock. Limit blue light (screen time) at night. Take magnesium before bed. Early to bed, early to rise—so if you have to be at work early or you have kids and they're up with the sun, go to sleep early!

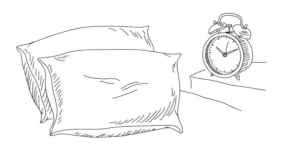

○ STRESS: Find healthy coping mechanisms, because we're eating for nourishment, not comfort. For me, it's working out. Maybe for you it's knitting, long baths, yoga, adult coloring books, video games. Whatever floats your boat. Know how to let off steam in a way that does not include detrimental behaviors.

○ SELF-CARE: Make time for you. Everyone needs moments of peace. Sitting in a garden, watching a movie alone, getting a massage, going for a walk. If you've been on the computer all day, take your shoes and socks off and go stand on dirt, grass, or sand, turn your phone off, and take a few deep breaths. Remember to schedule yourself some alone time to recharge those emotional batteries.

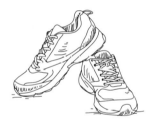

○ MOVEMENT: It's not about weight loss, it's about health! Sedentary lifestyles are killing us. Move at least twenty minutes a day. Walk, dance, shake it out. Set a timer to remind you to get up from your desk once an hour. Take a little stroll, jump around. If you can't move around, do a little chair dance, wiggle your toes, laugh till your belly hurts.

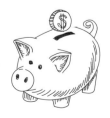

○ FAMILY: It can be hard when not everyone is on board with the changes you want to make in your eating habits. Step one, get over the fact that there might be foods around you that you can't eat. Actually, ditch the word *can't*—instead, think, *I choose not to eat these foods*. Remember *why* you are making this choice. Step two, especially if you are the one doing the cooking, when you make your food, make enough for everyone—everyone should be eating protein and vegetables. If you're living with sugar-burners, like me, make them a side dish. In my house, gluten-free pasta and white rice are the go-tos. I make a big batch once a week and heat some up for the boys around dinnertime. Ideally, we would all eat the same thing, but that's just not my reality, and it might not be yours either.

○ BUDGET: It can be done. When I first changed my way of eating we were a single-income military family living in Hawaii, where food is expensive. Budgeting is a must. I shop around a bit. Grass-fed ground beef is actually cheapest at our Whole Foods (I know, I was surprised too). Frozen wild-caught fish is affordable at Costco. Buy in-season produce. Stock up when free-range chicken is on sale and freeze it. Forget fancy supplements and packaged convenience foods; you don't really *need* them. All you need to eat keto is plants, animals, and good fats. The pricey stuff is always the pantry items. Build those up slowly: buy wholesale, bulk, and sale items. Ross, Home Goods, and other discount home stores often have random pantry items, like Himalayan salt and flax seeds, really cheap. Cut back on eating out, buying booze, and making other nonessential purchases. You don't have to spend more money overall to eat well, but you might have to reallocate some funds toward the grocery budget.

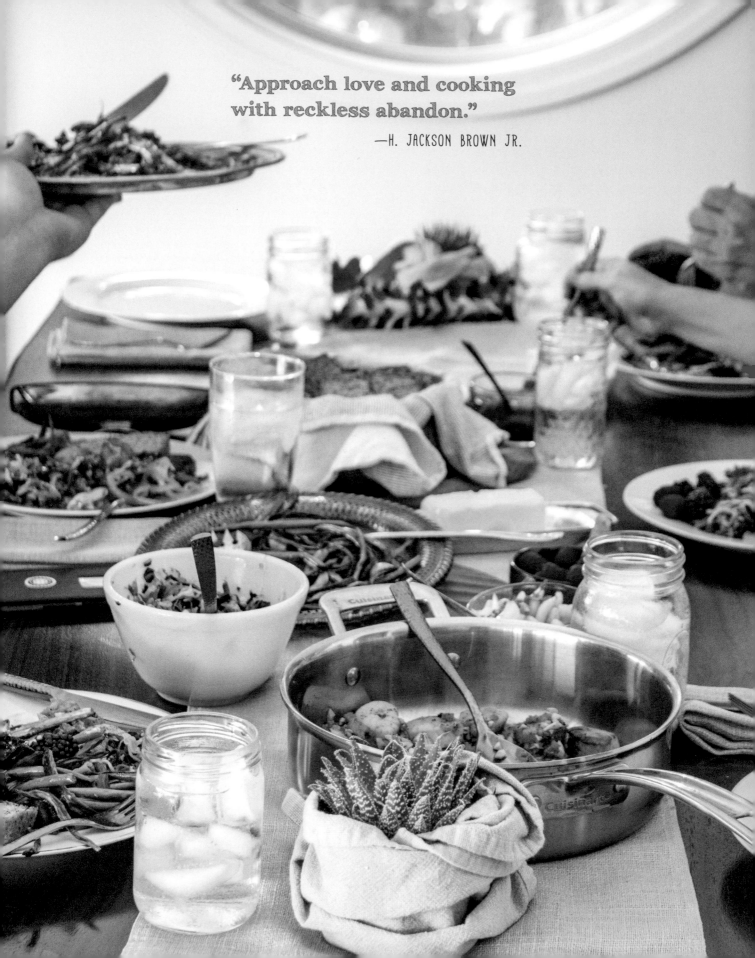

"Approach love and cooking
with reckless abandon."

—H. JACKSON BROWN JR.

Nourish

All of the food used in this book serves a purpose. To inspire, to evoke nostalgia, to create happiness. To fulfill a need, smash a craving. Each dish delivers a top-notch meal that tastes amazing and leaves you satisfied. So in this chapter, we'll explore exactly what you'll be cooking, eating, and, most of all, enjoying!

for the love of food

I said earlier that eating well is a way of respecting yourself. An inextricable part of eating well is cooking. Life can get pretty busy, but just as movement, self-care, and regular dentist appointments are priorities, cooking needs to factor in there, too. I'm not guilt-tripping you. If you've been resistant to cooking, I get it: No one taught you how, or you don't think you're any good. You work crazy hours and/or have a hectic household. Kids, pets, schedules, *life*. The chaos around us will always be there. Still, I urge you to spend time in the kitchen. The key to changing your eating habits begins with truly connecting with the food you eat.

Think of where food comes from. Animals and plants are sacrificed to nourish our bodies. The ingredients were once alive and we harvested them. We wash and prepare them. We change their chemistry. We chew, savor, and digest them. Food is broken down and metabolized to fuel our bodies on a cellular level. There is nothing more intimate than the relationship between our bodies and the food we eat.

I urge you to get to know your food. Cooking is a multisensory experience. Inhale the aroma of fresh herbs, feel the texture of raw meat, appreciate the sizzle in your cast-iron skillet. Whether you do all your meal preparation at once and cook just once a week, or you cook once for every two meals (see the meal plan that starts on page 402), enjoy the time you spend in the kitchen. I guarantee that the more comfortable you get in there, the more efficient you will be!

In this book, I will share with you all of my cooking wisdom, from what I learned from my mother to the knowledge I gained in restaurant kitchens. I want to share with you everything I know so that you can go forth with confidence. I will guide you through these recipes, from the sheet pan dinners to the labors of love. Mastering just a few simple recipes can be extremely empowering and open the door to a whole new world of home cooking.

It's time to slow down and stop looking for quick and easy fixes. Let us commit to learning, evolving, and cooking the foods that nourish us.

building your pantry

The list below of foods and ingredients used in this book looks extensive, but this isn't meant to be your weekly shopping list. It's here to give you an idea of where you can find different ingredients and help you keep an eye out for sales.

I recommend buying dried goods, pantry items, and cooking fats in bulk when you can, so you're only purchasing them every other month or so. Some ingredients might last you a whole year!

The produce you can buy once every ten to fourteen days, especially if you get it really fresh. Purchase protein by what you plan to cook, what you're in the mood for, or what you can find for a good price.

If you're starting from scratch, it may take some time to build up your collection of spices and herbs, but all the ingredients in this book are used more than once, so if you buy something you will use it again.

Once your pantry is stocked and you have all your produce, pick your proteins and you can cook out of any page of this book!

WHERE TO BUY THE FOODS USED IN THIS BOOK

○ *Grocery store (Safeway, Kroger, etc.)*

◐ *Health-food/specialty stores (Whole Foods, Down to Earth, etc.)*

◉ *Wholesale (Costco, Sam's Club, etc.)*

◔ *Online (Amazon, Thrive Market, Barefoot Provisions, Vitacost, etc.)*

VEGETABLES

Arugula ○○●

Asparagus ○○●

Broccoli and/or broccolini ○○●

Brussels sprouts ○○●

Butternut squash (frozen or fresh) ○○●

Cabbage ○○●

Carrots ○○●

Cauliflower (frozen or fresh) ○○●

Celery ○○●

Cremini mushrooms ○○●

Cucumbers ○○●

Garlic ○○●

Ginger root ○○●

Green beans ○○●

Green onions ○○●

Kale and/or collards ○○●

Lemongrass ○○●

Lettuce ○○●

Ong choy or watercress (optional) ○○●

Onions ○○●

Radishes ○○●

Rainbow slaw (shredded veggies) ○○●

Spinach ○○●

Zucchini ○○●

Fresh herbs: basil, cilantro, oregano, parsley, thyme ○○

FRUIT

Berries, all kinds (fresh and/or frozen) ○○○○

Lemons ○○○○

Limes ○○○○

Oranges (for cooking) ○○○○

PROTEINS
MOST FREQUENTLY USED

Bacon (sugar-free) ○○

Chicken breast ○○●

Chicken thighs (regular and boneless, skinless) ○○●

Ground beef ○○●

Ground pork ○○

Ground turkey ○○

Jumbo shrimp (frozen or fresh) ○○○

Salmon (fresh and canned) ○○○○

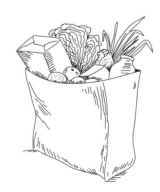

PROTEINS
USED IN A RECIPE OR TWO FOR VARIETY

Deli smoked turkey breast
Genoa salami
Ham steak
Pork chops (boneless)
Pork shoulder
Pork tenderloin
Prosciutto
Soppressata
Beef chuck roast (or another inexpensive cut)
Beef liver
Rib-eye steak (bone-in)
Sirloin steak
Skirt steak
Stew meat
Tri-tip steak
Calamari
Crab meat
Langostinos (optional)
White saltwater fish (cod, mahi mahi, sea bass)

COOKING FATS

Avocado oil
Butter
Coconut oil
Ghee
Lard
Olive oil (regular; use extra-virgin olive oil only for cold uses or as a finishing oil on a hot dish)

SEEDS

Chia seeds
Flax seeds
Pumpkin seeds
Sesame seeds
Shelled raw hemp seeds (aka hemp hearts)
Sunflower seeds

EGGS

Large pastured and/or organic eggs

PANTRY ITEMS

Apple cider vinegar
Baking soda
Canned pumpkin
Capers
Coconut aminos
Coconut butter
Coconut flour
Coconut milk (full-fat, canned)
Coconut vinegar
Coffee
Dark chocolate (stevia sweetened)
Dijon mustard
Fish sauce (I recommend Red Boat brand, which does not contain any sugar)
Kelp noodles or shirataki noodles
Liquid smoke
Matcha tea (optional)
Nori (dried seaweed; optional)
Nutritional yeast
Olives, black or green
Pastured collagen peptides (optional)
Pastured gelatin
Pure vanilla extract
Red wine vinegar
Sunflower seed butter
Sweetener(s) of choice (I use liquid stevia and granulated erythritol—see page 38)
Tahini (optional)
Unsweetened shredded coconut

SEASONINGS

Bay leaves
Chinese five-spice powder
Dried dill weed
Dried oregano
Dried parsley
Dried thyme
Fine Himalayan salt or fine sea salt
Garam masala
Garlic powder
Ground black pepper
Ground cardamom
Ground cinnamon (preferably Ceylon, see box)
Ground cumin
Ground ginger
Ground mustard seeds
Ground nutmeg
Ground turmeric
Italian herb blend
Onion powder

CEYLON CINNAMON

Most cinnamon found in the US is cassia cinnamon, but it's worth seeking out Ceylon cinnamon. It's more expensive and can be harder to find, but it's also sweeter and milder. More importantly, cassia cinnamon has much more coumarin, a blood thinner that can damage the liver and kidneys over time. One of the great things about cinnamon is that it helps keep blood sugar stable, so if you use it every day for that effect, make sure you're using Ceylon cinnamon!

Ceylon cinnamon   *Cassia cinnamon*

a quick guide to substitutions

While each recipe has its own variations and substitution instructions right there on the page, I've compiled all my knowledge of substitutions, conversions, variations, and so on here, so you have everything in one place. Some of what's here doesn't apply to this book—for instance, I've included information on nut flours because they're often used in place of gluten-containing wheat flour, but none of the recipes in this book call for nut flour because nuts contain antinutrients that can affect digestion, and because there are so many people with nut allergies out there. But I'm all about figuring out what works best *for you*, and if that includes nut flours or other ingredients not used in these recipes, you'll have everything you need to know about making substitutions right here.

grain-free flours

Finely ground almond flour, made from blanched almonds, and seed flours measure cup for cup like regular flour, but usually a second flour is needed to get the texture just right, especially for pancakes. For example, instead of 2 cups flour, I use 1¾ cups almond flour and ¼ cup MCT oil powder or 2 tablespoons coconut flour. Finely ground seed flours can be hard to find, with the exception of flaxseed meal, but you can use a high-powered blender or coffee grinder to grind your own raw seeds, like pumpkin seeds or shelled sunflower seeds, for a great nut-free flour alternative.

Coconut flour is a great substitute for wheat flour, but you need to use much less. For 2 cups regular flour or finely ground almond flour, you only need about ⅓ cup coconut flour. Because coconut flour is so absorbent, I often like to start with ¼ cup and add a tablespoon more at a time as needed.

MCT powder can be a great replacement for starches like tapioca or arrowroot in baked goods. Using nut and seed butters as a base can help cut carbs when baking; they become like dough when heated. And of course flourless treats are a good way to go (see, for example, the recipe for Flourless Brownies on page 372).

sweeteners

Erythritol is less sweet than sugar, honey, or maple syrup. For each cup of sugar used in a recipe, you will need to use 1⅓ cups granulated erythritol. However, I find that when you stick to whole foods and as you become fat adapted, your palate changes and very sweet foods aren't as palatable, so using erythritol cup for cup like sugar is just fine.

Liquid stevia is three hundred times as sweet as sugar, and you only need a few drops in recipes. The flavor changes from brand to brand, so you have to play around with it. I suggest sweetening to taste.

Pure monk fruit is gaining some popularity. It is very, very sweet; for ½ cup sugar, ½ teaspoon monk fruit is usually enough.

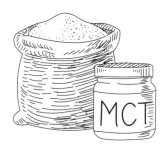

cooking fats

When a recipe calls for any kind of cooking fat, you can use or substitute butter, ghee, coconut oil, lard, and duck fat spoon for spoon—you can even use duck fat or lard to make dairy-free hollandaise.

In most recipes that call for melted butter or coconut oil, you can also use cold-pressed avocado oil. Olive oil may be used, too, but it could alter the flavor of the recipe.

milk

Full-fat canned coconut milk and coconut cream (which you can get by chilling a can of full-fat coconut milk overnight and then skimming off the separated cream) are king in the Paleo-keto world. If you can't do coconut milk, I think homemade cashew milk is second best in terms of performance.

If you can't do nut milk or coconut milk, other dairy-free options include hemp milk and tigernut milk.

In a pinch, if you don't have any Paleo-keto milk on hand, you can mix 1 tablespoon coconut butter or creamy seed or nut butter with ½ cup warm water until smooth for a homemade milk.

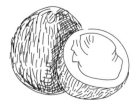

nightshades

In chunky sauces, stir-fries, and salsa, I like to use radishes in place of peppers. They have crunch, spice, and color, too!

In smooth sauces and soups, I like to use Roasted Beet Marinara (page 78) instead of tomato sauce or regular marinara. Unsweetened canned pumpkin also works as a substitute for tomato paste and canned tomatoes.

To give dishes the umami flavor tomatoes bring without, you know, the actual tomatoes, try adding mushrooms, a hit of fish sauce, or some nutritional yeast.

Steamed cauliflower is good at pretending to be white potato.

Use zucchini or summer squash in place of eggplant in your favorite recipes.

acids

Vinegar, lemon juice, pickle juice, and sauerkraut liquid can all be substituted for one another.

eggs

You can replace 1 large egg with:

○ 1 tablespoon water with 1 tablespoon flaxseed meal, OR

○ 1 tablespoon gelatin mixed with 1 tablespoon cold water, then vigorously mixed with 1 tablespoon hot water until white and foamy

If a recipe calls for more than two eggs, I don't recommend replacing the eggs. It would greatly alter the recipe and might result in failure.

nut and seed butters

Seed butters can replace nut butters spoon for spoon—and vice versa. I use unsweetened, unsalted versions. If you can't do nut or seed butters, you can use coconut butter in the same amounts.

cheese

For a sprinkled "cheese" topping, place 1 cup raw cashews and 2 tablespoons garlic powder in a food processor and grind to a crumble. For a nut-free version, use shelled raw hemp seeds or sunflower seeds in place of the cashews.

Nutritional yeast, which is a deactivated yeast that is gluten-free and AIP-friendly, has a lovely cheesy flavor and look! It's used to make Hard Cheese (page 70) and Cheesy Yellow Sauce (page 68).

In other recipes, such as Roasted Beet Marinara (page 78), you can use 1 tablespoon of fish sauce for each ¼ cup of nutritional yeast for an umami taste.

Mayo is a great replacement for cream cheese in baked goods, ounce for ounce.

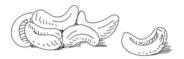

pasta

There are lots of options here, and you can use whichever you like best—they all work great!

Zoodles (zucchini noodles) are made by cutting fresh zucchini into long noodlelike strips. You can use a spiral slicer, julienne peeler, or regular vegetable peeler (which results in long, flat noodles). You can also use other veggies, like daikon radish, instead of zucchini.

Kelp noodles can be eaten raw, soaked, or sautéed, hot or cold. They're a great source of iodine.

Shirataki are made from konjac root. I don't fully understand the wizardry behind these, but they are said to have no carbs. They come in pouches of fluid that can have a weird smell, but rinsing them gets rid of it.

Shredded cabbage makes a great noodlelike food.

And finally, **spaghetti squash** is delicious and relatively low-carb at 10 grams of carbs per cup.

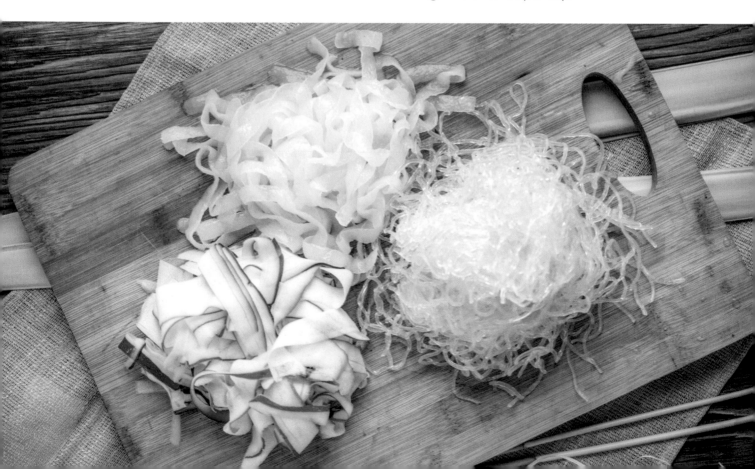

dried and fresh herbs

I use a lot of both dried and fresh herbs, but sometimes I have only dried when a recipe calls for fresh, or vice versa. I use this trick all the time: The rule of thumb is that dried herbs are more concentrated than fresh and therefore are three times as potent. If a recipe calls for 1 teaspoon dried parsley, for instance, you would use 3 teaspoons (1 tablespoon) minced fresh parsley. And to go in reverse: fresh herbs are one-third as potent as dried. If a recipe calls for 1 tablespoon minced fresh oregano, use 1 teaspoon dried oregano.

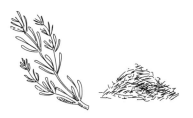

chocolate

If you can't use cocoa or cacao powder, use carob powder (it's AIP-compliant). Cocoa powder is just a more refined form of cacao powder. I like the latter, but cocoa powder has a more chocolaty taste. They can be substituted for each other cup for cup.

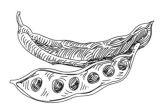

gelatin and collagen

Grass-fed or pastured gelatin is made from the bones of animals that were raised humanely. This bone dust is great for gut health, hair, skin, and nails. It also gels hot liquids when cooled, like Jell-O!

Collagen is the same thing as gelatin, except the protein is broken up to make the powder water soluble. This means that you can add collagen peptides to smoothies and cold beverages.

Both gelatin and collagen have the same nutritional benefits. However, I find gelatin to be more versatile. It's great to thicken sauces and add chewiness to cookies, for instance. If you have to pick one, pick gelatin.

If you don't do animal bones, agar, or agar-agar, powder is made from seaweed and has the same gelling effect, but you're missing out on the great nutritional benefits. Use 1 teaspoon agar powder to 1 tablespoon gelatin in recipes calling for gelatin. Note, however, that agar powder can't be used in place of collagen peptides, which are water soluble.

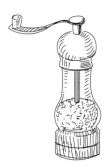

salt

You'll notice I use fine Himalayan salt in almost all of my recipes. I buy it in bulk at Costco or Ross at very good prices. You don't have to use Himalayan salt, but I don't recommend table salt, which usually has a bunch of fillers in it. Use fine sea salt if you can't find Himalayan salt. These natural salts deliver essential minerals that are lacking in table salt, and they also taste amazing.

kitchen intuition

I've had a lifetime of cooking, from my mother's kitchen, to her restaurant, to food trucks and catering. Experience is the best teacher, making mistakes and trying new things. There are things that I have picked up over the years that will make managing your Made Whole kitchen easier, more efficient, and more delicious—and I'll share them with you here so that you don't have to learn the hard way, as I did.

tools

◦ Heat your cast-iron and stainless-steel skillets over medium heat for several minutes and sprinkle a little water on them to test the temperature. When the water dances on the skillet, it's hot enough. Now put down the cooking fat, allow it to melt if applicable, then add the food. This will create a nonstick layer on the skillet. If you need the skillet to be hotter, you can now raise the temperature.

◦ If food gets stuck to your cast-iron or stainless-steel skillet, which usually happens when you cook something saucy or sticky, don't fret. Keep the skillet on the stove after you've removed the food and add ½ cup water. Bring it to a simmer, then use a spatula to gently lift the stuck food off. It's like deglazing the pan, but to clean it. Carefully pour everything out and wipe your skillet clean. If it's cast iron, oil it.

◦ If your cast-iron skillet has been neglected or run through the dishwasher (yes, my husband did that), scrape the skillet clean with coarse salt, rinse, and pat dry. Rub cooking oil all over it. Place it facedown in a hot (350°F) oven and put a sheet pan on the rack underneath to catch oil drippings. Bake it for 45 minutes. This is how you reseason your cast-iron skillets. They are never a lost cause.

◦ Dull knives cause more accidents and cuts than sharp knives. Sharpen your knives regularly.

◦ I use a whisk to break up ground beef when cooking. It works like a charm for perfect crumbly beef.

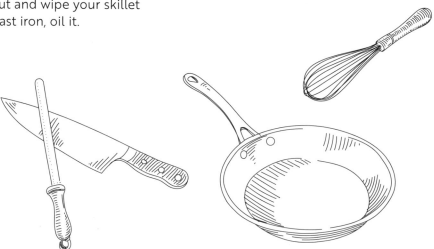

food prep

◦ If you open an unripe avocado by accident, leave it out. The cut area will cauterize, forming a matte brown skin or scab, but it will continue to ripen underneath. In a few days, check it again. When it gives a little as you gently squeeze it, it should be ready. Peel away that scab to find a creamy green avocado underneath.

◦ I like the smash-and-peel method for prepping garlic, but it can be tedious. When I can find it, I buy garlic in bulk, already peeled in bags. Then I make Garlic Confit (page 76), which is a great way to amp up the garlic flavor in any recipe.

◦ Mise en place! Before you start cooking, measure out and peel, chop, dice, and otherwise prepare all your ingredients. This will make for faster, smoother cooking. I love putting all my prepped ingredients in little ramekins and bowls around my workspace.

◦ You can grind large amounts of coffee beans in a high-powered blender. I like to grind enough beans for one or two days of coffee. You can also use a high-powered blender to grind your own cacao powder from cacao nibs and make your own coconut, nut, and seed butters.

◦ Save your onion peels and carrot and celery ends. I stash these odds and ends in freezer bags so I don't have to use whole vegetables when making bone broth.

◦ I keep a lot of cauliflower on hand. I steam one to two heads of florets at a time, until fork-tender, and then freeze them. Having steamed cauliflower ready to go makes a lot of my recipes easier, especially the sauces and smoothies. (See page 68 for steaming instructions.)

◦ Set your meats out to come to room temperature before cooking, especially thick steaks and roasts. The meat will cook more evenly. Thirty minutes is usually enough, longer for larger cuts of meat.

secret ingredients

◦ Add a tablespoon of finely ground coffee, like an espresso grind or even instant coffee, to your chocolate baked goods to really boost the chocolate flavor.

◦ A sweet component can often be missing in recipes, especially when cooking keto. Coconut aminos are great not only for replacing soy sauce but also for adding sweetness. Another good way to lightly sweeten dishes is to use cooked-down berries—frozen blueberries work well.

◦ If you're unsure of how to season a meat, start with 1 teaspoon of salt per pound. Then add ½ to 1 teaspoon of other seasonings. Salt, black pepper, garlic powder, and thyme are my go-to mix.

◦ Sauces are life. Keep a few good sauces on hand at all moments; they're the key to making meals interesting in a pinch.

◦ Chicken feet are super cheap and they make the jiggliest bone broth.

◦ After I slow cook pork or beef, I love to add chicken thighs to the liquid that is left behind in the pot. Cooking the chicken in that flavorful, fatty fluid gives it the most amazing flavor. Add some cauliflower rice at the end for an easy one-pot meal.

◦ A squeeze of lemon or lime juice goes a long way. Same goes for a splash of vinegar. Acidic touches tantalize the taste buds and give any dish that extra oompf!

cooking tips

○ Use your nose! Temperatures and cooking times can vary slightly from appliance to appliance. I always know my food is close to being done because I can smell it. Once something starts to smell like you want to eat it, go check on it!

○ Crispy fixes almost anything. At least for me it does. I like to reheat leftovers by crisping them up in a skillet or popping them under the broiler. If a dish is kind of meh, try adding a little cooking fat on top with a sprinkle of salt and then broiling until crispy.

○ Anytime you sear any protein on the stovetop, it's going to get smoky. Put the fan on and open a window.

○ Don't be afraid of high heat. You want to start cooking most things with a good sear. It keeps the flavor and juices in.

○ Find your favorite oven temp and roll with it. Mine is 400°F. I cook almost everything (except baked goods) at 400°F for 30 to 45 minutes. From veggies to chicken thighs, they turn out crunchy and delicious.

○ Taste food as you go—not raw meat or chicken, of course, but sauces and seasoning mixes. Lick the spatula when making brownies or cookies. Adjust flavors as you see fit. Don't be afraid to use taste buds, your nose, your eyes!

○ Don't be afraid to make changes to recipes. Cooking is part science, but it is mostly art, open to interpretation!

○ The most accurate way to measure flour, other than by weight, is to scoop it up using a dry measuring cup and then skim the extra off the top with the back of a knife.

○ If you have a fresh manicure, especially a light color, wear gloves before handling turmeric-rich foods, especially if you're getting your hands dirty tossing a marinade. The turmeric will stain your new paint job.

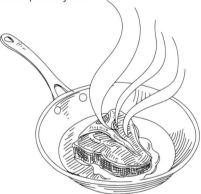

storage

○ Keep your fresh herbs in cups or jars of water in the fridge, loosely covered with a plastic bag. They will last much longer.

○ Don't keep your baked goods in the fridge—they will get dense and hard. But if you just *must,* make sure to let them sit out for an hour or so before eating.

○ Get a few of those cheap spray bottles from the drugstore and keep oils and vinegars in them to mist your food.

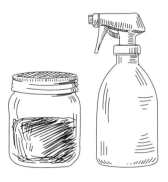

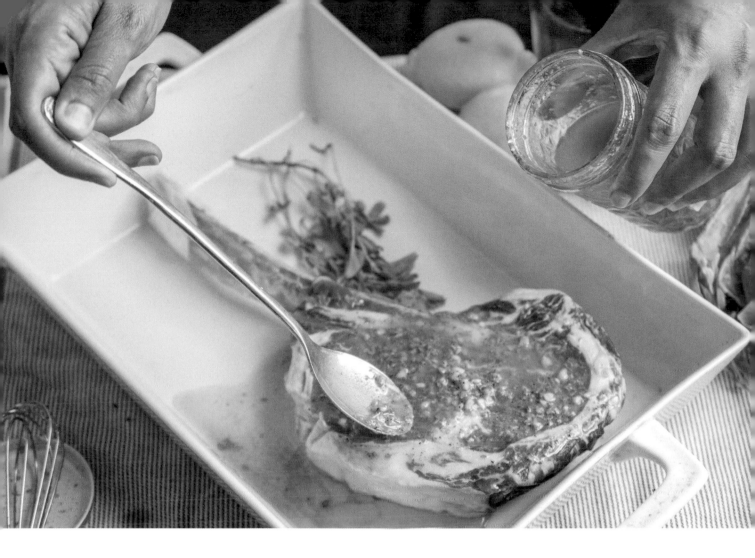

SECRETS FROM MY MOTHER'S KITCHEN

· Whenever I need to sauté onions I add a bay leaf, even if the recipe doesn't call for it. It enhances the flavor of the onions.

· A dash of cumin goes a long way when you are cooking any meat in a hurry. With butter, even better.

· Herbamare. We called it *polvito magico* (magic dust) growing up. It's a plant-based seasoning blend that makes everything taste better.

· Never leave behind the pan sauce. Reduce it, add some wine or broth, bring it to a simmer, and pour it over your food. It will always add welcome flavor!

· Throw a whole pound of raw spinach on a sheet pan and gently heat it in the oven for a couple of minutes. This wilting process brings out the flavor and makes it more manageable—fresh spinach is rather bulky, so when you want to stir it into a sauce or stir-fry, wilting it in the oven really helps. I like adding a little mound or touch of green to my dishes, and a bit of wilted spinach goes well with almost everything!

· Cook by color. If a meal is missing something, think of what will add a pop of color. It will surely add flavor, too.

tools of the trade
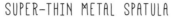

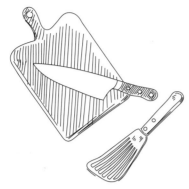

CHEF'S KNIFE AND CUTTING BOARD
A good knife and a safe cutting surface are a must for any cook. With these two you can mince, chop, and slice.

SUPER-THIN METAL SPATULA
Or *fish spatula,* which is the proper term. These ultrathin, bendy spatulas are my secret weapon for fried eggs and crispy seared fish!

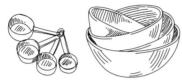

MIXING BOWLS, MEASURING CUPS AND SPOONS
You may be thinking "duh," but I know I did not have these essentials for many years, making it difficult to follow recipes properly.

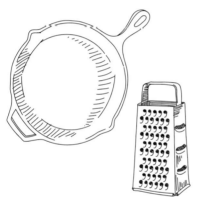

CAST-IRON OR STAINLESS-STEEL SKILLET
Sturdy, nontoxic, and affordable, these are my preferred skillets.

GRATER
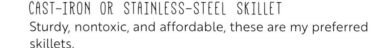
Get one that has large to fine grating. You can make anything from riced cauliflower to grated lemon zest with one handheld tool.

TWO SHEET PANS
Not those tiny little cookie sheets; you want a 17¾ by 13-inch pan with a 1-inch rim. These are actually called *half sheet pans* because they are half the size of the sheet pans restaurants use, but they're plenty big enough for a home kitchen (and anything bigger might not fit in your oven). These make roasting and sheet pan dinners a breeze!

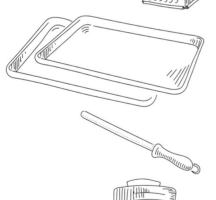

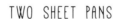

SHARPENING STEEL
Even cheap knives work better when honed with a sharpening steel. You just have to use the steel before each use.

BLENDER
I use a Vitamix. In general, I prefer high-powered blenders. They're used for way more than smoothies—a high-powered blender can grind seeds, make soup, and froth your coffee like no other. However, I understand not everyone has access to these machines. You can create all the recipes in this book with a regular blender, too.

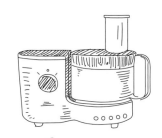

FOOD PROCESSOR
Generally less expensive than a high-powered blender, and while it's not as versatile, it's great for shredding cauliflower into rice, mincing veggies, and making sauces.

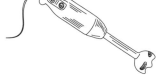

IMMERSION BLENDER
You can get these really cheap online, and you don't need a quality one, unless you plan to use it for soup. I only use mine for mayo, and it turns out beautifully every time. Worth every penny.

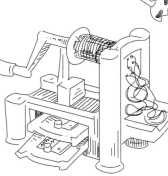

SPIRAL SLICER
I don't use mine that often, only to make zoodles. If you don't want to get a spiral slicer, you can always use a veggie peeler or julienne peeler to make zoodles.

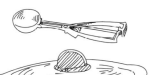

SCOOPS
Having spring-loaded scoops in a few sizes, from 4 inches to 2 centimeters, makes it easy-peasy to portion and shape burgers, meatballs, cookies, and more.

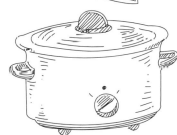

SLOW COOKER / PRESSURE COOKER
Any busy home cook will tell you these things save lives. Electric pressure cookers (like Instant Pot) both slow cook and pressure cook, which is much faster than slow cooking. All my slow cooker recipes in this book are adapted for both slow and pressure cooking.

MASON JARS
I use these to store leftovers, bone broth, sauces, and more. Sometimes they even double as water glasses!

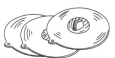

REUSABLE SILICONE LIDS
These reusable lids fit on opened jars and cans. They make storing half-full cans of coconut milk very easy.

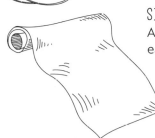

SILICONE BAKING MATS OR PARCHMENT PAPER
Always keep these on hand. They make cleanup much easier and will save your cookies in more ways than one.

how to use this book

AIP-FRIENDLY

COCONUT-FREE

EGG-FREE

SEED-FREE

First and foremost, enjoy it! Feel free to stock up with the handy list on pages 50 and 51 first and then do a flip-and-point random selection of a recipe. If you're more risk-averse or have very specific dietary needs, as most of us do, peruse the recipes for icons indicating if they're AIP-friendly, egg-free, coconut-free, and/or seed-free. If a modification is available for these, there will be an asterisk next to the icon—make sure to check out the notes for substitution information. (There's also an allergen index on pages 419 to 421 that lists the recipes and their allergen information.) Every recipe in this book is free of milk, cream, and cheese, and when butter or ghee are used, there are clearly marked substitutions. Nuts are not used at all.

The notes also offer tips and tricks for spicing up recipes, storage, meal prep, and more. There are also variations—recipe makeover tips.

Macronutrient information is provided for every recipe. If you track macros for medical or clinical reasons, however, please be sure to make your own calculations as variations will occur depending on the brands and ingredients used. Items that are for serving only are generally not included in the nutritional information.

The Staples chapter is, well, full of staples—building blocks for the recipes in later pages, like Hard Cheese (page 70), Garlic Confit (page 76), and a plethora of sauces that will make your meals pop. I've built the meal plans at the end of the book around a few staples each week. I suggest you do the same. Make a batch of Roasted Beet Marinara (page 78), for instance, and look up the recipes that feature it using the index on page 410. Having staples at the ready will make mealtime a whole lot easier.

After the Staples chapter, you will find Snacks + Small Bites, followed by Soups + Salads, two chapters filled with lighter fare perfect for appetizers or small meals, from post-workout nutrition to party-ready finger food.

The entrées are divided into sections for eggs, poultry, beef and lamb, pork, and seafood and fish. I didn't include a breakfast chapter because many people on keto skip breakfast—it happens naturally when you're fat adapted. However, you will find plenty of breakfast-friendly meals in these pages, from Pork Sausage (page 280) to Eggs Benny (page 176).

There are many entrée recipes that also include side dishes. For those that don't, or if you want to change things up, you can find delicious sides in the Sides + Beverages chapter, along with drinks like Korean Cinnamon Tea (page 356) and Coconut Butter Matcha Latte (page 358).

The Treats chapter has a well-curated selection of delicious indulgences, made with thoughtful ingredients so you can splurge a bit without feeling bloated, tired, or off your game.

Feel free to mix and match sides and entrées as you see fit. Change the sauces. Experiment. The spirit of adventure is woven into these pages, and I want to encourage you to make my recipes your own!

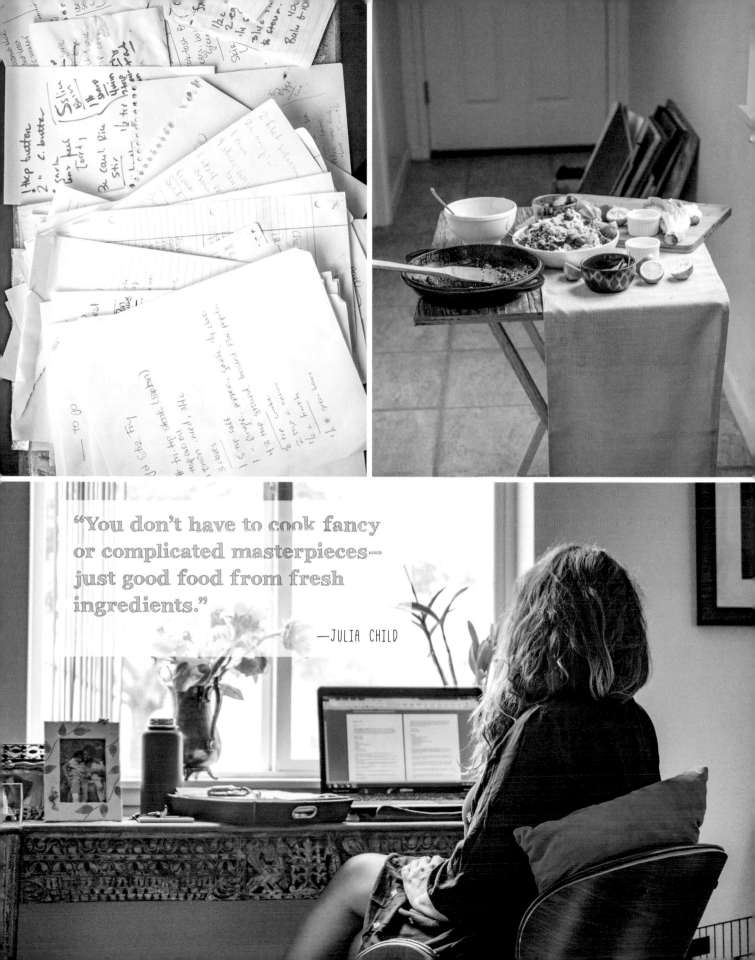

"You don't have to cook fancy
or complicated masterpieces—
just good food from fresh
ingredients."

—JULIA CHILD

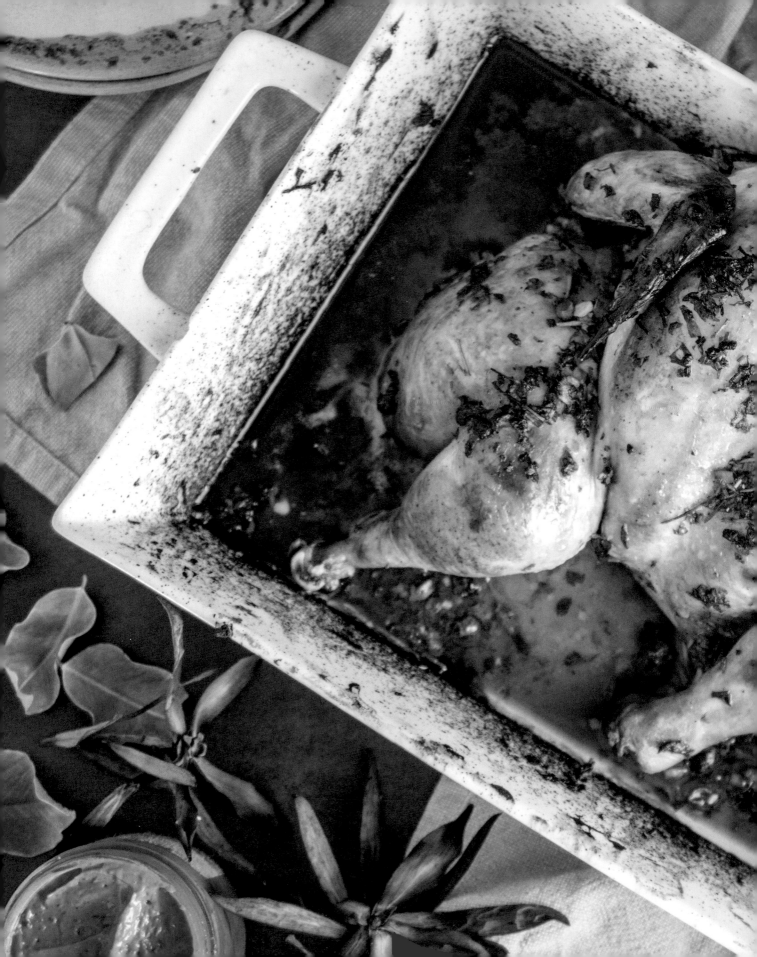

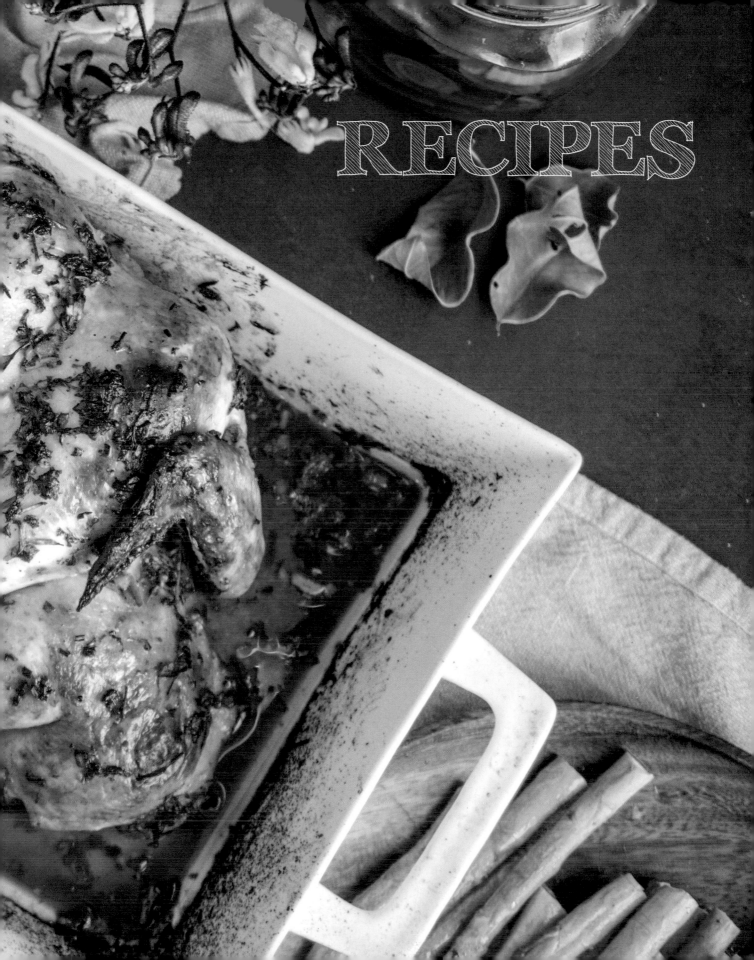

RECIPES

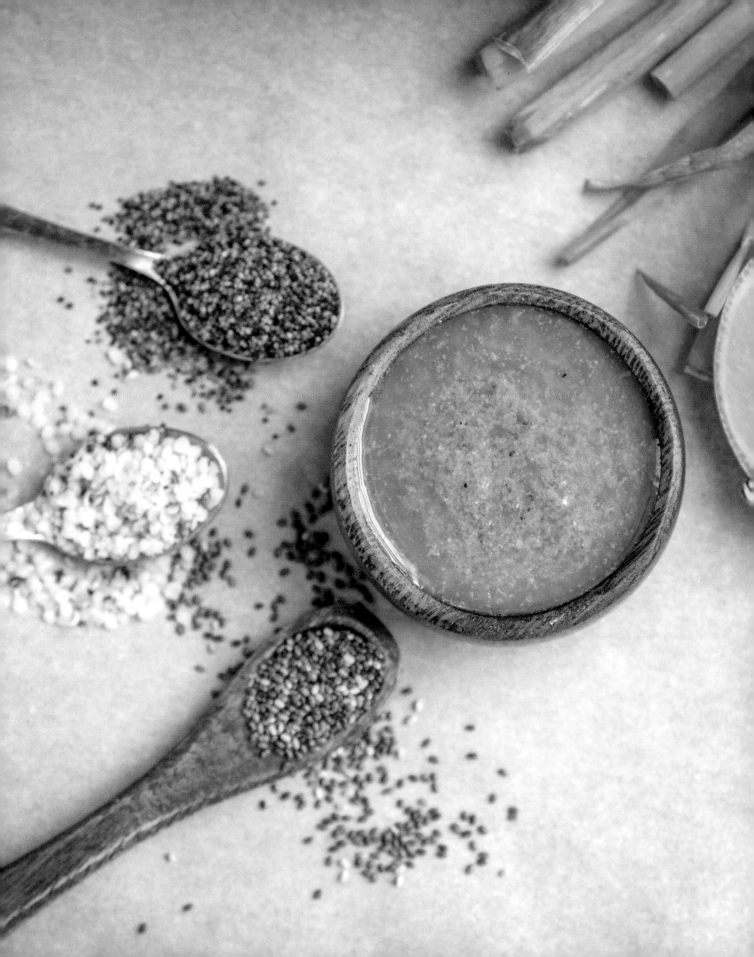

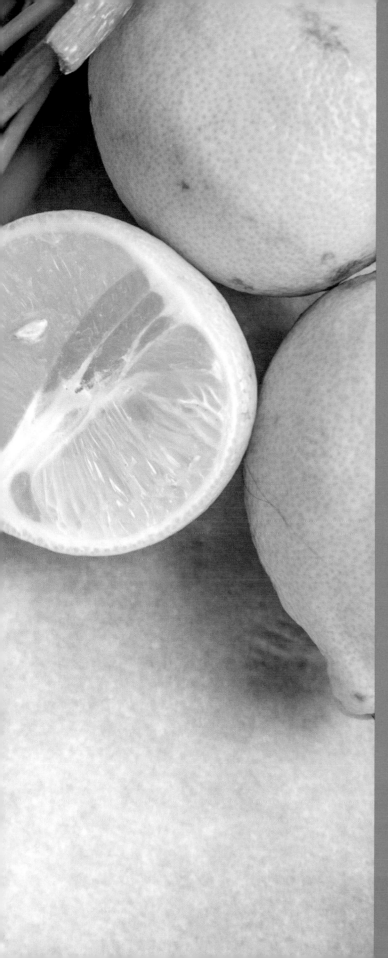

STAPLES, SAUCES + DRESSINGS

These staples are the building blocks of many of the recipes to come. I've been a sauce connoisseur as long as I can remember, always sneaking back in the kitchen to pour pan sauce over my dish or licking the Alfredo off the plate. And keeping a few good staples like Garlic Confit (page 76) or Roasted Beet Marinara (page 78) around the kitchen can quickly take your meals from boring to exciting. My goal for this chapter is to arm you with enough options to keep your taste buds tingling! As they say, the secret is in the sauce.

cheesy yellow sauce

This is an old Paleo trick: MacGyvering a combination of seasonings, acidity, and umami to trick your taste buds into believing they're getting some nacho cheese goodness when really, you're eating a super nutrient-dense addition to your meals. Use this delicious sauce to turn kelp noodles into Creamy Kale Noodles (page 320), spoon it over Beef Carnitas (page 246), or serve it as a dip with Prosciutto Chips (page 118).

1½ cups steamed, mashed cauliflower florets (about 1 small head), hot (see Notes)

½ cup full-fat coconut milk

½ cup nutritional yeast

1 tablespoon unsalted butter, ghee, or lard

1½ teaspoons coconut vinegar

1 teaspoon fine Himalayan salt

1 teaspoon garlic powder

Makes 2 cups (½ cup per serving)
PREP TIME: 15 minutes

◦ Place all of the ingredients in a blender. Cover and blend on low, slowly bringing the speed up to high.

◦ Continue blending until the sauce is completely smooth. Taste for seasoning and add a little more salt and/or garlic powder if you like.

◦ Store in an airtight container in the refrigerator for up to 1 week. Warm in a saucepan on the stovetop over medium heat, stirring occasionally.

CHEF'S NOTES: To steam cauliflower, cut the head of cauliflower into florets. Fill a saucepan with about an inch of water and bring to a boil. Place the cauliflower florets in a steamer basket and place over the boiling water. Cover and steam for about 8 minutes, until the cauliflower is fork-tender. (It's a good idea to keep a bunch of steamed cauliflower in the freezer—it comes in handy for all kinds of uses.)

This is best made with freshly steamed or reheated cauliflower because the heat from the cauliflower helps to melt the fat. If you make it with leftover refrigerated cauliflower, you will need to run the blender longer, until it heats up the sauce to melt the fat. If using refrigerated, already steamed cauliflower, reheat it in the microwave before using it in this recipe.

SUBSTITUTIONS: Use lard, duck fat, or suet in place of the butter or ghee to make this AIP-compliant. If you can't use coconut milk, you can omit it; simply double the amount of butter (or other fat) and add a little more mashed cauliflower. In place of coconut vinegar, you can use red wine vinegar or apple cider vinegar.

PER SERVING: Calories **185** · Fat **11g** · Total Carbohydrate **15g** · Dietary Fiber **7.5g** · Protein **11g**

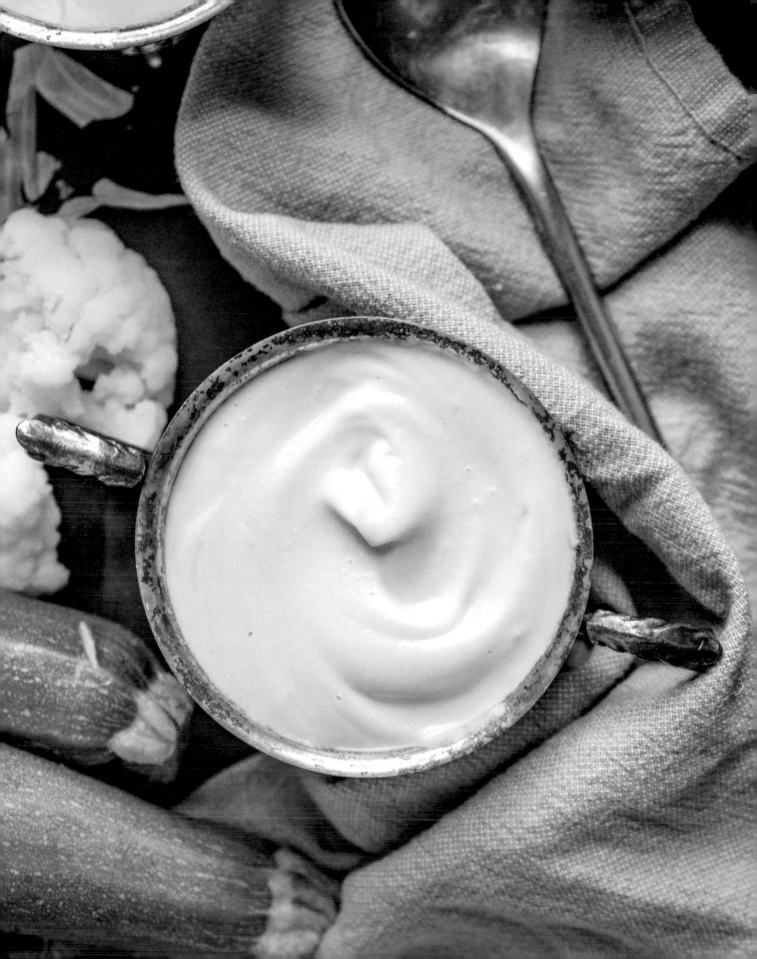

hard cheese

A few tweaks and a little pastured gelatin and you can turn Cheesy Yellow Sauce (page 68) into a firm, sliceable, meltable, spreadable cheese. It's a fantastic option when you want to make a pizza-shaped meal or a panini! Melt between two slices of Nut-Free Keto Bread (page 324) and dip in Roasted Beet Marinara (page 78) for a keto take on grilled cheese and tomato soup. It's easy to make and yummy to have on hand, especially if you're missing cheese.

Makes one 8½ by 4½-inch loaf (about 12 slices)
PREP TIME: 15 minutes, plus 4 hours to set

1 cup steamed, mashed cauliflower florets (about ¾ pound cauliflower), hot (see Note, page 68)

⅔ cup full-fat coconut milk

½ cup nutritional yeast

2 tablespoons coconut vinegar

2 tablespoons Italian herb blend

1 tablespoon unsalted butter (softened), ghee, or lard

2 teaspoons fine Himalayan salt

1 teaspoon garlic powder

2 tablespoons unflavored grass-fed beef gelatin

○ Line an 8½ by 4½-inch loaf pan with parchment paper.

○ Place all of the ingredients except the gelatin in a blender and blend on high until a thick, smooth paste forms. Stop and scrape down the sides with a spatula as necessary. When it's completely smooth, add the gelatin and blend on low until just combined.

○ Transfer the mix to the prepared loaf pan and place in the fridge to set for at least 4 hours.

○ Remove the cheese from the pan and cut it in half for storage. Store in airtight containers in the refrigerator for up to 10 days.

VARIATIONS: You can omit or amp up the herbs in this cheese to change the flavor. I really like adding chives and dill, too! For the taste of a fermented cheese, use Coconut Yogurt (page 96) in place of the coconut milk—it really gives it that dairy flavor.

If you want a cheese that has some stretch to it, like mozzarella, add 3 to 4 tablespoons tapioca starch to the mix. Add 1 teaspoon turmeric powder for a bright yellow color. For a harder cheese, use up to ¼ cup gelatin total—the more gelatin, the harder the cheese.

SUBSTITUTIONS: To make this AIP-friendly, use lard instead of butter. If you can source bone marrow, try that—not only is it more nutritious, but it also gives it a more authentic flavor. For coconut-free, omit the coconut milk and double the mashed cauliflower, and in place of coconut vinegar, use red wine vinegar or apple cider vinegar.

PER SLICE: Calories **50** · Fat **2.2g** · Total Carbohydrate **2.2g** · Dietary Fiber **2g** · Protein **3g**

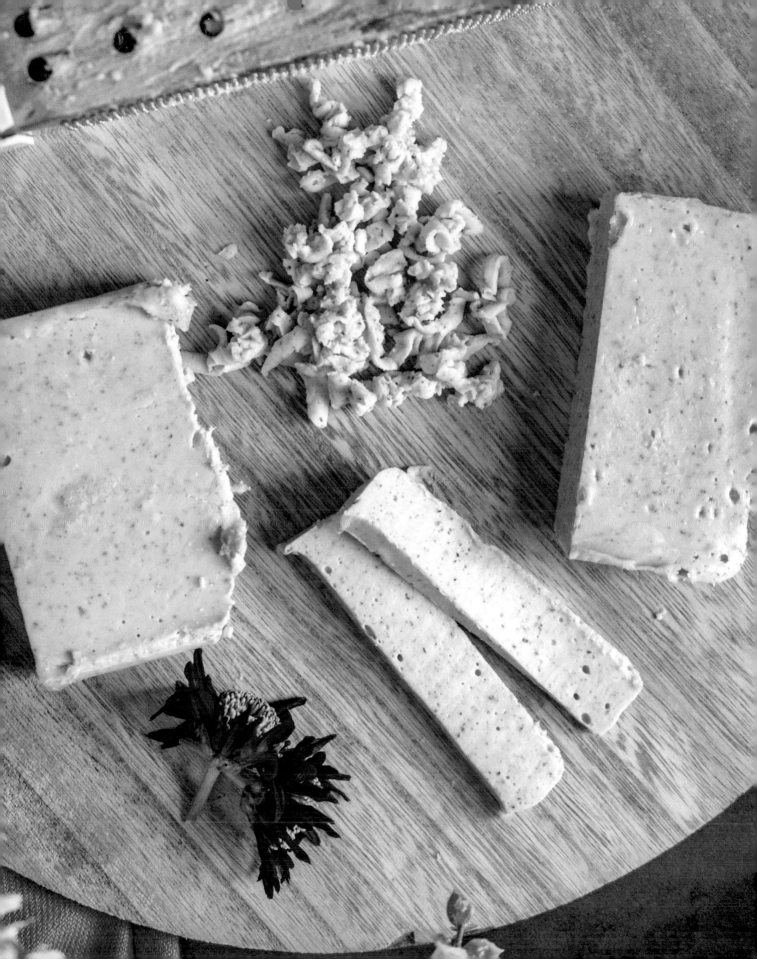

toum

This creamy sauce may look like mayo, but it's made with only five ingredients: lemon, garlic, olive oil, salt, and water. Yep! It's that simple. I first had toum at Daily Bread, a Middle Eastern market and deli in Miami. My friend Jallyn and I used to get there early to score a shawarma platter or the all-too-elusive moussaka, which was only served on weekends and disappeared ever so quickly. I just love the tangy, warm flavors of Lebanese food. The pickled red onions, the parsley in the tabbouleh, the garlicky toum, and the spiced beef. What beautiful food!

Toum can be a little tricky to make: if it doesn't emulsify, you have a great marinade, but not a sauce you'd want to slather on everything. Don't fret, I will walk you through my method, and I have a very high success rate. My trick? I chill the oil! Toum is traditionally made with sunflower or grapeseed oil, but I like to use olive or avocado oil for those good healthy fats. Use extra-virgin oil for a smooth taste that won't skew the flavor of the sauce.

Best of all, this is the perfect mayo substitute for all of my egg-free friends!

2 cups extra-virgin olive oil or avocado oil

10 cloves garlic, smashed with the side of a knife and peeled

⅓ cup lemon juice (about 2 lemons)

1 teaspoon fine Himalayan salt

CHEF'S NOTE: The color of the sauce will vary depending on the oil you use, from very white to yellowish.

VARIATION: You can always add black pepper or fresh herbs at the end to mix up the flavor profile.

Makes 3 cups (2 tablespoons per serving)
PREP TIME: 10 minutes, plus 5 to 30 minutes to chill the oil

⊙ Place the oil in a Pyrex measuring cup and put it in the freezer for about 5 minutes or in the fridge for 30 minutes. (Be careful not to chill it for too long; eventually it will solidify. If that happens, leave it out on the counter just until it liquefies but is still chilled.)

⊙ Meanwhile, place the garlic cloves, lemon juice, and salt in a food processor. Blend until the mixture is almost smooth. You may need to stop the food processor and use a spatula to scrape down the sides a few times.

⊙ With the food processor running, begin to drizzle in the chilled oil in a needle-thin stream. (If you don't have a steady hand, use a squeeze bottle. Some food processors come with an accessory that fits into the opening and has a small hole at the bottom, perfect for this kind of thing.)

⊙ Once all of the oil is incorporated and the sauce has magically become creamy, continue to run the food processor until the sauce has thickened to a creamy, smooth consistency. This should take a few extra seconds, nothing more. Stop the food processor, then taste and add more salt as desired.

⊙ Serve immediately or store in an airtight container in the refrigerator for up to 1 month. The sauce will become even thicker after being refrigerated. To return it to its original consistency, let it sit out for about 10 minutes; if you let it sit out too long, it will thin out to a dressing-like consistency.

PER SERVING: Calories **164** · Fat **18g** · Total Carbohydrate **1.2g** · Dietary Fiber **0g** · Protein **0.2g**

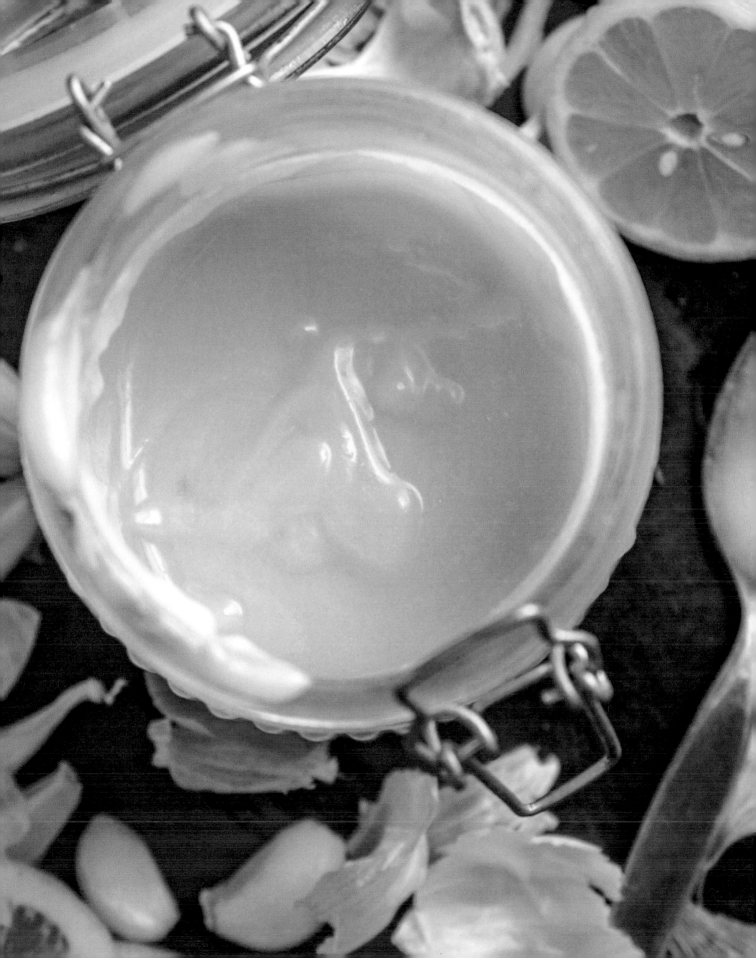

pistou

Pistou is a French herb sauce that's essentially just like pesto but without the pine nuts. Originally it was made with a mortar and pestle, with fresh basil ground to a paste and mixed with minced garlic and grated cheese. To make this a quick affair, I use my blender. (Ghastly, I know.) I've also ditched the cheese for hemp seeds. I love these little seeds because they are oh-so-rich in fiber and pack in all nine essential amino acids. This sauce is perfect for meatballs, zoodles, or chicken kebabs, or stirred into some cauliflower rice.

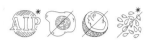

3 packed cups fresh basil leaves

6 cloves garlic, peeled

¾ cup avocado oil

½ cup shelled hemp seeds (aka hemp hearts)

1 teaspoon fine Himalayan salt

1 teaspoon garlic powder

1 teaspoon ground black pepper (optional)

Makes 1½ cups (¼ cup per serving)
PREP TIME: 10 minutes

○ Place all of the ingredients in a blender or food processor. Pulse until all of the basil and garlic is minced.

○ Blend on low for 20 to 30 seconds to smooth it out just a bit and bring the texture of the sauce together. Use a spatula to scrape it all out into a glass jar with a lid. Store in the fridge for up to 10 days.

SUBSTITUTIONS: To make this AIP-compliant, omit the black pepper and the hemp seeds and use ½ cup diced avocado instead. The pistou won't last as long, but avocado adds a great creaminess to herb-based sauces while keeping them nut- and seed-free. You may use extra-virgin olive oil instead of avocado oil; it has a more robust flavor but is still delicious.

PER SERVING: Calories **490** · Fat **47g** · Total Carbohydrate **4.5g** · Dietary Fiber **3g** · Protein **14g**

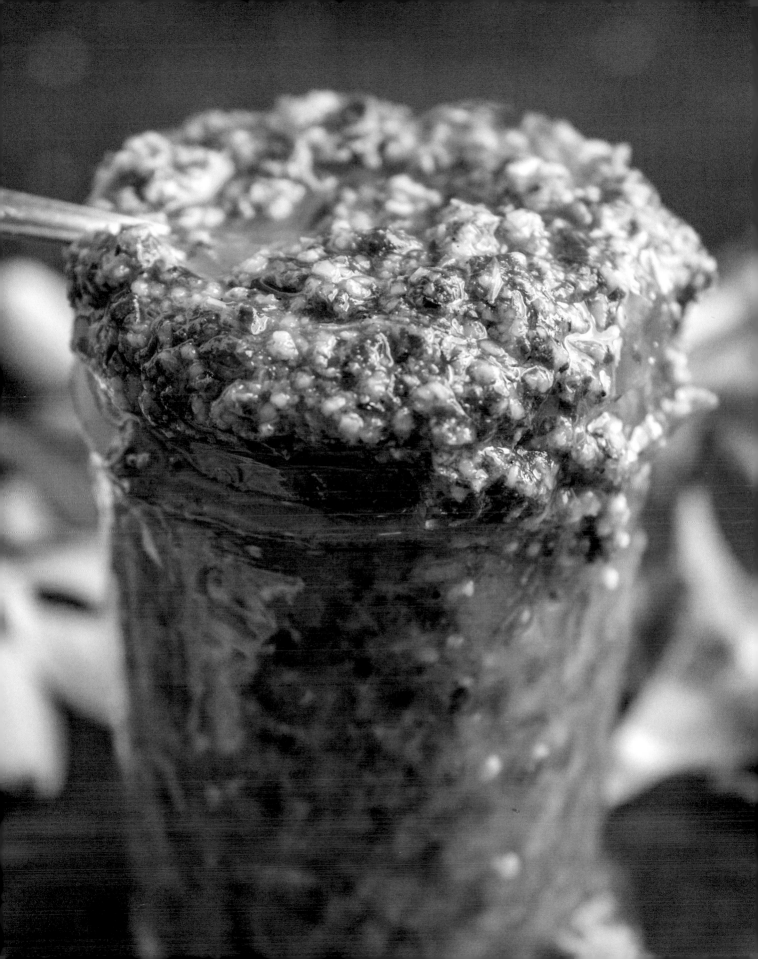

garlic confit

Don't be fooled by the fancy name; this recipe is as simple as it gets: garlic cloves submerged in oil and slowly baked to tender perfection. Keep a jar of this in the fridge for months; it's perfect to spoon over your proteins and salads or to blend into sauces. Get all the cancer-fighting, antioxidant benefits of eating garlic with these sweet and tender cloves, so soft you can spread them like butter! Oh, now that's a good idea!

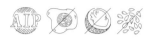

Garlic cloves, peeled (see Tip)

Olive oil or avocado oil

Himalayan salt

Fresh herb sprigs, such as thyme, rosemary, oregano, or sage

Makes ½ cup per head of garlic
PREP TIME: 5 minutes   COOK TIME: 1 hour

◦ Preheat the oven to 250°F.

◦ Put as many garlic cloves as you like in a small baking dish with a lid (a cocotte is perfect for this), leaving at least an inch of space at the top.

◦ Pour in the olive oil until the garlic is just submerged. Sprinkle in a little salt and place a few sprigs of herbs on top. Cover with the lid and place on a sheet pan to prevent a mess.

◦ Pop it in the oven and bake for 1 hour, or until you can easily pierce the garlic cloves with a fork. Remove from the oven and let it cool to room temperature.

◦ Transfer all of the garlic with the oil and herbs to an airtight glass or ceramic storage container. Store in the fridge for up to 3 months. Always use a clean spoon to remove garlic cloves or oil.

TIME-SAVING TIP: If you are strapped for time or dislike peeling garlic, buy prepeeled whole cloves. I think the fresher the garlic, the better the flavor, but I too will use a shortcut when needed.

CHEF'S NOTE: This oil is divine on meats, and the garlic can be spread like butter on a hot steak. When only a few cloves are left, let the jar sit at room temperature until the oil is fluid. Use the remaining cloves and infused olive oil to make garlic mayo, using the recipe on page 82. Because the oil is not heated past 390°F (olive oil's smoke point), it is safe to use for cooking in this instance.

PER 2 TABLESPOONS: Calories **169** · Fat **18.5g** · Total Carbohydrate **1.5g** · Dietary Fiber **0g** · Protein **0.2g**

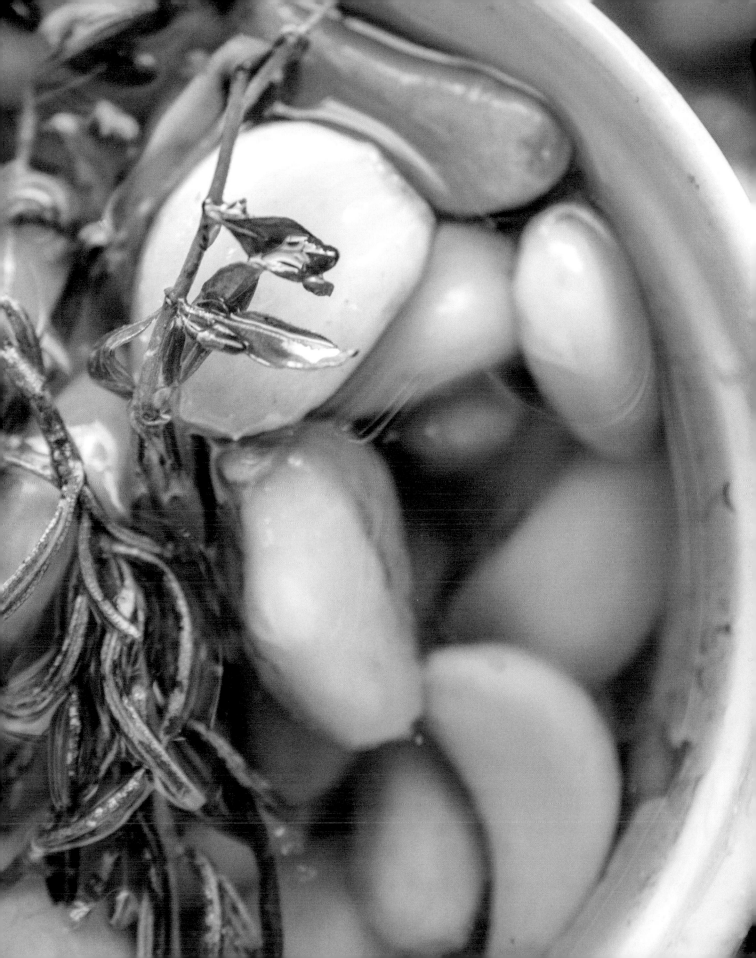

roasted beet marinara

I won't go into why this marinara doesn't have tomatoes—tomatoes are a nightshade, and I've explained why I avoid nightshades on page 25. I will, however, tell you that the roasted beets that go into this sauce come out of the oven tasting like candy. They're then blended with bone broth, herbs, and olive oil to create a robust and delicious sauce. I love adding beets to sauces for color and flavor, but also for their amazing nutritional properties. They contain vitamins A, B, and C, B9 (yup, folic acid), and fiber, and those nutrients keep us looking beautiful and feeling fantastic! Add this sauce to eggs, smear it on some toasted Nut-Free Keto Bread (page 324), mix it with kelp noodles, or use it as a dip with Prosciutto Chips (page 118) for a delicious meat-and-hidden-veggie combo!

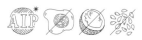

2 medium beets

2 teaspoons ghee or lard, melted

⅓ cup red wine vinegar, divided

2 cups bone broth (page 100)

¼ cup nutritional yeast

2 tablespoons Italian herb blend

2 tablespoons olive oil

2 teaspoons fine Himalayan salt

2 teaspoons granulated garlic

2 teaspoons onion powder

1 teaspoon ground black pepper

Makes 4 cups (½ cup per serving)
PREP TIME: 10 minutes   COOK TIME: 25 minutes

○ Preheat the oven to 400°F.

○ Slice the beets into ¼-inch-thick rounds and place on a sheet pan. Pour the ghee and half of the vinegar over the beets. Toss to coat the beet slices, then arrange them so they are all lying flat. Roast for 25 minutes, until they have caramelized, darkened in color, and become sticky, sweet, and toasted on the edges.

○ Remove from the oven and use a spatula to carefully transfer the beets to a blender. Add the remaining vinegar along with the rest of the ingredients and blend until smooth.

○ Pour the beet mixture into a skillet over medium-low heat to warm and serve with meatballs and/or noodles, or as desired. If you are not using all of the sauce at once, store the leftovers in an airtight container in the fridge for up to 10 days. You may also freeze the sauce for up to 3 months. (I recommend freezing in portion-sized silicone molds.) Thaw and reheat in a skillet over medium heat.

SUBSTITUTIONS: To make this recipe AIP-compliant, omit the black pepper. If you can't have nutritional yeast, omit it and use 1 tablespoon fish sauce instead. If you're avoiding vinegar or you don't have any on hand, you can use lemon juice; it will greatly change the flavor of the sauce, making it very tangy, but it will still be delicious.

CHEF'S NOTE: If you are using this sauce for dunking purposes, simmer it over medium heat for about 10 minutes, until reduced by half. Reducing the sauce will make it thick and turn it a fabulous shade of burgundy!

PER SERVING: Calories **90** · Fat **5g** · Total Carbohydrate **7.7g** · Dietary Fiber **2.5g** · Protein **4.5g**

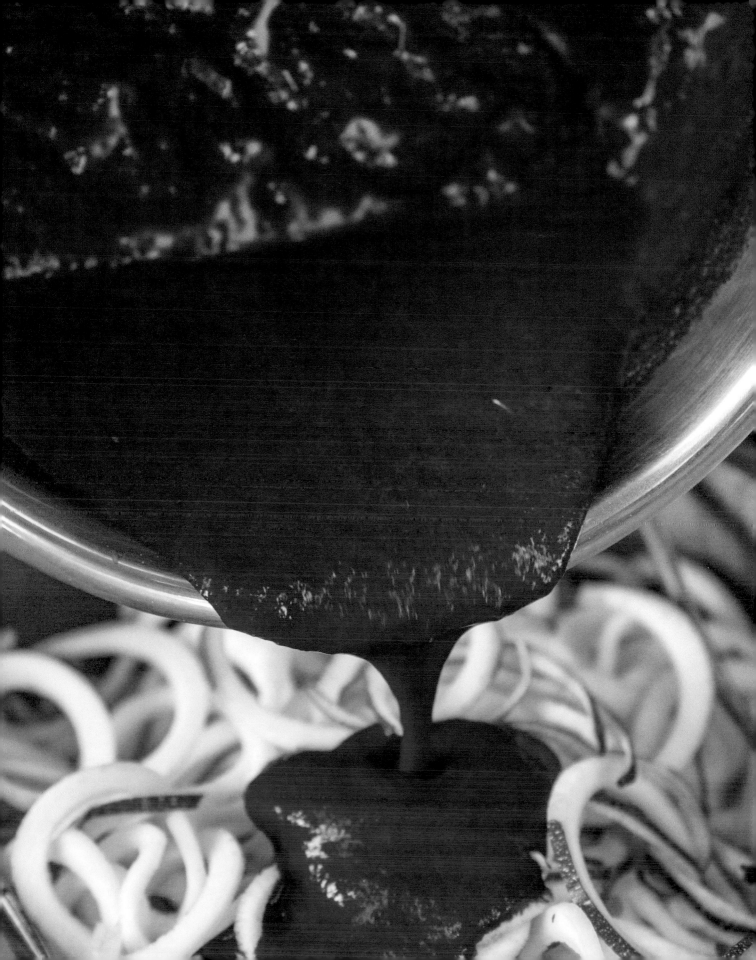

chimichurri

When I was growing up in Miami, a melting pot of Latin cultures, chimichurri was a staple. From Nicaraguan steak houses to backyard barbecues, when there was churrasco (skirt steak)—and there always was—there was chimichurri. Oh yes, chimichurri and churrasco are like peanut butter and jelly. But chimichurri is also fantastic on almost everything, from grilled seafood to crispy eggs. It's my put-on-all-things sauce. The recipe varies from region to region, household to household, and it is said the word chimichurri has its roots in Basque and means "several things mixed in no particular order."

1 cup minced fresh parsley

½ cup minced fresh cilantro

¼ cup minced fresh mint leaves

2 tablespoons minced fresh oregano leaves

¼ cup minced garlic (about 6 cloves)

1 teaspoon fine Himalayan salt

½ cup red wine vinegar

Juice of 1 lemon

1 cup olive oil or avocado oil

Makes 2 cups (2 tablespoons per serving)
PREP TIME: 15 minutes

◦ In a medium-sized mixing bowl, combine the herbs, garlic, and salt. Add the vinegar and lemon juice and let it sit for a few minutes, then whisk in the olive oil. You're not trying to emulsify the mixture, just thoroughly combine it.

◦ Transfer the mixture to a glass jar with a tight-fitting lid and seal. Store in a cool, dark place, such as a pantry. Mix or shake before using.

◦ Chimichurri gets tastier with age, though it becomes less pretty— the bright-green color it has when it's freshly made will turn dark. I don't think your chimichurri will last long enough to go bad, but use your judgment.

TIME-SAVING TIP: Instead of mincing the herbs and garlic, pulse them a few times in your food processor, then whisk in the olive oil.

VARIATIONS: You can make this with only parsley or only cilantro—as long as you have one of these two main herbs, it's chimichurri. But I like using the combination of herbs here for a special flavor. You can also add ground cumin or black pepper in place of the red pepper found in traditional chimichurri; it's very flexible and fun to experiment with.

CHEF'S NOTE: Because chimichurri keeps for a long time, it's great to make in big batches. I like to mix it into creamy sauces like mayo or ranch when I want to change things up. Mix up a double batch during your next meal prep.

PER SERVING: Calories **251** · Fat **27.1g** · Total Carbohydrate **4.1g** · Dietary Fiber **0.3g** · Protein **0.4g**

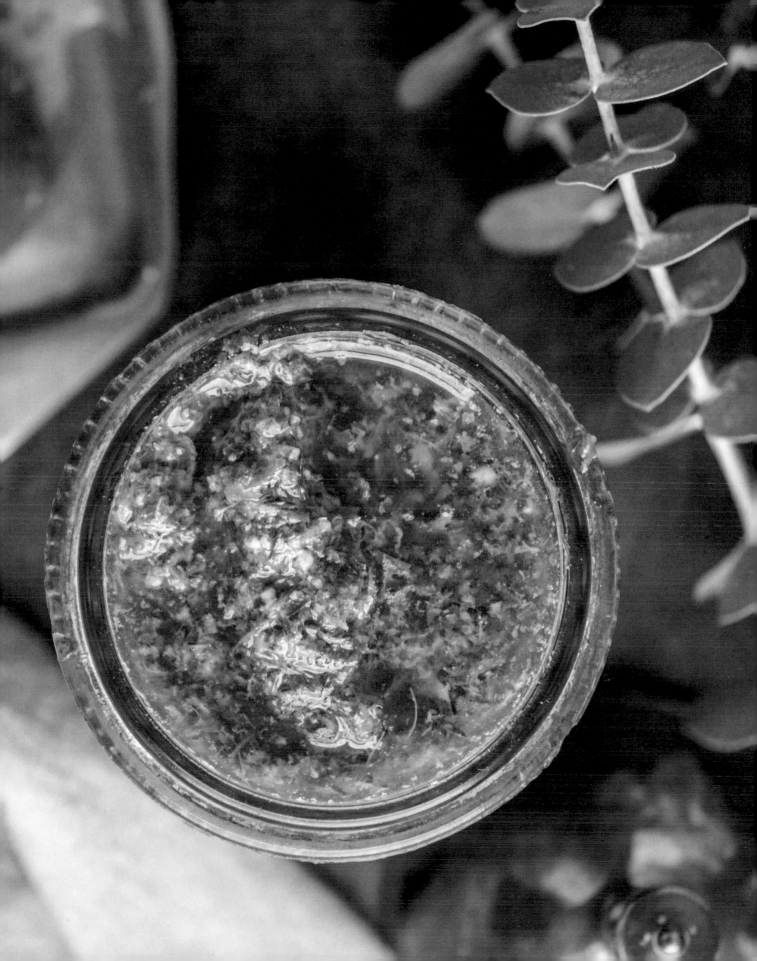

homemade mayo

My love affair with mayonesa casera (homemade mayonnaise) began about twenty years ago in the kitchen of my mother's first restaurant, Yerba Buena, which made a rosemary-and-olive-oil mayonnaise that was to die for. Before that, I thought those jars at the store were real mayonnaise. Not even close. There is nothing quite like homemade mayo, and it's a fantastic opportunity to omit unwanted additives and vegetable oils from your diet. Yes, sad to say, most store-bought brands of mayo have less-than-admirable ingredients. While better options are becoming available, homemade is more cost-effective, and with this no-fail recipe, it's a breeze to make!

3 tablespoons coconut vinegar

1 teaspoon dried thyme leaves

½ teaspoon granulated garlic

½ teaspoon dry mustard

½ teaspoon fine Himalayan salt

3 large egg yolks

1 cup avocado oil

Special equipment:
Immersion blender

Makes 1 cup (2 tablespoons per serving)
PREP TIME: 5 minutes

○ Place the vinegar and seasonings in a 16-ounce measuring cup or quart-sized mason jar. Gently add the egg yolks and then the avocado oil.

○ Insert the immersion blender into the mixture, turn it on high, and move it up and down slightly until the mix is completely emulsified. Use a spatula to scrape all of the mayonnaise off of the blender and then to transfer the mayonnaise to a jar or other container with a tight-fitting lid.

○ Store in the refrigerator for up to 10 days, and always use clean utensils when serving.

VARIATIONS:

Beet Mayo. Add 2 tablespoons minced fresh beets, which will produce a sweeter, bright-pink mayo.

Garlic Mayo. Add ¼ cup Garlic Confit (page 76), which will produce a rich, garlicky flavor. You can also substitute garlic-infused oil for the avocado oil.

Herb Mayo. Add ¼ cup Chimichurri (page 80) for a quick and tangy herb mayo.

CHEF'S NOTES: I use a lot of mayo, and not only in typical dishes like Castaway Chicken Salad (page 164)—I find it to be the perfect condiment for dipping anything! For example, try it with Chicken Kofta Kebabs (page 206) or Vietnamese Crispy Chicken (page 214).

If Mercury is in retrograde or you're having an off day and for some reason the mayo doesn't come together, add the egg whites and keep blending to thicken it up. I prefer egg yolk mayo because adding the egg whites blocks some of the nutritional benefits of the yolk, but when you have to troubleshoot a recipe, do what you have to do!

SUBSTITUTIONS: If you can't find coconut vinegar or don't have any on hand, you can use apple cider vinegar or red wine vinegar instead. Extra-virgin olive oil is an acceptable substitute for the avocado oil.

PER SERVING: Calories **262** · Fat **30g** · Total Carbohydrate **0g** · Dietary Fiber **0g** · Protein **1g**

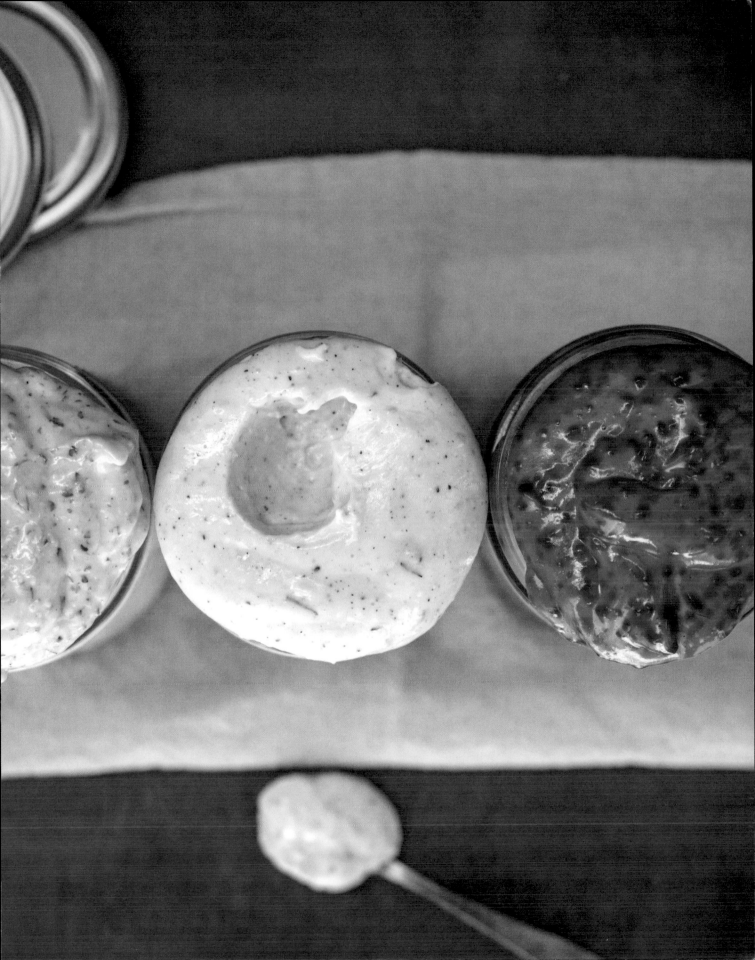

everything bacon

Everything bagel seasoning on bacon, roasted to crispy perfection. You can eat these bacon slices on their own, like chips, or with eggs, or chop them up and sprinkle them on a salad. There is really no wrong way to enjoy these delicious, slightly addicting strips.

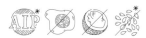

10 slices bacon

1 teaspoon dried dill weed

1 teaspoon onion powder

1 teaspoon poppy seeds

1 teaspoon toasted sesame seeds

¼ teaspoon fine Himalayan salt

Makes 5 servings (2 slices per serving)
PREP TIME: 5 minutes   COOK TIME: 20 minutes

○ Lay the slices of bacon flat on a sheet pan. Sprinkle the seasonings evenly over the bacon. The higher up you sprinkle from, the more evenly the bacon will be seasoned.

○ Place the sheet pan in the oven and set the temperature to 375°F. (Note: Don't preheat the oven! You want to start with a cold oven.) Bake until the oven comes to temperature, then for 10 to 15 minutes more. (I like to make this bacon extra crispy; if you prefer softer bacon, take it out of the oven sooner.) Keep an eye on it for the last few minutes. When it's ready, it will be dark brown and firm, and your home will smell of bacon.

○ Remove from the oven and lay the bacon slices on a cooling rack until they're room temperature and crisp.

○ Store flat in an airtight container in the fridge for up to 8 days. Bring to room temperature before adding to salads or snacking on, and heat in a warm skillet before adding to hot dishes.

VARIATIONS: You can change up the flavor of these quite easily by loading them up with your favorite seasonings. Switch out the poppy seeds and sesame seeds for 1 teaspoon smoked salt and 1 tablespoon granulated erythritol for sticky, sweet, and smoky bacon!

SUBSTITUTIONS: To make these AIP-compliant, omit the seeds; add your favorite herbs or some lemon zest instead for delicious, seed-free crispy bacon.

PER SERVING: Calories **214** · Fat **16.5g** · Total Carbohydrate **1.3g** · Dietary Fiber **0.2g** · Protein **14.4g**

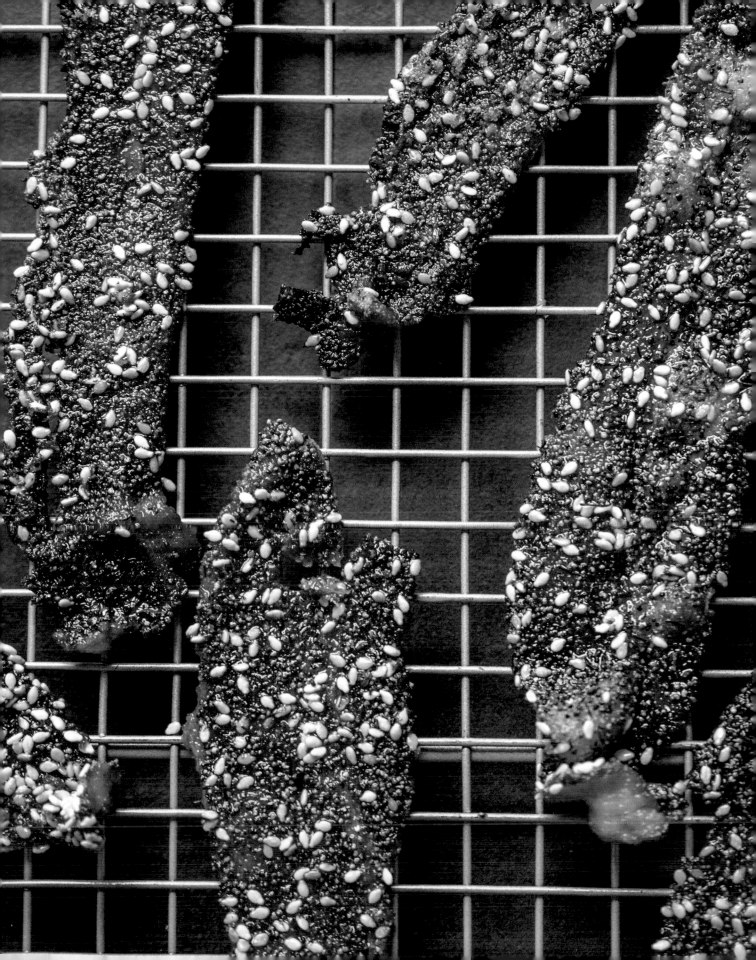

cauliflower alfredo

Can a sauce feel decadent yet simple at the same time? I think this one does. It's warm and creamy, with a gentle flavor. It's easily tweaked to work any time you need a savory cream sauce: add an egg yolk to make it more like a béchamel, reduce it to make it thicker, or add broth to water it down. It's the perfect addition to casseroles, noodles, or soup bases! Who needs heavy cream when you have this vegetable-loaded option?

   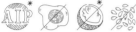

3 cups cauliflower florets

5 cloves garlic, peeled

1 cup full-fat coconut milk

3 tablespoons salted butter, ghee, or lard

1 tablespoon fish sauce

1 tablespoon red wine vinegar

1 teaspoon fine Himalayan salt

1 teaspoon ground black pepper

Makes 2 cups (½ cup per serving)
PREP TIME: 10 minutes   COOK TIME: 12 minutes

⊙ Fill a saucepan with about an inch of water and add the cauliflower and garlic. Heat the pan over medium-high heat and bring to a boil with the lid on. Cook for about 8 minutes, until the cauliflower is fork-tender. Remove from the heat and drain.

⊙ Place the cauliflower, garlic, and remaining ingredients in a blender. Puree until smooth.

⊙ Store in an airtight container in the fridge for up to 10 days. To reheat, bring to a simmer in a saucepan over medium heat.

VARIATIONS: If you want to really boost the flavor of this sauce, steam the cauliflower and garlic with bone broth (page 100) instead of water, or add a bouillon cube to the water while steaming. If you do all right with alcohol, add a splash of white wine to the recipe—it creates a rich flavor, reminiscent of little Italian trattorias. Use Garlic Confit (page 76) instead of raw garlic for a sweeter flavor!

SUBSTITUTIONS: To make this sauce AIP-compliant, omit the black pepper and use lard instead of butter. You can also make it coconut-free: omit the coconut milk and add an extra cup of cauliflower florets to compensate.

PER SERVING: Calories **250** · Fat **24g** · Total Carbohydrate **9g** · Dietary Fiber **3.4g** · Protein **3.5g**

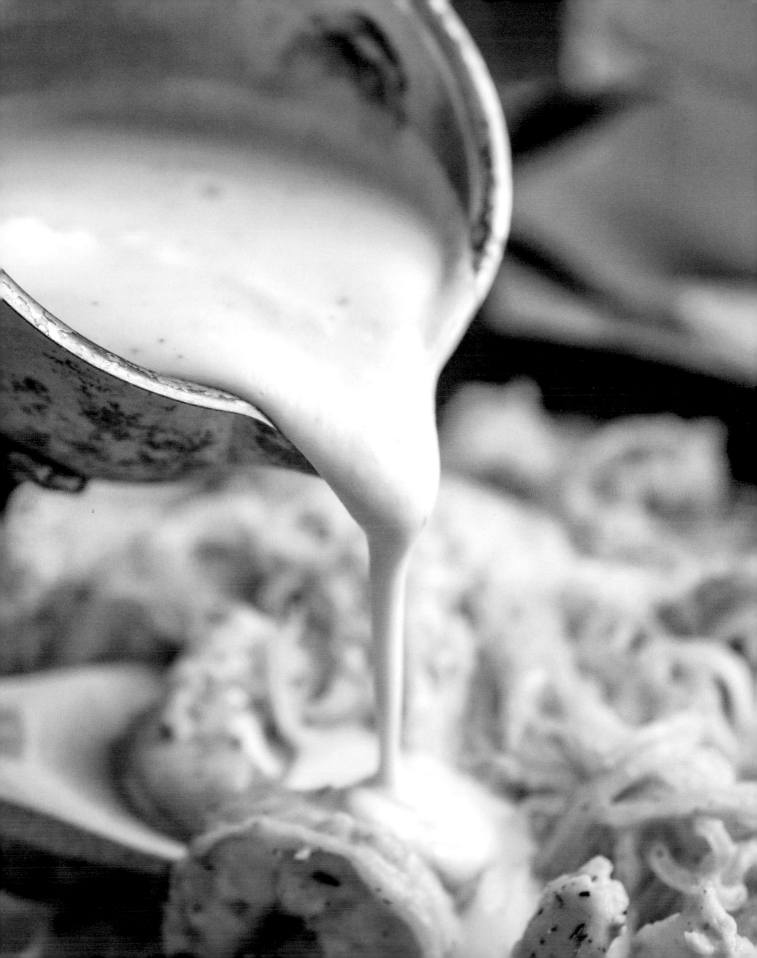

pickled red onions

These are a game changer. Add them to salads or put them on a juicy steak, tacos, or crispy chicken—pickled red onions are a welcome addition to any dish, providing color, crunch, and tang. I first discovered these when working on a food truck in San Diego. I was leaving the job because I was pregnant and was training my replacement. Little did I know the chef replacing me was way more experienced, a New Orleans restaurant veteran with more than twenty years under her belt. Marguerite's first creation was a very impressive taco combination that included pickled red onions, and I was hooked. Now I make these regularly and put them on everything.

2 cups filtered water

1 cup apple cider vinegar

1 teaspoon fine Himalayan salt

1 teaspoon granulated erythritol or other low-carb sweetener (optional; see Note)

2 bay leaves

2 red onions, thinly sliced and cut into half-moons

Special equipment:

3-cup or larger glass or ceramic container with a tight-fitting lid

Makes 4 cups (¼ cup per serving)
PREP TIME: 5 minutes, plus 30 minutes to steep   COOK TIME: 10 minutes

⦾ Combine the water, vinegar, salt, erythritol (if using), and bay leaves in a small saucepan over medium heat. Bring to a light simmer and cook for about 8 minutes. Stir to make sure the salt and sweetener have dissolved.

⦾ Put all the onion slices in a jar with the bay leaves and then pour the hot brine over the onions until they are fully submerged. Let the onions steep for 30 minutes at room temperature before using. Seal the jar and store in the fridge for up to 1 month.

VARIATIONS: Peppercorns, cloves, thyme sprigs, garlic, and even sliced radishes are a welcome addition to these pickled onions. You can really play around with the brine.

CHEF'S NOTE: The sweetener is not necessary, especially if you like your onions extra tangy. If you do use sweetener, use a low-carb one like erythritol or monk fruit (see page 38 for more on these). If you're okay having a little bit of sugar, maple syrup or coconut palm sugar also work well.

PER SERVING: Calories **5** · Fat **0g** · Total Carbohydrate **2g** · Dietary Fiber **0.2g** · Protein **0g**

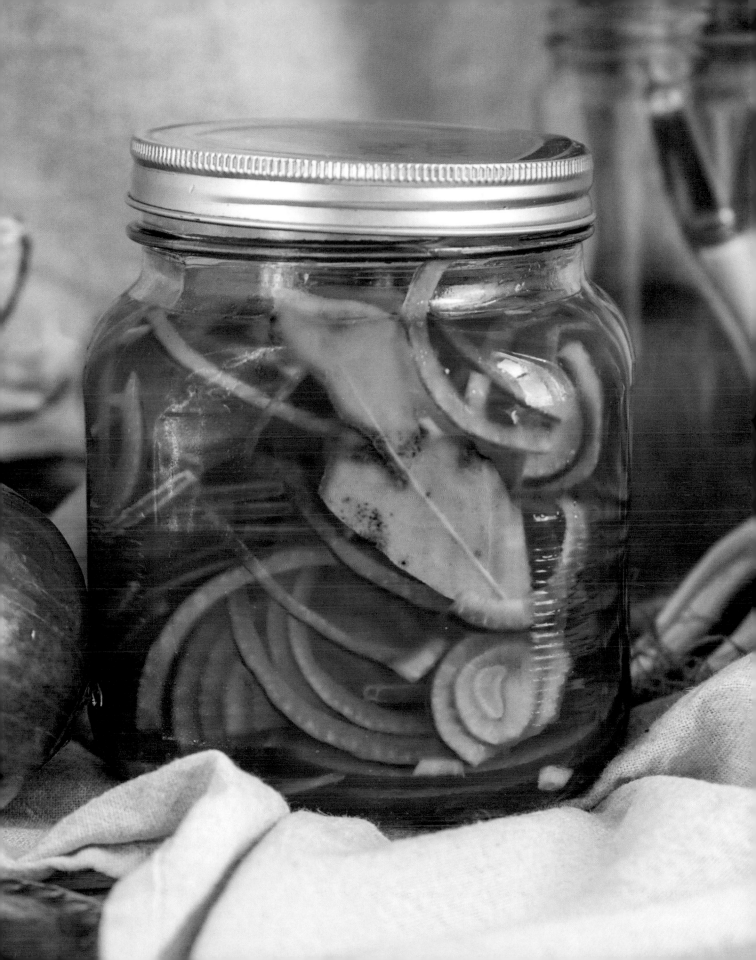

fiesta guacamole

Crunchy and spicy radishes, sweet strawberries, crispy green onions, and creamy avocado: this colorful take on guac is a veritable party in your mouth. It's perfect for scooping up with crunchy veggies and spooning over salads or ground beef, and absolutely necessary when making tacos (see page 246). You won't even miss the nightshades, I promise! Here's a tip for when you're making a dish, like guacamole, that will yield a lot of food trash: keep an extra bowl or bag on the counter to throw your peels, seeds, and scraps in. It saves a few trips to the garbage or keeps the food scraps separate for your compost!

Makes 3 cups (½ cup per serving)
PREP TIME: 15 minutes

3 medium Hass avocados, halved, pitted, and peeled

3 small radishes, sliced

3 large strawberries, diced

3 cloves garlic, minced

1 green onion, sliced

½ bunch fresh cilantro (about 1½ ounces), minced

Juice of 2 lemons

2 teaspoons fine Himalayan salt

1 tablespoon extra-virgin olive oil

⊙ Place all the ingredients in a large bowl. Use a whisk or pestle to mix and mash them together until you have a chunky guacamole.

⊙ If it's not all going to be consumed right away, transfer it to an airtight container, drizzle olive oil on it, set a sheet of plastic wrap on the top so that it sticks directly to the guacamole—this will help keep the avocado from turning brown—and then put the lid on. Store in the fridge until ready to enjoy, but no more than 4 days.

PER SERVING: Calories **215** · Fat **18g** · Total Carbohydrate **15g** · Dietary Fiber **9g** · Protein **4g**

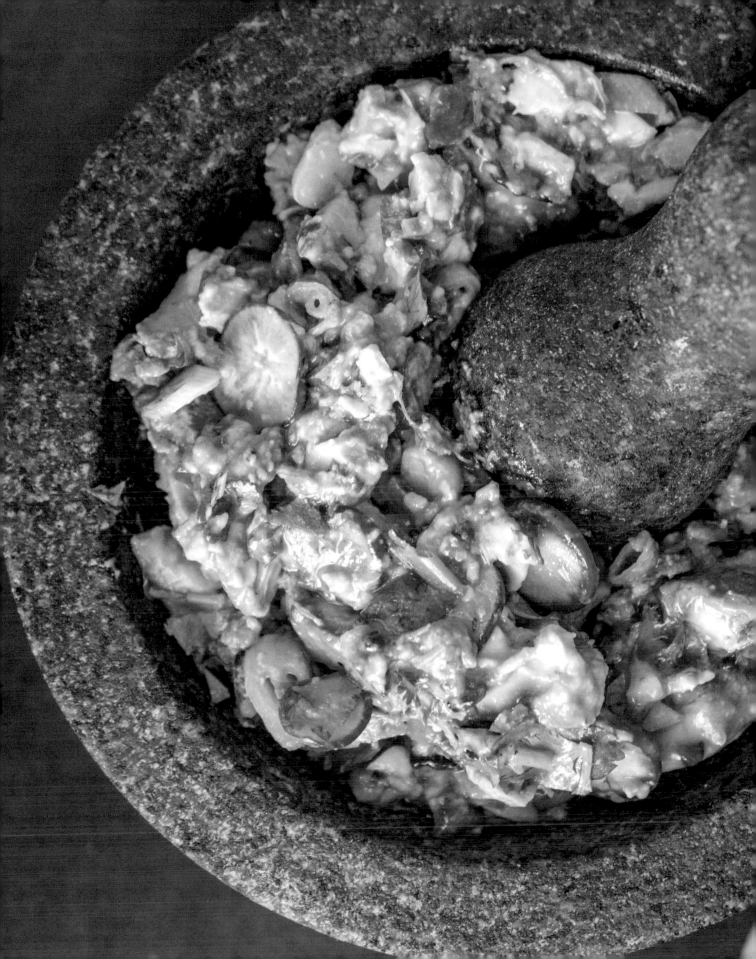

pie crust

Just by changing the amount of coconut flour, the dough for Crispy Thin Flatbread (page 134) becomes an excellent pie crust dough that you can knead and simply press into a pie pan. This recipe makes enough crust for one 8-inch pie or four empanadas. This is a versatile recipe for savory or sweet dishes—it has your low-carb pie needs covered. It even makes a great tart, baking up beautifully in a springform pan with a nice tall crust that holds up wonderfully (see Coconut Citrus Tart, page 366).

4 large eggs, cold

½ cup melted coconut oil, not hot

¼ teaspoon fine Himalayan salt

1 teaspoon granulated erythritol or other low-carb sweetener (see page 38) (optional; use only if making a sweet pie)

⅓ cup plus 1 tablespoon coconut flour

Makes 1 (8-inch) pie crust
PREP TIME: 20 minutes   COOK TIME: 15 minutes

◦ Preheat the oven to 400°F.

◦ In a small bowl, whisk the eggs as you slowly pour in the coconut oil—it will become creamy. Then add the salt and granulated erythritol (if using) and stir to combine. Add the coconut flour and fold until a dough forms.

◦ Transfer the dough to an 8-inch pie pan and use your fingers to gently press it into the dish, bringing it 1 inch up the sides. Pie crust is all about patience and finesse. Work slowly; aim to make the thickness even throughout, and make sure the 1-inch crust on the sides is level all around.

◦ Use a fork to poke a few holes in the bottom of the crust. Bake for 15 minutes, or until golden with browned edges.

◦ Use to make a pie right away, or wrap it up in the pie pan and freeze for up to 30 days. To thaw and heat, bake in a preheated 400°F oven for 15 minutes.

TIME-SAVING TIP: To save time when making dishes that use this pie crust, bake the pie crust ahead of time and wrap it tightly in plastic wrap. Refrigerate for a few hours or freeze overnight or until you're ready to use it. When you're ready to use it, pull it out, fill it up, and pop it in the oven.

CHEF'S NOTE: I love using this dough to make empanadas with leftover Crispy Kalua Pork (page 282) or Carne Molida (page 244). I add a spoonful of Homemade Mayo (page 82) or Cheesy Yellow Sauce (page 68) to the filling for a nice moist empanada. Make the dough as instructed, then roll out eight 3-inch circles between parchment paper, four for the bottoms and four for the tops. Transfer the four bottoms to a parchment paper–lined sheet pan, add the filling, then top with the remaining crusts and use wet fingers to seal the edges shut. Use a fork to poke a few holes in the top, then bake in a preheated 400°F oven for 15 minutes, or until golden and brown at the edges.

PER ¼ CRUST: Calories **411** · Fat **35.7g** · Total Carbohydrate **14.4g** · Dietary Fiber **8.8g** · Protein **9.8g**

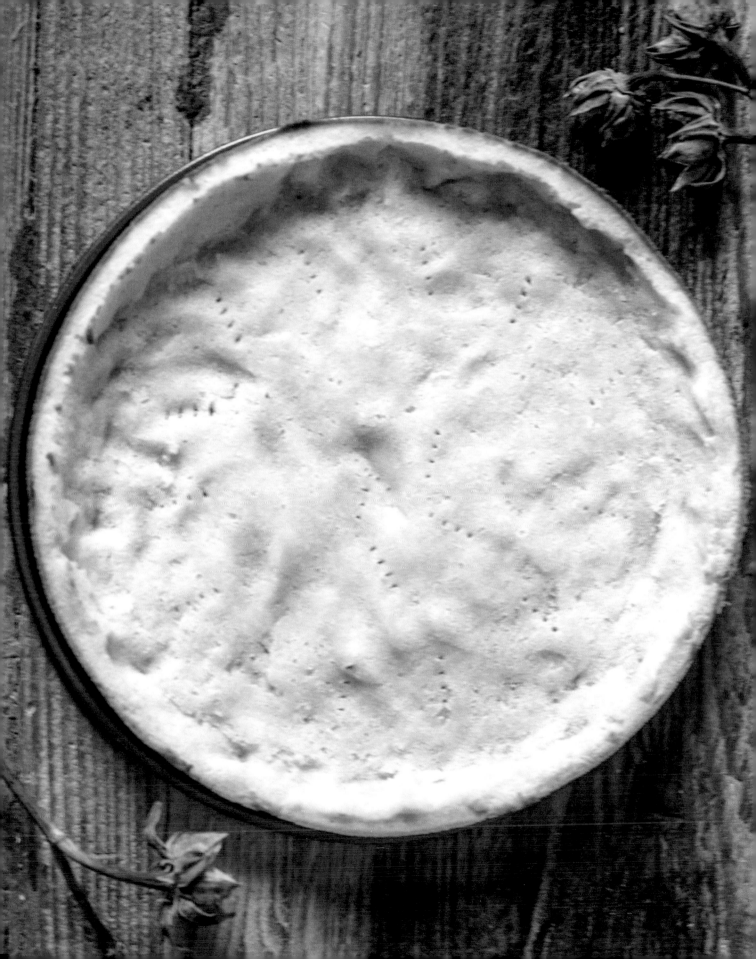

ranch dressing

A good creamy salad dressing is a must-have in your sauce arsenal, and ranch is a great go-to. Ranch dressing is like everyone's favorite uncle: always welcome, makes everything more fun, and gets along with everyone. Ranch makes salads amazing, but it's pretty life changing when paired with proteins or pizza. This rendition uses hemp seeds and little coconut milk in lieu of eggs and cream.

½ cup filtered water

½ cup full-fat coconut milk

½ cup shelled hemp seeds
(aka hemp hearts)

2 tablespoons red wine vinegar

1 tablespoon coconut aminos
(optional)

1 tablespoon Dijon mustard

2 teaspoons dried dill weed

1 teaspoon dried parsley

1 teaspoon fine Himalayan salt

1 teaspoon fish sauce

1 teaspoon garlic powder

1 teaspoon onion powder

1 teaspoon ground black pepper

Makes 1½ cups (¼ cup per serving)
PREP TIME: 5 minutes

○ Place all of the ingredients in a blender and blend until smooth.

○ Store in an airtight glass or ceramic container in the fridge for up to 10 days. Set out at room temperature to soften for a few minutes before using, and shake or stir to mix well.

SUBSTITUTIONS: To make this AIP-compliant, use half a Hass avocado instead of hemp seeds, omit the black pepper, and replace the mustard with 1 teaspoon horseradish. It won't last as long, but it will be so good, you won't have to worry about that.

CHEF'S NOTE: Here's a tip for you ranch lovers: mix up a big batch of the dry seasoning in this recipe to have ranch flavor ready to go anytime to make Party Meatballs (page 260), sprinkle over your soups and salads, or season any protein for a quick flavor boost.

PER SERVING: Calories **225** · Fat **18g** · Total Carbohydrate **4g** · Dietary Fiber **2.2g** · Protein **10.7g**

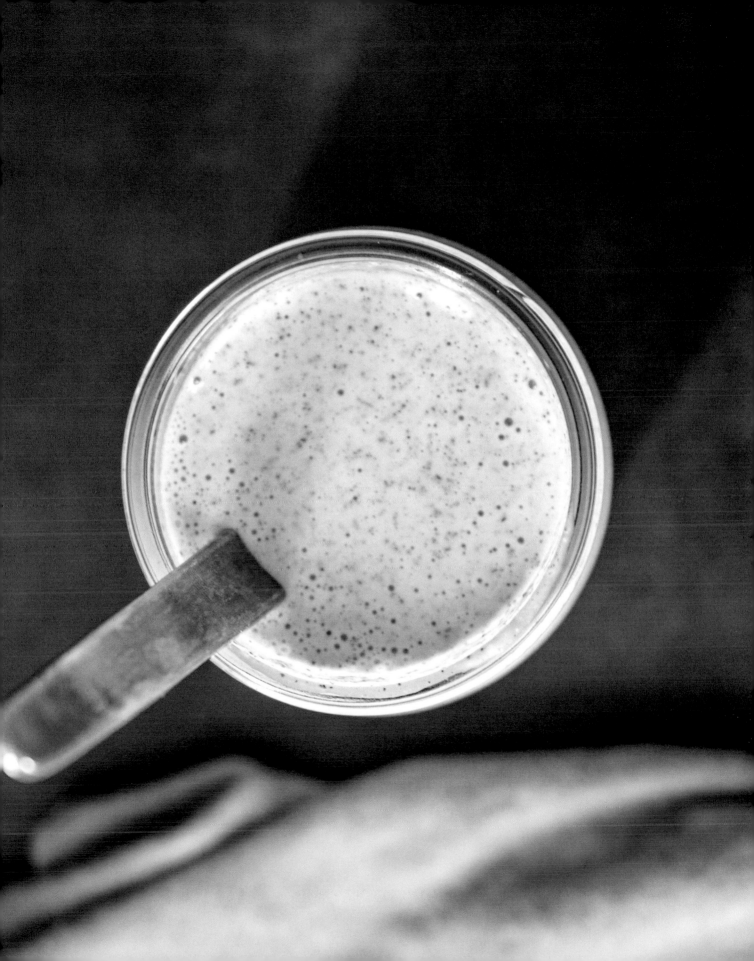

coconut yogurt

I'm a little obsessed with Greek yogurt. I love its thick and creamy texture and tart flavor. So I was ecstatic when this coconut yogurt turned out to be just as good as my favorite store-bought Greek yogurt. It is absolutely divine—the tartness is dairy-mimicking perfection. With just ten minutes of hands-on time required, there's no excuse not to make this yogurt. Store-bought options always have fillers or emulsifiers or cost a fortune. This recipe? It's got just three ingredients and zero shenanigans. I love to cook with this, too—it makes an appearance in a few of the recipes in this book, so keep some on hand.

3 cups full-fat, additive-free canned or frozen coconut milk (see Note)

2 capsules dairy-free, live-culture probiotics

2 teaspoons unflavored grass-fed beef gelatin

Special equipment:

Sterilized quart-sized mason jar or two 12-ounce jars with lids (see sterilizing instructions below)

Makes 3 cups (½ cup per serving)
PREP TIME: 10 minutes, plus at least 12 hours to ferment and 4 hours to chill

○ Preheat the oven to 100°F. (If it will not go that low, set it to the lowest possible temperature and watch it until it reaches 100°F, then turn it off.) If using frozen coconut milk, defrost it in the refrigerator.

○ Gently heat the coconut milk in a saucepan over medium-low heat just until lukewarm. Fill the sterilized jar(s) with the warm coconut milk. Empty the probiotic capsules into the milk and add the gelatin. Using a scrupulously clean whisk or fork, whisk until completely smooth and thick.

○ Place the jar(s) on the middle rack of the oven, close the oven, and turn on the oven light. Do not open the oven for 12 to 24 hours. The longer the yogurt ferments, the more tart it will become.

○ Remove the yogurt from the oven and whisk until smooth. Seal the jar(s) with a tight-fitting lid(s) and chill in the fridge for at least 4 hours. Now it's ready to enjoy. There will be some separation; just stir to combine. (*Note:* If the yogurt has pink or gray spots, toss it and make a new batch, making sure you have properly sterilized the jars—see the instructions below.)

○ Store in the fridge for up to 1 week.

CHEF'S NOTE: While garden-variety canned coconut milk is fine to use in most of my recipes, this one truly works best with additive-free milk, which means no guar gum. There are options available at most health-food stores or online. My absolute favorite additive-free brand is Hawaiian Sun Frozen Coconut Milk. If you use coconut milk with guar gum, you will need to add an additional teaspoon of gelatin to achieve the consistency of a thick Greek-style yogurt.

HOW TO STERILIZE A JAR: This step is necessary because if the jar is not sterilized, bad bacteria can grow during the fermenting process. There are two methods for sterilizing jars: the traditional (and more time-consuming) method uses boiling water, and the shortcut method (my preferred way) uses the microwave. For both methods, start by washing a quart-sized mason jar (or two 12-ounce jars) in warm soapy water and rinsing well.

To sterilize in water, place the clean jar in a large pot. Cover with water by at least 1 inch and bring to a boil; continue to boil for 15 minutes, then remove the jar and let air-dry, upside-down, on a clean towel.

Alternatively, microwave the clean jar on high for 45 seconds, or until bone dry. This is the most efficient way of sterilizing jars I have found.

PER SERVING: Calories **280** · Fat **28.6g** · Total Carbohydrate **6.7g** · Dietary Fiber **2.6g** · Protein **4.3g**

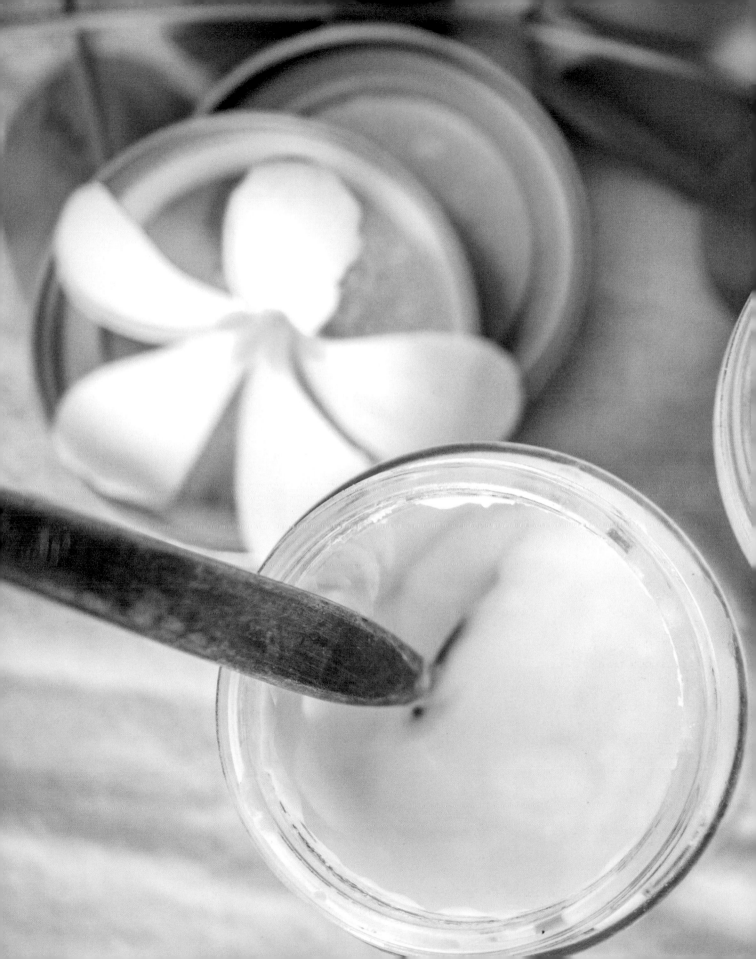

tzatziki

This is my husband's favorite sauce—well, apart from hot sauce, which he douses everything in. I stopped taking it personally a few years ago, but every now and then I twinge as I see my works of art being drowned in fiery fluid. It's interesting to me that he loves tzatziki so much because this Mediterranean sauce is anything but hot. Served chilled and made with cucumber, yogurt, lemon, and dill, it's the epitome of cool. Some tzatzikis have a chunky texture; I like this smooth rendition. Made easy-peasy using the blender, dried dill weed, and seedless cucumber, tzatziki is no longer a labor of love—although, I assure you, you will fall head over heels for it.

Makes 2 cups (¼ cup per serving)
PREP TIME: 8 minutes

2 cups roughly chopped seedless cucumber (1 large cucumber)

⅔ cup Coconut Yogurt (page 96)

⅓ cup olive oil

2 cloves garlic, peeled

Juice of 2 lemons

1 tablespoon dried dill weed

1½ teaspoons ground black pepper

1 teaspoon fine Himalayan salt

○ Place all of the ingredients in a blender and blend until smooth.

○ Store in a glass jar with a tight-fitting lid in the refrigerator for up to 1 week. Shake well before using.

SUBSTITUTIONS: Omit the black pepper to make this recipe AIP-compliant. If you do not have coconut yogurt on hand, use ⅔ cup coconut cream (see Note, page 144) instead; the sauce won't have as much tang, but it will still be delicious.

PER SERVING: Calories **132** · Fat **13.5g** · Total Carbohydrate **2.9g** · Dietary Fiber **0.2g** · Protein **0.5g**

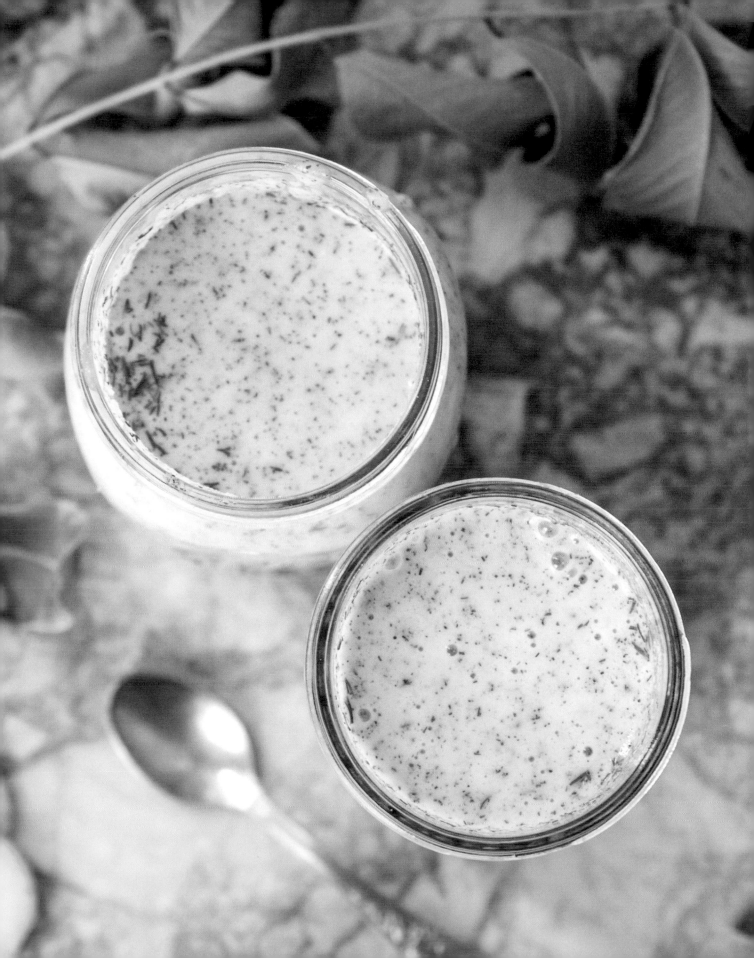

bone broth

These days it's quite easy to purchase quality bone broth. However, homemade broth is not only extremely cheap to make, it also reduces waste. I squirrel away all my vegetable scraps and chicken bones, stashing them in freezer bags and saving them for the day I have enough scraps to make a good, flavorful broth. I like bold flavors, so naturally, I like a strong broth, something delicious enough to sip when I'm feeling under the weather and yet versatile enough that it's a welcome addition to any recipe. Kick it old-school, and let's make some broth.

   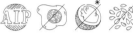

Makes 6 cups (1 cup per serving)
PREP TIME: 15 minutes   **COOK TIME:** 40 minutes, plus 48 hours in a slow cooker

5 pounds pastured animal bones, such as chicken, beef, turkey, and/or pork

3 cups vegetable scraps (see Notes)

2 sprigs fresh oregano

2 sprigs fresh sage

1 red onion, quartered but not peeled

2 large carrots

4 ribs celery

2 teaspoons fine Himalayan salt

5 cups filtered water

1 tablespoon coconut vinegar

2 bay leaves

○ Preheat the oven to 400°F.

○ Place all of the bones on a sheet pan and arrange the vegetable scraps around them. Place the fresh herbs on the bones and add the onions, carrots, and celery. Sprinkle the salt over everything. Roast for 40 minutes.

○ Remove from the oven and transfer to a slow cooker. Pour the water and vinegar over the bones and vegetables and add the bay leaves. Cook on low for 48 hours.

○ After 48 hours, remove the broth from the slow cooker and strain to remove the solids. Pour into storage containers. You can freeze cubes of it in silicone molds or ice cube trays, or store in glass jars in the refrigerator for up to 1 week.

CHEF'S NOTES: I like a good variety of vegetable scraps. Onions, celery, carrots, and vegetable peels from garlic, butternut squash, and beets are fantastic. Don't use more than 2 cups of cruciferous vegetables (such as broccoli, Brussels sprouts, cauliflower, etc.) or the flavor will be overpowering.

If you're going to use the broth for sweet dishes (and there are some sweet recipes in this book that do), skip the vegetables and herbs for a mild-tasting broth that can blend in with any flavors.

SUBSTITUTIONS: For coconut-free, replace the coconut vinegar with red wine vinegar or apple cider vinegar.

PER SERVING: Calories **60** · Fat **6g** · Total Carbohydrate **1g** · Dietary Fiber **0g** · Protein **4.8g**

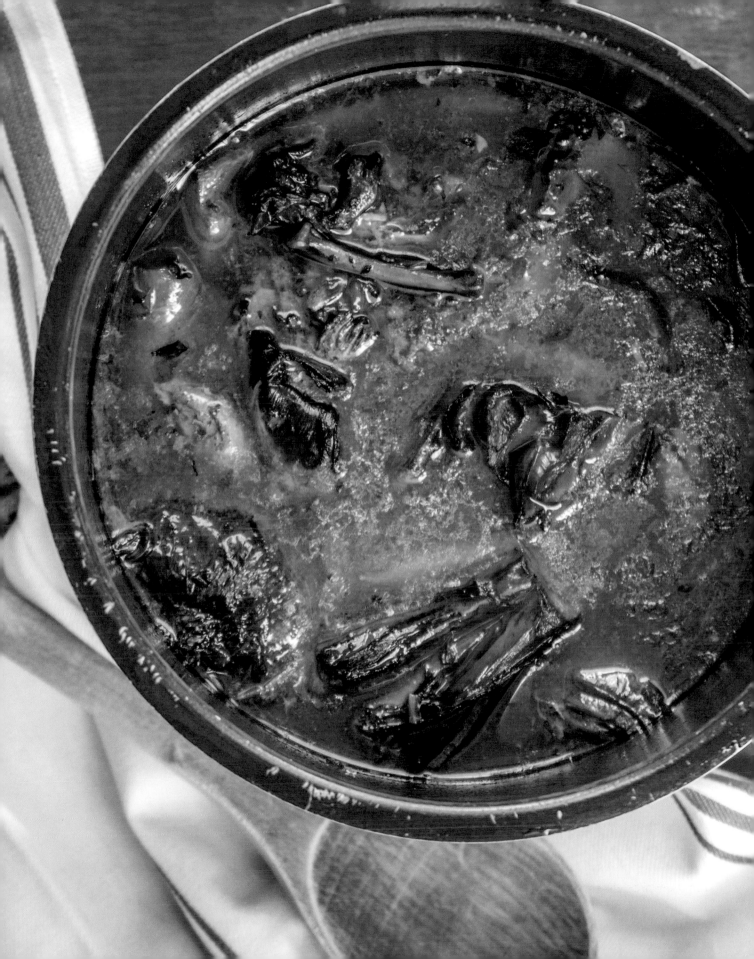

ginger sauce

My favorite thing about this sauce is its versatility. Good on everything from salads to steaks, this flavorful sauce is one you will be licking off of plates for years to come.

½ cup full-fat coconut milk

¼ cup coconut aminos

¼ cup peeled and minced fresh ginger

4 cloves garlic, peeled

2 tablespoons coconut vinegar or red wine vinegar

2 tablespoons sesame oil

1 tablespoon Dijon mustard

1 tablespoon fish sauce

1 teaspoon minced lemongrass or grated lemon zest

Makes 1½ cups (¼ cup per serving)
PREP TIME: 10 minutes

○ Place all of the ingredients in a blender and blend on high until the mixture is smooth and light brown. You can also make this sauce in a jar with an immersion blender.

○ Store in an airtight container in the refrigerator for up to 10 days. Shake before using.

SUBSTITUTIONS: To make this dressing AIP-compliant, omit the sesame oil and Dijon mustard and add 2 tablespoons more coconut milk and two more garlic cloves.

PER SERVING: Calories **113** · Fat **9.6g** · Total Carbohydrate **6.2g** · Dietary Fiber **0.6g** · Protein **0.9g**

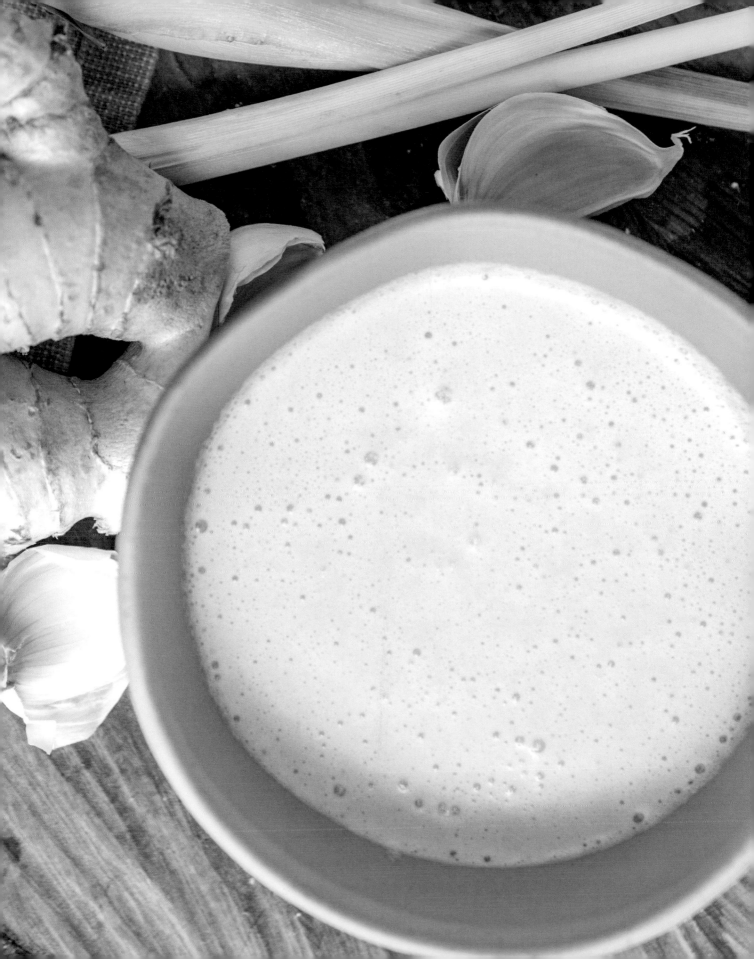

raspberry vinaigrette

As I write this recipe, raspberries are at the peak of their season. Sweet as candy and oh-so-cheap! It's late summer, when the sun still sets after 7 p.m. and your weekends consist of long days that leave you sun-kissed and exhausted—these are my favorite days. The days you come home too tired to cook and nothing sounds good but a big easy salad, thrown together with leftovers. This colorful and lightly sweet dressing is just the thing for a salad like that.

1 cup raspberries

1 cup avocado oil

½ cup chopped red onions

¼ cup chopped fresh parsley

¼ cup red wine vinegar

1 teaspoon fine Himalayan salt

1 teaspoon ground black pepper

1 teaspoon peeled and minced fresh ginger

10 drops liquid stevia, or 1 teaspoon granulated erythritol (optional)

Dash of ground cinnamon

Pinch of ground nutmeg

Makes 2 cups (2 tablespoons per serving)
PREP TIME: 10 minutes

○ Place all of the ingredients in a blender and blend on high until smooth. The mixture will go from bright red to a dull dark pink. It will be creamy, piquant, and a little sweet.

○ Store in an airtight container in the refrigerator for up to 10 days. Shake before using.

VARIATIONS: If you're not into stevia, use 1 teaspoon raw honey instead or omit the sweetener altogether. Strawberries or blueberries would also work in this recipe instead of raspberries.

SUBSTITUTION: To make this recipe AIP-compliant, omit the pepper and stevia.

PER SERVING: Calories **130** · Fat **14g** · Total Carbohydrate **2g** · Dietary Fiber **1g** · Protein **0g**

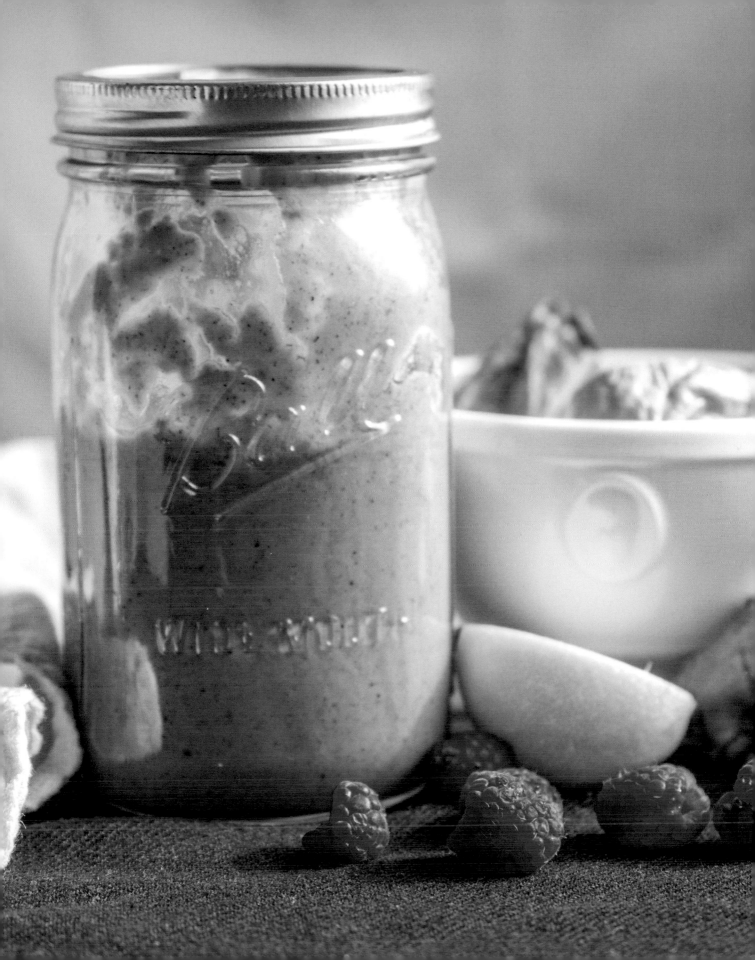

green goddess dressing

Akin to the ranch dressing on page 94, this is a loose adaptation of classic green goddess dressing for those who can't have eggs or nuts. Also, it's a super-easy version. This dressing is a vibrant hue of green and packs in three kinds of seeds, which give it a lovely thick texture, and a whole lot of chives for a whole lot of flavor! I love this dressing with big savory bowls—drizzled over avocado, berries, and sprouts, snuggled up to some protein, or piled over a bed of baby greens. Beautiful!

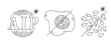

4 cloves garlic, peeled

½ cup minced fresh chives or green onions

¼ cup lemon juice

2 tablespoons coconut aminos

1 tablespoon Dijon mustard

1½ teaspoons fine Himalayan salt

1 teaspoon chia seeds

1 teaspoon ground black pepper

1 teaspoon poppy seeds

1 teaspoon shelled hemp seeds (aka hemp hearts)

5 drops liquid stevia (optional)

1 cup avocado oil

Makes 2 cups (2 tablespoons per serving)
PREP TIME: 10 minutes

○ Place all of the ingredients except the oil in a blender and pulse to combine. Drizzle in the avocado oil slowly while the blender runs, until the sauce comes together creamy and smooth.

○ Store in an airtight container in the refrigerator for up to 10 days. Shake before using.

VARIATIONS: If you've got extra herbs in the fridge that are wilting, you can add them to this dressing. A handful of cilantro and parsley are a welcome addition but not necessary.

SUBSTITUTIONS: If you're out of lemon or short on time, you can use ¼ cup coconut vinegar or apple cider vinegar instead of lemon juice. The stevia is optional—omit it if you're off sweeteners. To make this dressing AIP-compliant, omit the seeds, black pepper, and stevia; use ¼ cup coconut butter instead.

PER SERVING: Calories **128** · Fat **14.3g** · Total Carbohydrate **1g** · Dietary Fiber **0g** · Protein **0.3g**

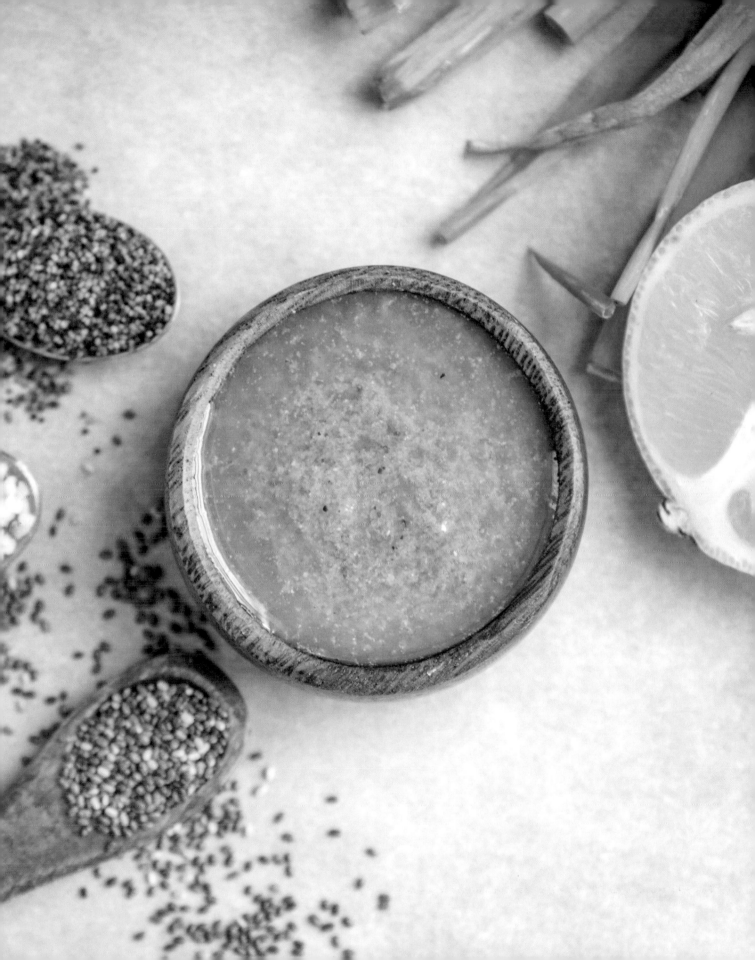

greek marinade + dressing

Simple, clean, and classic, this is a great dressing for greens but also a killer marinade for steak or chicken—having a jar of this in your fridge will always come in handy. You can make this dressing old-school and mince everything by hand, combine it all with the lemon juice, and then whisk in the oil. I'm sort of married to my blender, so I use it for everything. The choice is yours; all in all, it takes about the same amount of time.

Makes 1½ cups (2 tablespoons per serving)
PREP TIME: 10 minutes

3 cloves garlic, minced

1 cup extra-virgin olive oil or avocado oil

Juice of 3 lemons (about ½ cup)

2 tablespoons minced fresh oregano leaves

1 teaspoon ground black pepper

1 teaspoon onion powder

½ teaspoon fine Himalayan salt

○ Place all of the ingredients in a blender and blend on medium speed until the dressing has emulsified and is a light-brown color and the garlic is almost smooth.

○ Store in an airtight container in the fridge for up to 10 days. This dressing separates very quickly, so shake or stir before using.

SUBSTITUTIONS: To make this dressing AIP-compliant, omit the black pepper.

PER SERVING: Calories **150** · Fat **17g** · Total Carbohydrate **1g** · Dietary Fiber **0.1g** · Protein **0.2g**

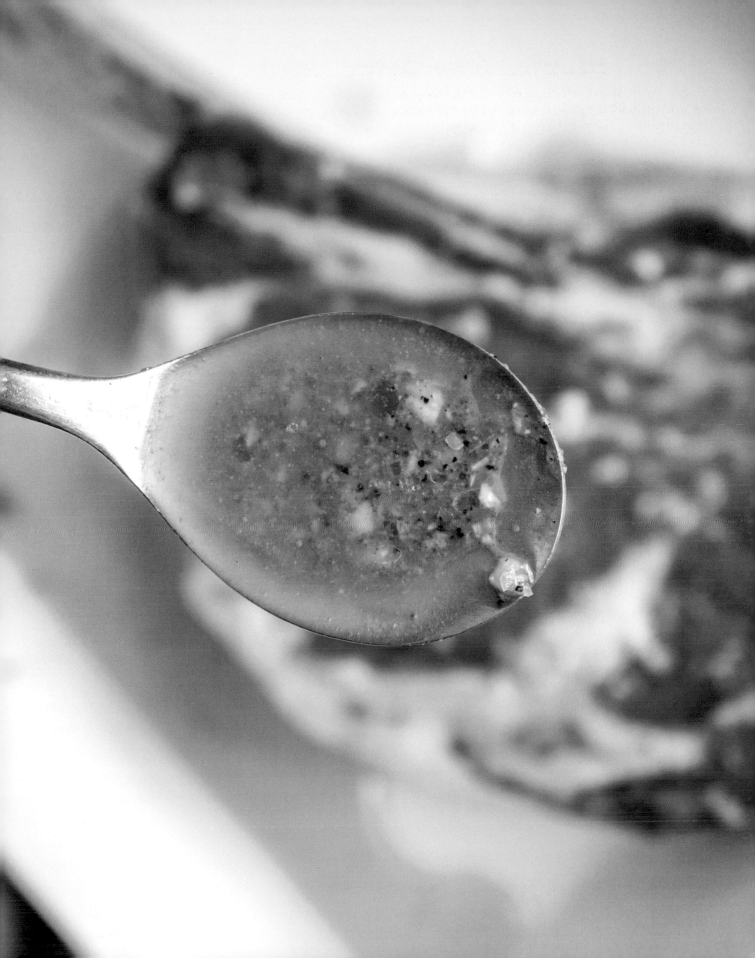

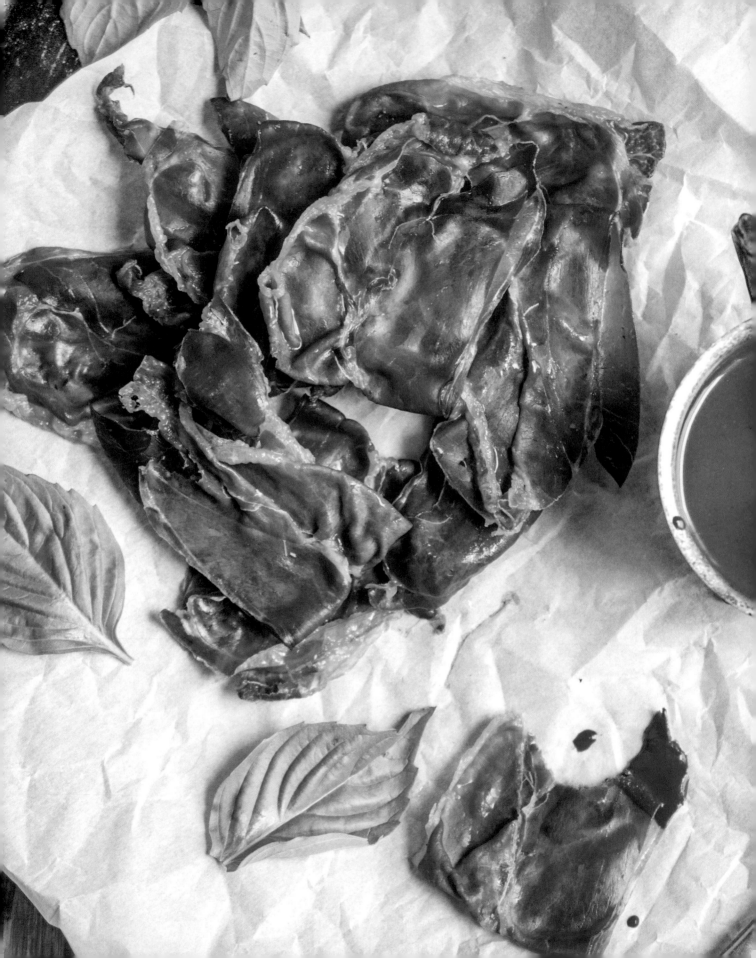

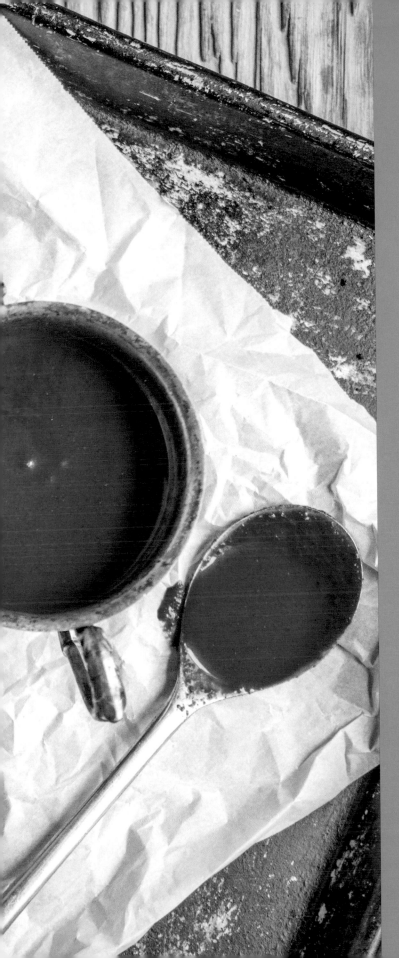

SNACKS + SMALL BITES

Sometimes all you need is a little snack. From quick and simple between-meal bites to the perfect appetizer or potluck finger food, here you'll find fun foods for every occasion.

croquetas de jamón

When I was growing up, croquetas de jamón were a staple. When you grow up Cuban, Dad doesn't go out to get donuts on the weekend; he gets a box of pastelitos and croquetas, and don't forget the cafecito. In Miami, you can pick up these fried goodies at almost any corner boasting a bodega or diner. La Carreta was our regular place when I was a kid; my dad would make a pit stop for a shot of espresso and my sisters and I would get some snacks. Croquetas are traditionally made with a ham paste and béchamel sauce that's mixed into dough, breaded, and deep-fried. I've simplified the recipe and cleaned it up a bit for a little taste of nostalgia without the canola or carbs.

1 pound boneless ham steak, diced

½ cup full-fat coconut milk

3 large eggs

1 teaspoon dried parsley

1 teaspoon onion powder

Pinch of ground nutmeg

⅔ cup plus 1 teaspoon coconut flour, divided

1½ cups coconut oil, or more if needed, for frying

CHEF'S NOTE: I like to use my cast-iron Dutch oven to fry these up. When 5 or 6 croquetas are in the oil, it rises enough to cover just the bottom half. After 3 minutes, the bottom halves will be a deep golden brown and firm if you slide a slotted spoon under them and give them a flip. If your pot is too big or you don't use enough oil and the sides are not submerged when frying, they will be much more difficult to flip—so make sure you're deep-frying, not pan-frying.

VARIATIONS: You can make these with chicken, too! Smoked chicken breast would be best, but any leftover cooked chicken meat will work.

Makes 20 croquetas (2 per serving)
PREP TIME: 20 minutes   COOK TIME: 30 minutes

○ Line a baking sheet with parchment paper.

○ Place the ham in a food processor and pulse to mince. Add the coconut milk, eggs, dried parsley, onion powder, nutmeg, and 1 teaspoon of the coconut flour. Blend until a moist dough forms.

○ Heat the coconut oil in a 5-quart Dutch oven or cast-iron skillet over high heat. The oil should be approximately 2 inches in depth; add more if necessary.

○ While the oil heats, prepare the croquetas: Pour the remaining ⅔ cup of coconut flour on a plate. Use wet fingers to scoop about 2 tablespoons of the ham paste out of the food processor and shape it into a ball about the size of a lime, then gently flatten it into an oval. Dredge it in the coconut flour, gently toss it between your hands to shake off the extra flour, and place it on the prepared baking sheet. Repeat with the rest of the ham paste. You should end up with about twenty croquetas.

○ Insert the end of a wooden spoon handle in the oil; if it sizzles, the oil is ready. Place five or six croquetas in the oil at a time; the oil should cover about the bottom half of the croquetas. Fry for 3 minutes, then carefully turn over using tongs or a slotted spoon and fry for another 3 to 4 minutes, until the croquetas are deep golden brown all over. Remove the croquetas from the oil with a slotted spoon and place on a cooling rack. Repeat with the remaining croquetas.

○ Let cool to room temperature before serving. They're definitely best served right away.

○ Store leftovers in an airtight container in the refrigerator for up to 1 week. Reheat in the oven or toaster oven at 400°F for 5 to 8 minutes.

PER SERVING: Calories **445** · Fat **40.3g** · Total Carbohydrate **11.6g** · Dietary Fiber **6.3g** · Protein **11.8g**

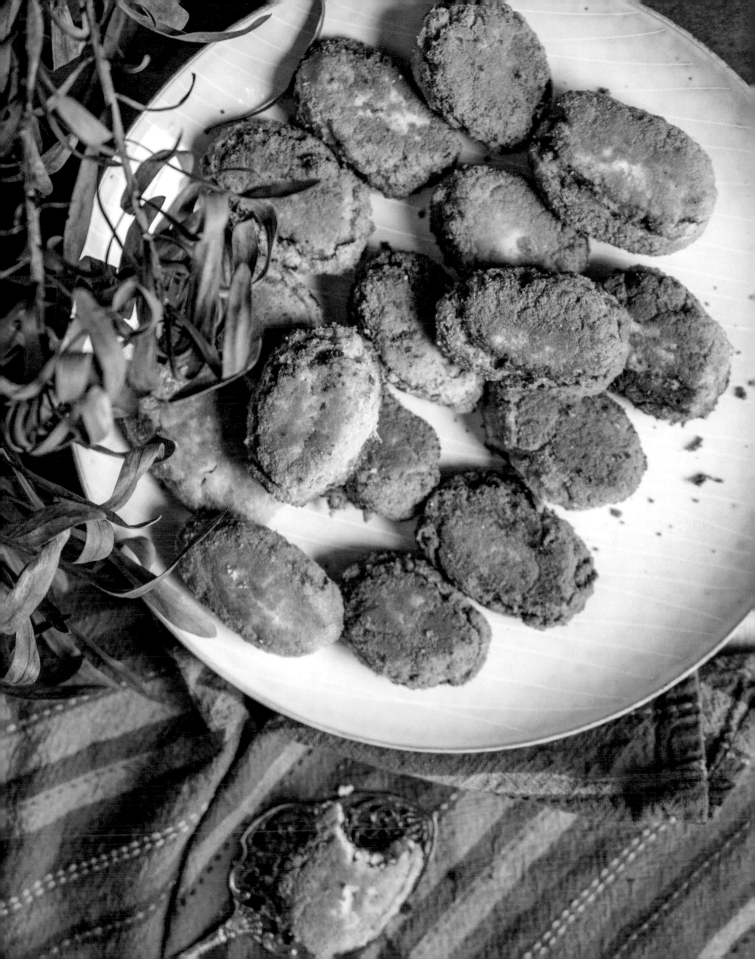

deli skewers

The Earl of Sandwich would have approved of these! After all, he had his supper between bread so as not to leave the gambling table, and these sandwich-style skewers are perfect for one-handed eating, entertaining, or brown-bagging lunch. I love the Genoa salami in these; their saltiness and fattier texture is a welcome companion to the lean turkey. Any dressing will do for these, but I'm partial to my Green Goddess Dressing (page 106). The recipe makes four skewers, the perfect snack for a pair, but it's easily multiplied to feed a crowd.

  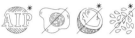 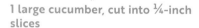

Makes 4 skewers (2 per serving)
PREP TIME: 10 minutes

1 large cucumber, cut into ¼-inch slices

4 slices smoked turkey breast, cut into twelve ½-inch-wide strips

12 slices Genoa salami

½ large Hass avocado, cut into 8 pieces

½ cup Green Goddess Dressing (page 106)

Special equipment:

Bamboo, wooden, or metal skewers

○ Thread a slice of cucumber onto the first skewer. Roll a strip of turkey lengthwise and thread it on the skewer. Fold a slice of salami and follow suit.

○ Repeat this sequence twice more, so there are three cucumber slices, three strips of turkey, and three slices of salami on the skewer. Finish the skewer with two pieces of avocado and one last slice of cucumber. Repeat for the rest of the skewers.

○ Serve with green goddess dressing on the side or drizzled over the skewers. Wrap in foil or trim the ends of the skewers and store in an airtight container in the fridge for up to 2 days.

SUBSTITUTIONS: To make this recipe AIP-compliant, use the AIP-compliant version of the dressing and replace the salami with prosciutto. To make it coconut-free and seed-free, replace the dressing with Greek Marinade + Dressing (page 108).

PER SERVING: Calories **343** · Fat **27.9g** · Total Carbohydrate **3.9g** · Dietary Fiber **0g** · Protein **19.1g**

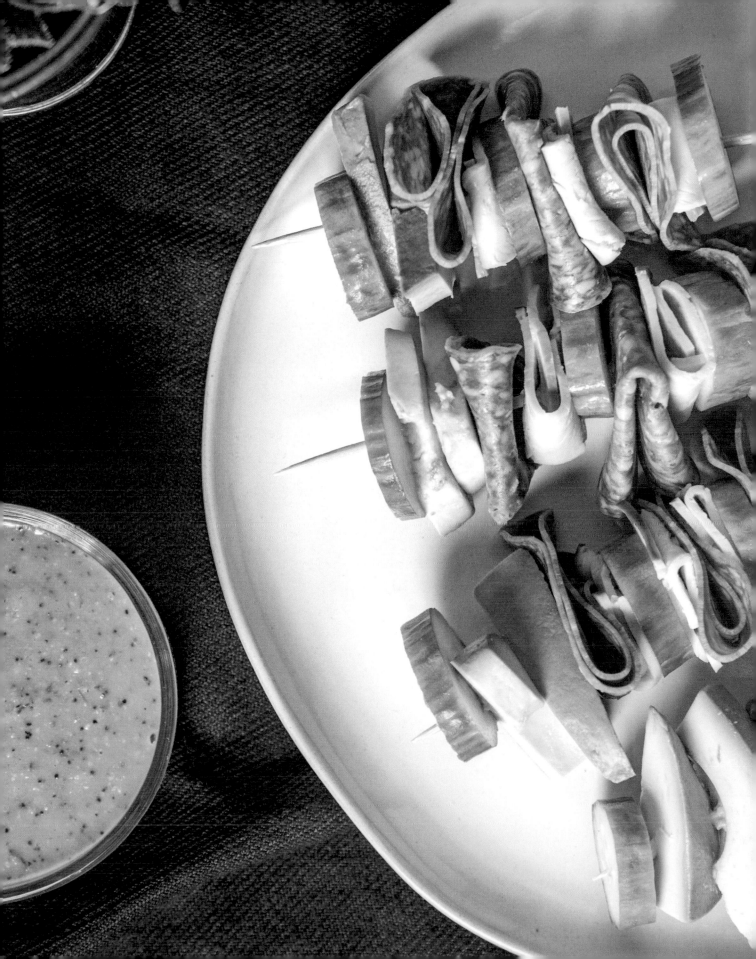

fried hard-boiled eggs

The first time I saw this dish was on my Instagram feed in a post from Mary Shenouda, The Paleo Chef, and I had one of those aha moments! Hard-boiled eggs are so easy to make ahead, but I never made them in big batches because I don't like them cold. No sir, cold eggs are not my thing, and these crispy boiled eggs were the answer! I just boil the eggs in advance, keep them in the fridge, and fry up a pair to order when I'm ready to eat. I like to cook my eggs so the yolks are a great jammy consistency; this way, after they're pan-fried, the yolk is still bright yellow and never chalky. I'll walk you through the boiling and peeling process, too, so you get the perfect egg every time!

12 large eggs

2 tablespoons avocado oil

1 teaspoon black sesame seeds

½ teaspoon fine Himalayan salt

½ teaspoon garlic powder

½ teaspoon ground black pepper

Makes 1 dozen eggs (2 per serving)
PREP TIME: 10 minutes   COOK TIME: 15 minutes

○ Bring a large pot of water to a rapid boil. One at a time, add the eggs to the boiling water. Boil the eggs for 8 minutes, then quickly drain all the water from the pot and cover the eggs with ice and cold water. Let them sit for 2 minutes.

○ Peel the eggs under the cold water or under a fine stream of running water. Make sure to remove that fine film under the shell; this ensures that the whites won't break off. Store the peeled eggs in the fridge for up to a week.

○ When you want a crispy egg, heat a cast-iron skillet over medium heat. As the skillet heats, toss two hard-boiled eggs with the oil, sesame seeds, salt, garlic powder, and black pepper in a shallow bowl.

○ When the skillet is hot, tip the eggs and all of the seasonings and oil into the skillet. Let the eggs cook for 2 to 3 minutes, then flip them over and cook the opposite side for 2 to 3 minutes.

○ Remove the eggs from the skillet. Cut them in half and spoon the avocado oil and sesame seeds from the skillet over them. Sprinkle with a little more salt. Enjoy!

CHEF'S NOTE: You can get really creative with these crispy eggs—a number of flavors would go well with them. Add garam masala, turmeric powder, furikake, nutritional yeast... Serve with Roasted Beet Marinara (page 78), Chimichurri (page 80), or Pistou (page 74)!

PER SERVING: Calories **411** · Fat **39g** · Total Carbohydrate **2.2g** · Dietary Fiber **0.1g** · Protein **14g**

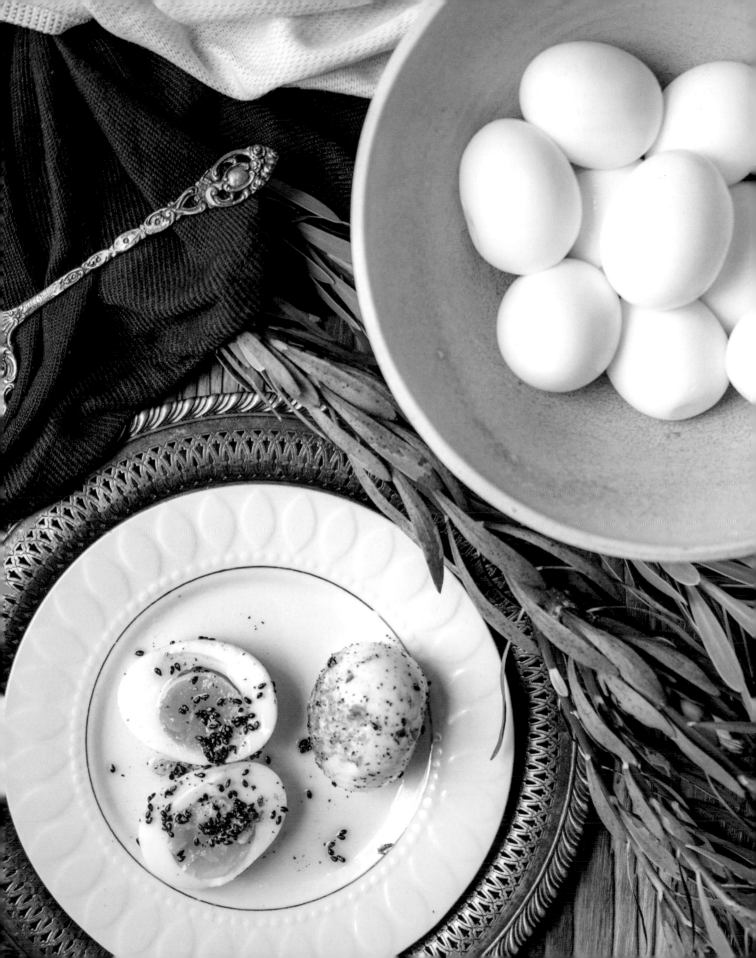

prosciutto chips

Oven-baked in just a few minutes and dipped in deliciously tangy Roasted Beet Marinara (page 78), this is a snack you can really get behind. Make a big batch once a week and keep them in the fridge for easy access!

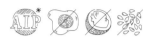

20 slices prosciutto di Parma

½ cup Roasted Beet Marinara (page 78), for serving

Makes 20 chips (4 per serving)
PREP TIME: 5 minutes   COOK TIME: 15 minutes

○ Preheat the oven to 350°F.

○ Place a cooling rack over a sheet pan. Carefully fold each slice of prosciutto in half and place on the rack. Use as many slices as you wish to make, or as many as you can fit on the rack without overlapping.

○ Bake for 12 to 15 minutes, until lightly browned and crispy. Remove from the oven and let them cool to room temperature.

○ Serve right away with the marinara for dipping, or store in an airtight container in the fridge for up to 5 days.

CHEF'S NOTE: These chips make a great party dish, garnish, or quick snack. I love them with Tzatziki (page 98) as well as the marinara—both cool and sweet sauces play nicely against the salty meat chips

SUBSTITUTIONS: To make this recipe AIP-compliant, use the AIP-compliant version of the marinara.

PER SERVING: Calories **212** · Fat **12g** · Total Carbohydrate **1.5g** · Dietary Fiber **0.2g** · Protein **20.2g**

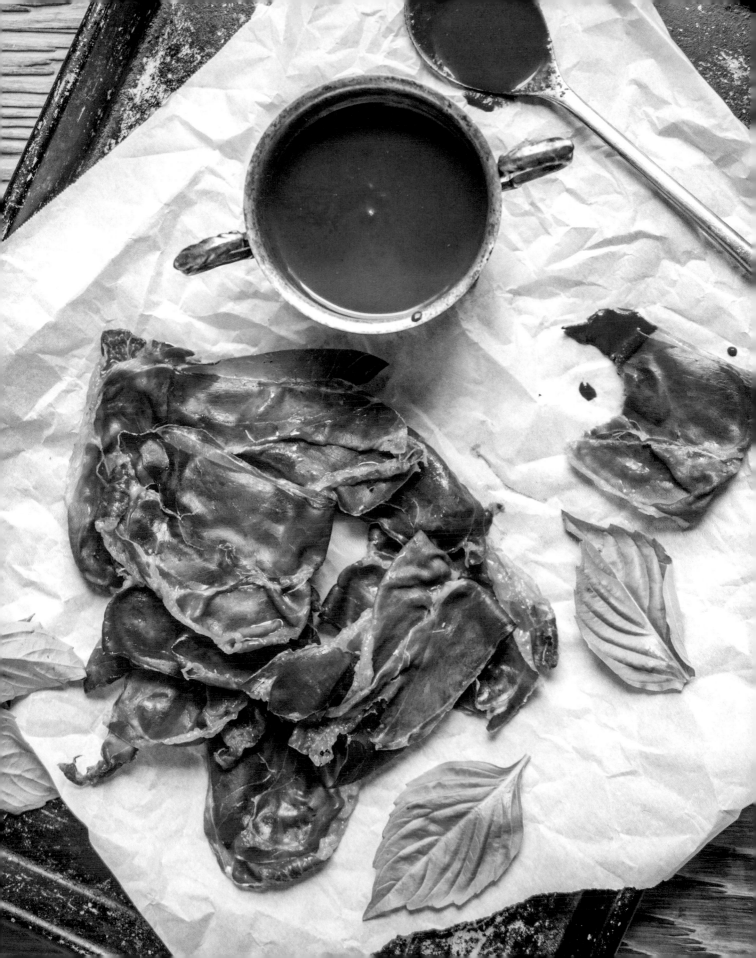

zucchini latkes

The trick to crispy latkes made of zucchini is getting as much water out of the zucchini as possible. I like to take a two-step dehydration approach: salt and squeeze. It takes a little more time on the front end, but you can prep the zucchini a day ahead—which I highly recommend. That way, when it's time to fry these up and serve them, you're not held up with all the legwork. After all, these are meant to be served at gatherings and celebrations, and you want to enjoy the party!

2 medium zucchini, grated (about 3 cups)

1 teaspoon fine Himalayan salt, divided

2 tablespoons grated onions

2 large eggs

2 tablespoons coconut flour

½ teaspoon garlic powder

½ cup coconut oil, or more if needed, for frying

Coconut Yogurt (page 96), Pistou (page 74), or Roasted Beet Marinara (page 78), for serving (optional)

Makes 10 latkes (2½ per serving)
PREP TIME: 40 minutes   COOK TIME: 12 minutes

○ Place the grated zucchini in a colander and sprinkle with ½ teaspoon of the salt. Let it sit for 30 minutes in the sink or over a bowl, as it will release water. Drain the zucchini by tossing it in the colander, then transfer it to a nut milk bag or clean kitchen towel and squeeze out as much water as possible—it should release somewhere between ¾ and 1 cup of water. You should end up with approximately 1½ cups of dehydrated grated zucchini.

○ Place the grated zucchini in a large bowl. Add the onions (be sure to pat it dry first to soak up any excess liquid they may have released during grating). Add the remaining ½ teaspoon of salt, eggs, coconut flour, and garlic powder to the bowl and mix to combine. It will create a moist dough. If there is liquid pooling, sprinkle in a little more coconut flour and fold until the liquid is absorbed.

○ In a large skillet over medium heat, heat the coconut oil. It should be about ½ inch deep. When a wooden spoon inserted into the coconut oil sizzles, it's ready for frying.

○ Form the latke batter into ten 1-inch balls. Working in batches (don't overcrowd the skillet), add them to the oil one at a time, gently flattening them with the back of a spoon as you go. Fry for 3 minutes, gently flip them with a spatula, and fry on the other side for another 3 minutes. Remove the latkes from the oil and place on a cooling rack. Repeat with the remaining latkes.

○ Serve immediately with coconut yogurt, pistou, or marinara, or freeze immediately. (I do not recommend eating these as leftovers, as they will get soggy.) To freeze, set the latkes on a sheet pan, rack, or plate and freeze for 2 hours, then transfer to a freezer bag. They will keep in the freezer for up to 3 months. To reheat, bake in a preheated 400°F oven for 10 minutes.

VARIATIONS: Frying these in coconut oil doesn't give them a coconut oil flavor, but other great options include duck fat and bacon fat. Although it seems wrong to pair a traditional Jewish dish with pork, I did make mini kalua pork sliders with these, and they were glorious! (See the recipe for Crispy Kalua Pork on page 282.)

PER SERVING: Calories **320** · Fat **31g** · Total Carbohydrate **8.2g** · Dietary Fiber **3.7g** · Protein **5.5g**

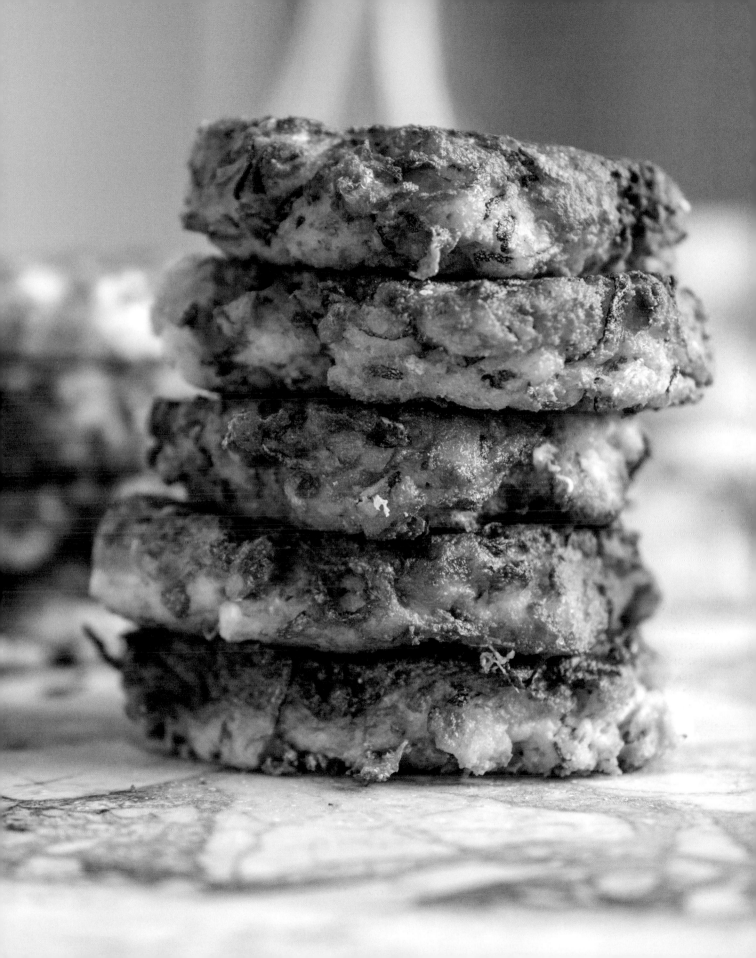

protein porridge

Doesn't the word porridge *remind you of "Goldilocks and the Three Bears"? It does me! And I thought a good porridge would be much better than yet another "n'oatmeal" recipe. This high-protein porridge has the warm, creamy, nutty consistency that you love about hot cereal, but it's made with eggs and seeds! An absolutely satisfying dish that is perfect when you're cutting your fast short or having breakfast for dinner. Adding frozen blueberries is a little mom trick: it's the perfect way to garnish your porridge and cool it down at the same time.*

½ cup water or mild bone broth (page 100)

½ cup full-fat coconut milk

1 large egg, beaten

1 tablespoon granulated erythritol or other low-carb sweetener (see page 38)

1 teaspoon ground cinnamon

1 teaspoon pure vanilla extract

¼ cup shelled hemp seeds (aka hemp hearts)

1 tablespoon chia seeds

1 tablespoon flaxseed meal

1 tablespoon shredded coconut (optional)

5 to 10 drops liquid stevia (optional)

¼ cup frozen blueberries, for garnish (optional)

Makes 2 servings
PREP TIME: 10 minutes   COOK TIME: 15 minutes

○ Place the water and coconut milk in a small saucepan and bring to a simmer over medium-high heat. Slowly pour in the beaten egg, whisking the mixture as you pour—as with egg drop soup, you want the egg to cook as it hits the simmering liquid.

○ Continue to whisk and add the erythritol, cinnamon, vanilla extract, hemp seeds, chia seeds, and flaxseed meal. Simmer, stirring often, until the porridge begins to thicken, about 4 minutes. Stir in the shredded coconut (if using).

○ Continue to cook until the porridge reaches the desired consistency. I like mine very thick, so I let it simmer until there is no more pooling liquid, about 6 minutes.

○ Taste the porridge and, if desired, add stevia to sweeten it to your liking. If desired, garnish with frozen blueberries, which will turn the porridge purple when stirred in!

○ Store leftover porridge in small jars in the fridge for up to 3 days. To reheat, microwave on high for 1 minute.

VARIATIONS: This recipe can be as simple or as complex as you like. Add a scoop of your favorite protein powder and top with all sorts of goodies, like pepitas, sunflower seed butter, or chocolate chips! Use Coconut Yogurt (page 96) instead of the coconut milk for a nice tangy flavor.

SUBSTITUTIONS: For an egg-free option, combine the water, coconut milk, cinnamon, vanilla, sweetener, and seeds in a saucepan over medium-high heat and simmer until thickened. The chia seeds and flaxseed meal with become sticky and give the porridge body.

PER SERVING: Calories **374** · Fat **32g** · Total Carbohydrate **16.5g** · Dietary Fiber **9.2g** · Protein **12.8g**

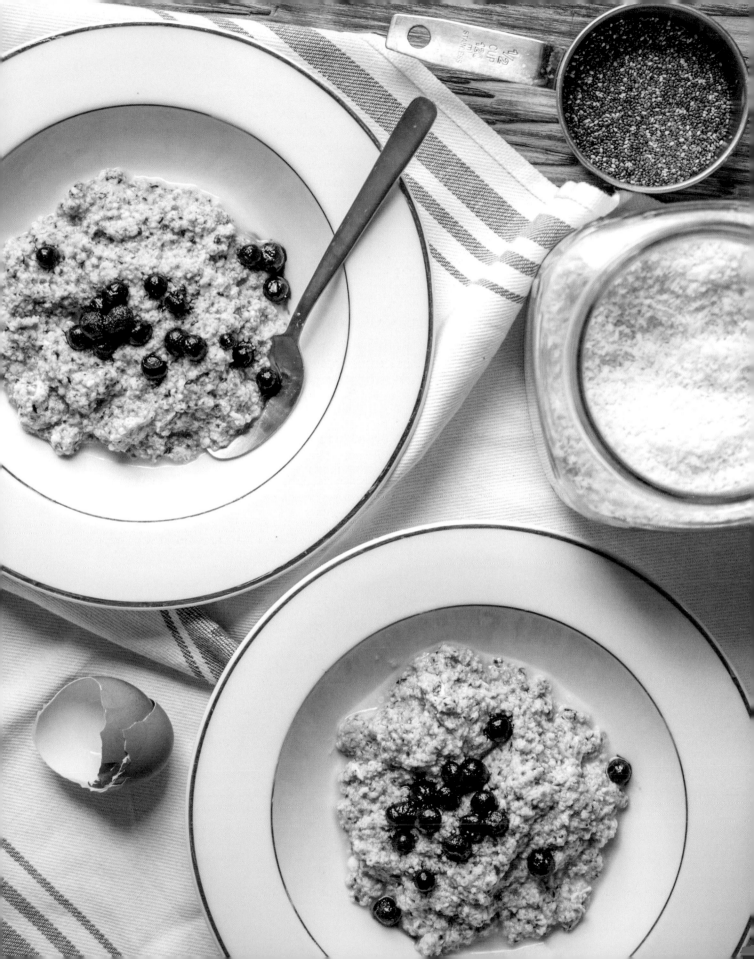

smooth chia pudding

This chocolaty pudding might look like dessert, but it's packing serious nutrition. I know bone broth and cauliflower seem like unlikely ingredients for a sweet recipe, but once you let go of conventional ideas about how certain foods should be used, it really opens the door for some creative and delicious options. Case in point: jars of creamy, sweet chocolate pudding made with bone broth and cauliflower! With a great balance of protein and carbs and a little less fat, this pudding is a great option for post-workout nutrition. It's also toddler approved—I love to pack a jar in Jack's lunch box! To get a smooth, creamy texture, you'll need a high-powered blender, but this recipe works equally well as a tapioca-style pudding, made with a regular blender (see Variation below).

Makes 4 servings
PREP TIME: 10 minutes, plus 4 hours to chill

1 cup mild bone broth (page 100) (see Note)

1 cup full-fat coconut milk

1 cup water

¼ cup cocoa powder

¼ cup steamed and then frozen cauliflower florets (about 3 florets) (see Note, page 68)

¼ cup granulated erythritol, or 20 drops liquid stevia

3 tablespoons chia seeds

Pinch of fine Himalayan salt

Fresh blackberries, for garnish (optional)

◦ Place all of the ingredients in a high-powered blender. Blend on high until the chia seeds are pulverized and the mix is completely smooth and thick.

◦ Pour the mixture into four 6-ounce jars with lids, cover, and refrigerate for at least 4 hours to thicken. Garnish with blackberries before serving, if desired. Store in the refrigerator for up to 1 week.

CHEF'S NOTE: I like to use beef bone broth, whether homemade from the recipe on page 100 or store-bought. However, any kind of broth will work.

VARIATION: This recipe works best with a high-powered blender, which will completely pulverize the chia seeds. You can still make this recipe with a regular blender, but you'll end up with a pudding that's more like tapioca. To make, blend all of the ingredients except the chia seeds in the blender until smooth. Then pulse in ¼ cup of chia seeds.

SUBSTITUTIONS: If you can't do coconut, replace the coconut milk with 2 tablespoons butter or ghee and ½ cup warm water.

PER SERVING: Calories **295** · Fat **24.5g** · Total Carbohydrate **15.6g** · Dietary Fiber **7.6g** · Protein **7.5g**

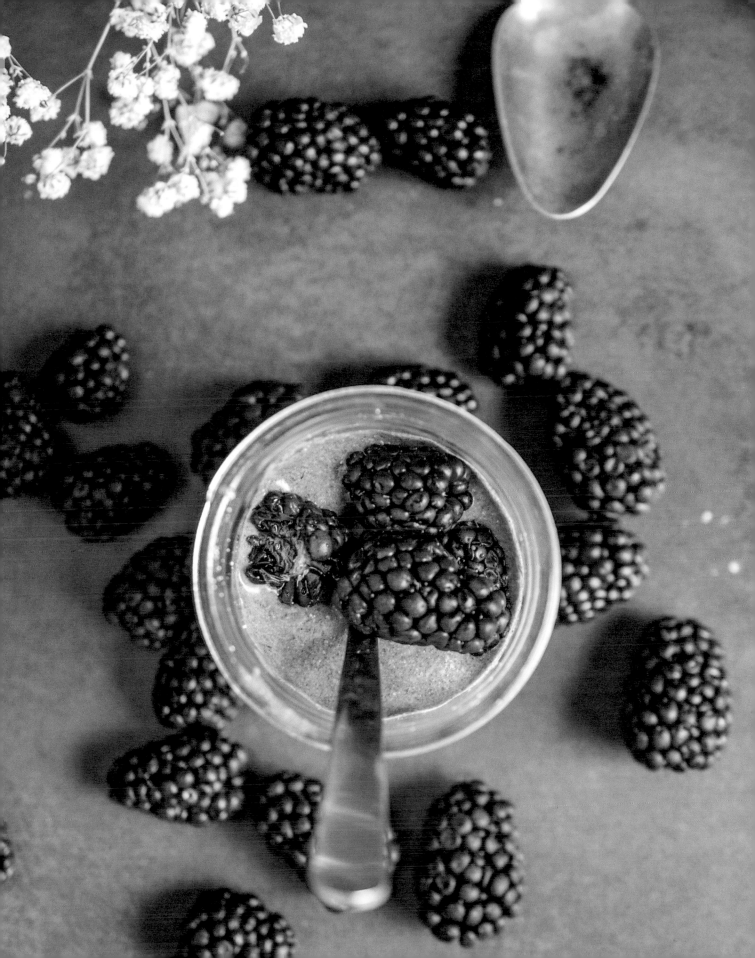

ceviche

Fishing off of the Florida Keys and making ceviche with your fresh catch right on the boat was a rite of passage when I was growing up in South Florida. The key to a great ceviche is fresh fish! Firm white saltwater fish are ideal. Since I live in Hawaii, I like blue marlin (kajiki here), but you can use sea bass, grouper, or flounder, too. Ask your fishmonger for the freshest catch and make the ceviche that same day or the next. If you're feeding a crowd, this works really well served in lettuce cups or shot glasses.

Makes 6 servings
PREP TIME: 20 minutes, plus 40 minutes to marinate

1 pound fresh wild-caught white fish

8 lemons, halved

5 limes, halved

1 cup minced red onions

½ cup minced fresh cilantro

1 teaspoon fine Himalayan salt

1 teaspoon ground black pepper

1 teaspoon peeled and minced fresh ginger

3 cloves garlic, minced

½ medium Hass avocado, peeled, pitted, and diced

○ Cut the fish into ½-inch cubes and place in a large glass or ceramic mixing bowl. Put a fine-mesh sieve over the bowl and squeeze all of the lemons and limes over the fish, using the sieve to catch the seeds.

○ Flatten the fish so it is submerged in the citrus juice. Place the squeezed lemon and lime halves cut side down on top of the fish. Cover and set in the fridge for 40 minutes.

○ While the fish marinates, in a small bowl, mix the onions, cilantro, salt, pepper, ginger, and garlic.

○ Remove the fish from the fridge and add the onion mix to the bowl. Use a wooden spoon to combine.

○ Just before serving, add the diced avocado. Enjoy right away or store in a covered glass container in the fridge until the following day.

CHEF'S NOTE: The citrus juice with all the onions and herbs that's left behind is called *leche de tigre* and is rumored to improve vitality. It's also delicious!

VARIATIONS: If you want to add more fat to this snack, add a glug of avocado oil.

SUBSTITUTION: To make this AIP-compliant, omit the black pepper and double the fresh ginger.

PER SERVING: Calories **150** · Fat **4g** · Total Carbohydrate **12.9g** · Dietary Fiber **2.1g** · Protein **18.3g**

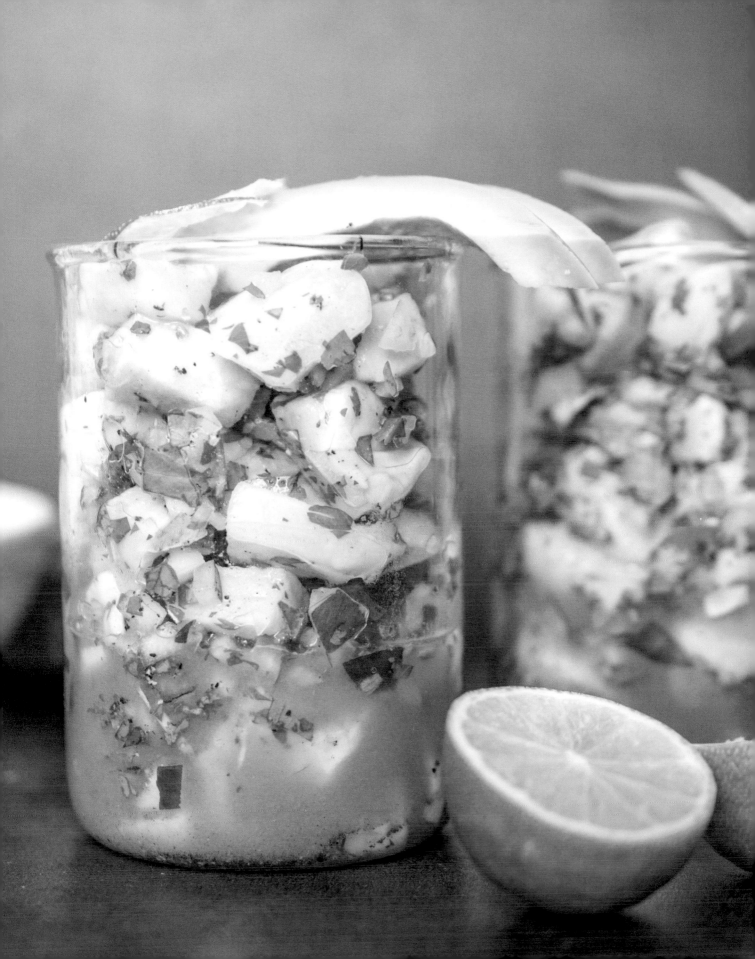

cold soup smoothie

Nutrition on the go! This smoothie is just like those fancy beverages at your local health-food store—but better, because it doesn't cost ten dollars a serving. I love this as a post-workout meal, but it also works really well when you need food ASAP. You can make it with bone broth (page 100) or collagen peptides; you can drink it cold or warm it up. You can enjoy it as is or beef it up with leftover Crispy Kalua Pork (page 282), a fried egg, or diced avocado.

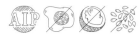

FOR THE FROZEN VEGGIE MIX:

(makes enough for 5 smoothies)

2 cups diced butternut squash

1 cup broccoli florets

1 cup diced onions

4 cloves garlic, peeled

3 cups water

FOR THE SMOOTHIE:

1 (1-cup) bag steamed and then frozen mixed veggies (from above)

1½ cups bone broth (page 100) or water

2 tablespoons collagen peptides (optional)

1 tablespoon MCT oil or MCT oil powder (optional)

2 teaspoons apple cider vinegar

½ teaspoon dried thyme or oregano, or a combination

½ teaspoon fine Himalayan salt

½ teaspoon turmeric powder (optional)

Makes 1 serving
PREP TIME: 15 minutes, plus 1 hour to freeze   COOK TIME: 15 minutes

○ Make the frozen veggie mix: Place all of the veggies in a large skillet with a tight-fitting lid. Add the water and bring to a boil. Cover and steam for 15 minutes, or until the butternut squash is fork-tender. Remove from the heat, drain, and let cool.

○ Divide the cooled vegetables into five resealable plastic bags, about 1 cup per bag. Seal and pop in the freezer for at least an hour before making your smoothie.

○ When you're ready to make a smoothie, place 1 bag (1 cup) of frozen veggies in a blender, add the smoothie ingredients, and blend until smooth. Drink up! Store any leftovers in the fridge in an airtight container for up to 4 days.

TIME-SAVING TIP: Buy frozen veggies, steam according to the instructions, and refreeze—it will save you time on the front end with all the dicing. You can also make this with steamed and frozen cauliflower for a creamy white soup smoothie.

CHEF'S NOTE: When you prep these veggies, steam and freeze a bunch of cauliflower, too (see Note, page 68). It comes in real handy for smoothies and sauces.

PER SERVING (with collagen + MCT oil): Calories **304** · Fat **18g** · Total Carbohydrate **9g** · Dietary Fiber **2.2g** · Protein **20.4g**

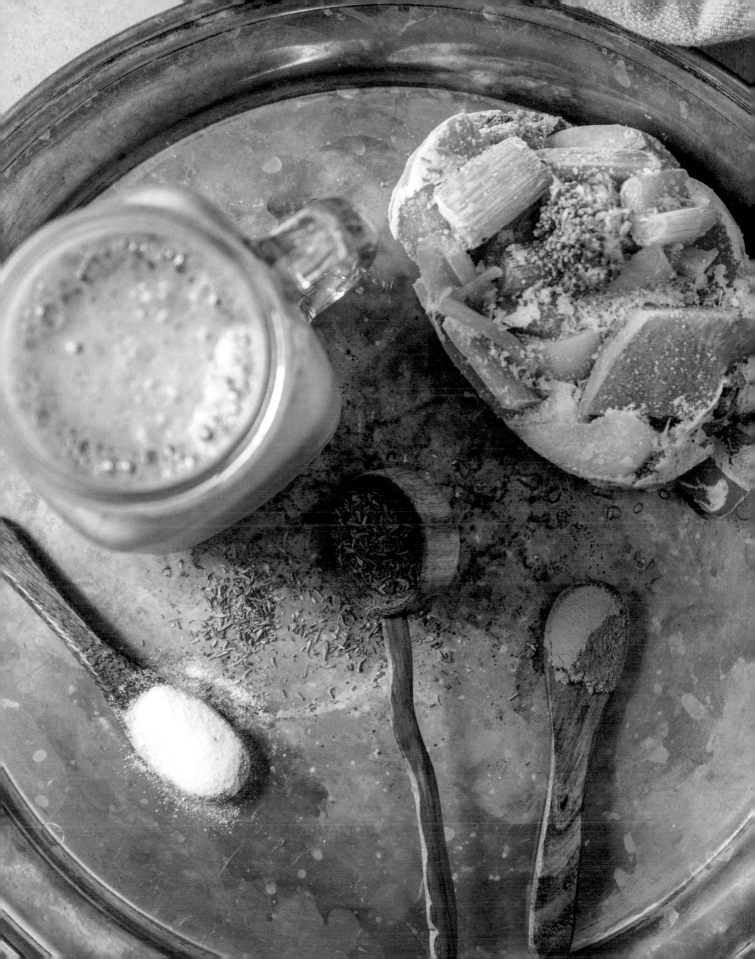

parfaits

Layers of thick Coconut Yogurt (page 96) with fresh berries and a quick skillet granola: these parfaits are squeaky-clean but taste like dessert! Make them ahead of time and store them in the fridge for quick grab-and-go nutrition you can take to work or play.

FOR THE GRANOLA:

(makes ½ cup)

½ cup shelled hemp seeds (aka hemp hearts)

1 tablespoon granulated erythritol or other low-carb sweetener (see page 38)

1 teaspoon ground cinnamon

⅛ teaspoon fine Himalayan salt

FOR THE PARFAITS:

1 cup fresh berries (I like to use ½ cup strawberries and ½ cup blueberries)

½ cup granola (from above)

2 cups Coconut Yogurt (page 96)

Makes 4 parfaits
PREP TIME: 5 minutes   COOK TIME: 8 minutes

◦ Make the granola: Combine the hemp seeds, erythritol, cinnamon, and salt in a small skillet over medium-high heat. Cook for 5 minutes, or until the seeds begin to smell toasty, stirring occasionally. Then flatten the mix down on the skillet, lower the heat to medium-low, and cook for another 3 minutes. Remove from the heat and let cool.

◦ Use a spoon or spatula to scrape and chip at the hemp seed granola, crumble it up, and transfer it to a jar with a lid. Store for up to 15 days in the pantry.

◦ Make the parfaits: Put ¼ cup fresh berries in each of four jars or cups. Sprinkle 1 tablespoon granola over the berries. Layer ½ cup yogurt on top of the granola. Sprinkle another tablespoon of granola on the yogurt and garnish with 1 or 2 more berries.

◦ Enjoy right away or store in the fridge to enjoy within a day or two.

VARIATIONS: The possibilities are endless with these. You can add any combination of seeds to the skillet granola, or shredded coconut, or even crunchy bacon or dark chocolate.

PER PARFAIT: Calories **415** · Fat **37.4g** · Total Carbohydrate **13.4g** · Dietary Fiber **6.2g** · Protein **11.2g**

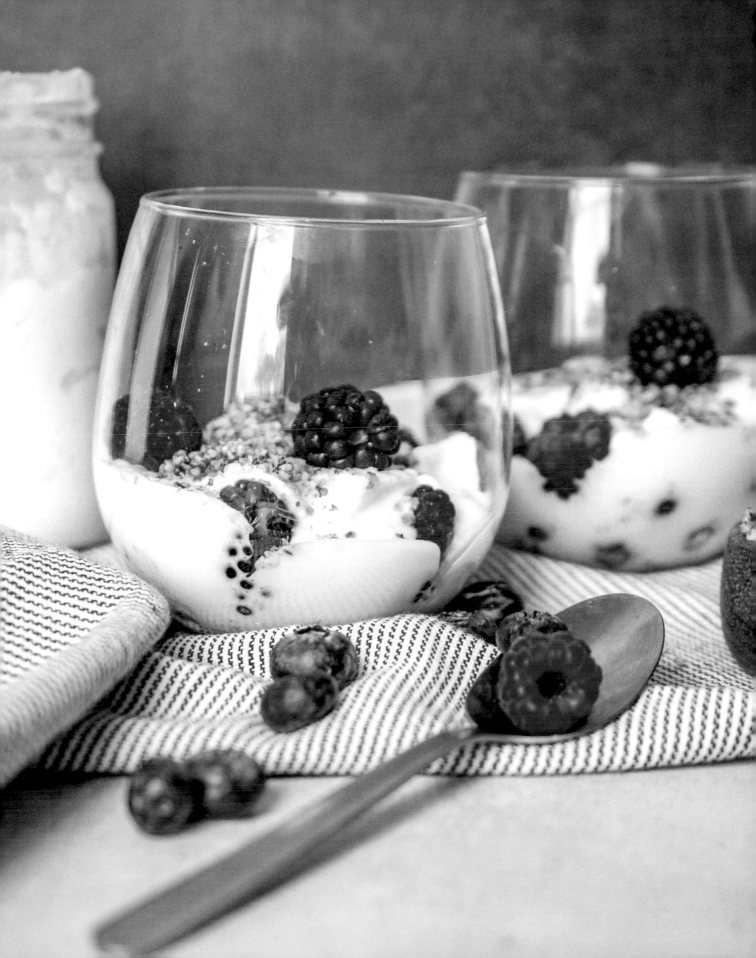

chocolate shake

Cauliflower that's steamed and then frozen is a smoothie game changer. You get the thick, cold, creamy texture without having to add loads of coconut or frozen banana. Trust me—it works.

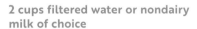

2 cups filtered water or nondairy milk of choice

1 cup steamed then frozen cauliflower florets (see Note, page 68)

¼ cup collagen peptides

2 tablespoons cacao powder

2 tablespoons MCT oil (optional)

1 tablespoon ground cinnamon

2 teaspoons powdered erythritol, or 20 drops liquid stevia

2 teaspoons maca root, coffee grounds, or pure vanilla extract (optional)

Pinch of fine Himalayan salt

Makes 2 servings
PREP TIME: 5 minutes

○ Place all of the ingredients in a blender. Blend until smooth.

○ Store any leftovers in a jar in the fridge for up to 4 days. Shake before drinking as separation may occur.

SUBSTITUTIONS: To make this AIP-compliant, use carob powder instead of cacao powder and use an AIP-compliant sweetener (see page 23).

You can use either powdered or granulated erythritol in this recipe. Some people prefer powdered because it has less of a cooling effect than granulated, but I haven't noticed a difference. In fact, this goes for all my recipes—if you have powdered erythritol, feel free to use it in place of granulated!

VARIATIONS: Use coconut milk instead of water for a fatty meal replacement shake.

PER SERVING (with MCT oil + maca root): Calories **174** · Fat **8.2g** · Total Carbohydrate **15.1g** · Dietary Fiber **5.2g** · Protein **15.7g**

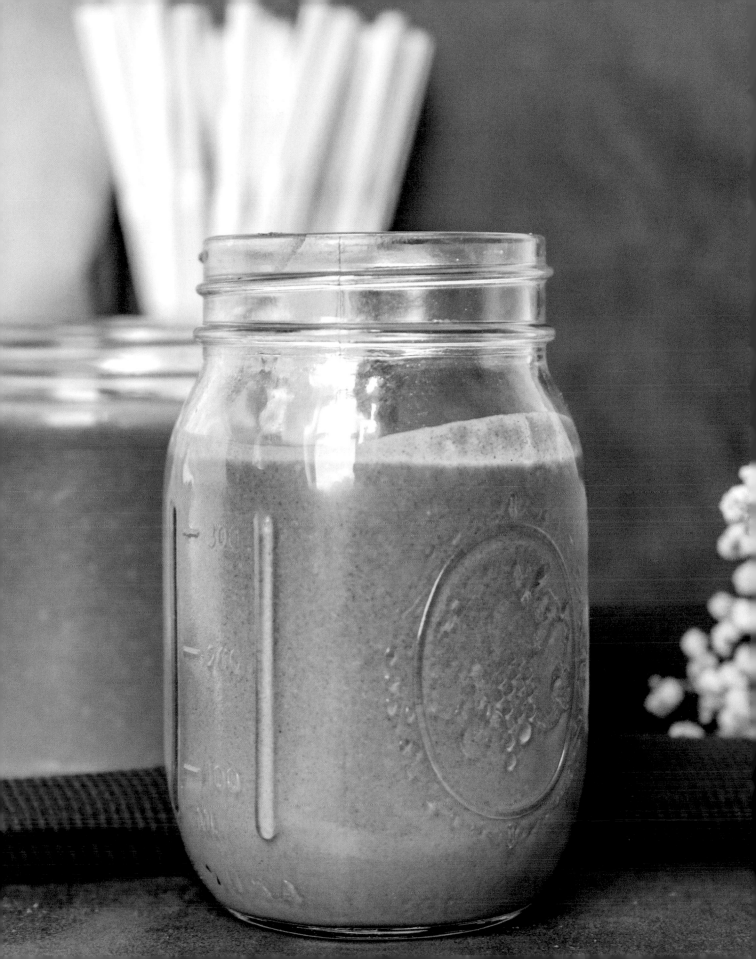

crispy thin flatbread

This multipurpose flatbread recipe is a more pliable version of the pie crust recipe on page 92. This combination of fat, eggs, and coconut flour bakes up crispy in various shapes and sizes. Bake it until firm, pile on toppings, slice it or stack it—the recipe is a blank slate. My favorite way to use this recipe is for easy prosciutto and arugula pizza: I make the crust ahead of time and keep it in the fridge, then just reheat it in the oven and top it with fresh arugula and thinly sliced prosciutto for a quick bite. Drizzle with olive oil and voilà—a gourmet snack for the whole family!

4 large eggs, cold

½ cup coconut oil, melted

½ teaspoon fine Himalayan salt

⅓ cup coconut flour, plus more if needed

Makes two 8-inch crusts (½ per serving)
PREP TIME: 10 minutes   COOK TIME: 20 minutes

○ Preheat the oven to 400°F. Line a baking sheet with parchment paper.

○ In a small bowl, whisk the eggs as you slowly pour in the coconut oil—it will become creamy. Then add the salt and stir to combine. Add the coconut flour and fold until a loose dough forms

○ The density of coconut flour can vary from brand to brand. If the dough does not take shape, add more flour a teaspoon at a time, waiting at least 30 seconds before adding the next teaspoon, until a pliable dough forms.

○ Separate the dough into 2 large balls. Use a spoon or spatula to spread each ball into a ¼-inch-thick, 8-inch round on the prepared baking sheet.

○ Bake for 15 to 20 minutes, until the center is firm and the edges are browned. Remove from the oven and let cool.

○ These flatbreads can be wrapped up tight and stored in the fridge for up to 4 days. To reheat, bake in a preheated 350°F oven for 8 minutes.

PER SERVING: Calories **395** · Fat **35.2g** · Total Carbohydrate **12.4g** · Dietary Fiber **7.5g** · Protein **9.3g**

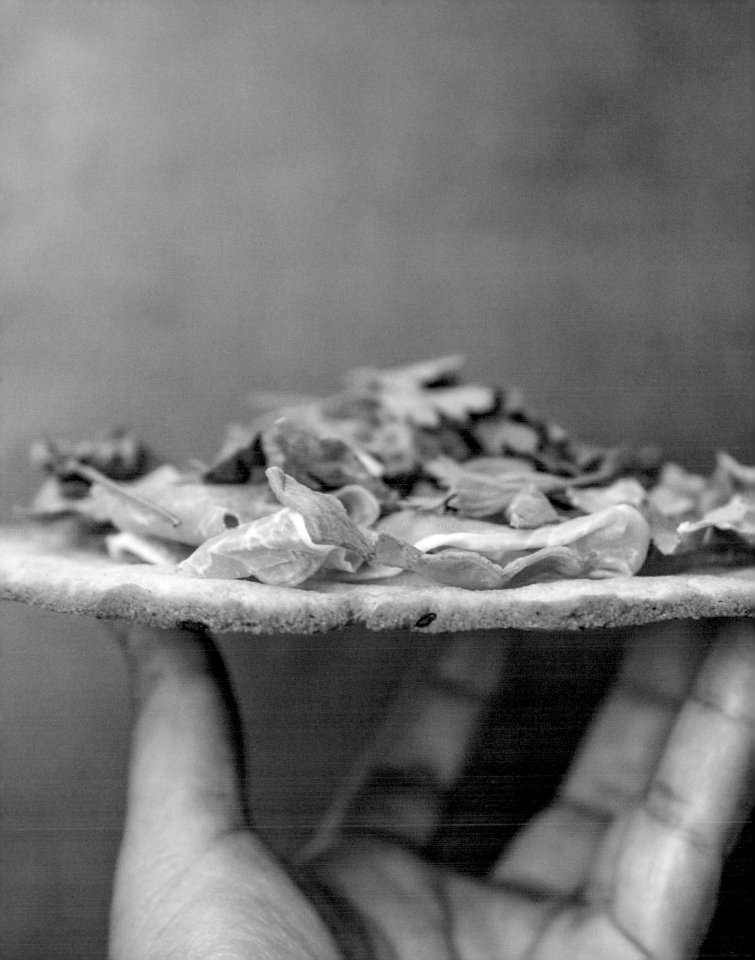

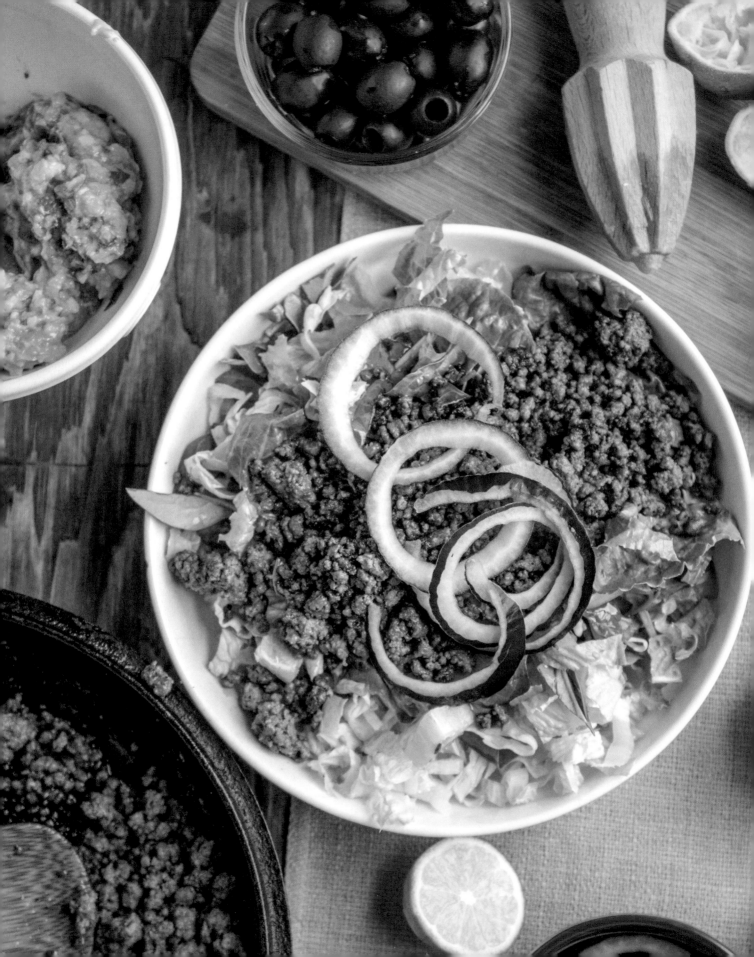

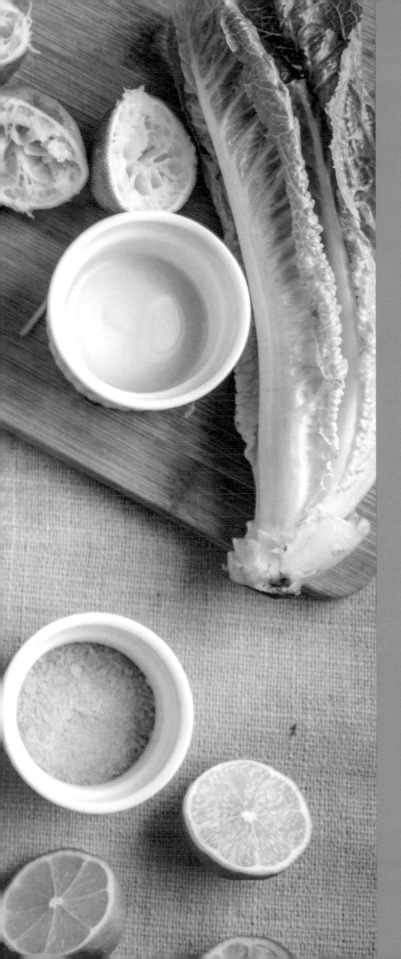

SOUPS + SALADS

Soups and salads are just the thing when you need something fast and simple or when you're craving something soothing. This chapter offers everything from no-cook heat-wave-weather meals to baby-it's-cold-outside soups. Amazing soups and beautiful salads are my mother's specialty, and she taught me well!

roasted vegetable soup

A make-it-your-own, add-what-you-like, easy, flexible, and warming meal. Perfect for when you're feeling under the weather, physically or emotionally. This soup replenishes my soul, is super easy on my tummy, and comes together with minimal hands-on time. This recipe includes the vegetables I use most often, but really, you can use anything you've got in the fridge.

2 medium carrots, peeled

1 cup baby Brussels sprouts

1 rib celery

¼ medium head cabbage

2 teaspoons fine Himalayan salt, divided

2 tablespoons coconut oil

2 cups bone broth (page 100)

½ medium Hass avocado, peeled, pitted, and sliced

1 green onion, minced

4 sprigs fresh cilantro, minced

Makes 2 servings
PREP TIME: 10 minutes   COOK TIME: 30 minutes

○ Preheat the oven to 400°F.

○ Cut all of the vegetables into small pieces and spread out on a sheet pan. Sprinkle with 1 teaspoon of the salt and toss with the coconut oil. Roast for 30 minutes.

○ While the vegetables are roasting, heat the broth in a saucepan over medium heat.

○ When the vegetables are ready, divide them between two serving bowls. Add the avocado, green onion, and cilantro and sprinkle in the remaining teaspoon of salt. Divide the broth between the bowls.

○ Serve immediately. Store leftovers in an airtight container in the fridge for up to 4 days.

TIME-SAVING TIP: You can roast the veggies ahead of time, even days ahead, and then pour the hot broth over them for an even quicker meal.

VARIATIONS: Add leftover protein like meatballs (page 228, 248, 260, or 272) or roast chicken (page 202) to beef up this soup. Use extra carrots or add sweet potatoes to make this a carb-up meal (see page 39 for more on carb cycling). Drizzle in a little garlic-infused olive oil and some Garlic Confit (page 76) to really boost the flavor.

PER SERVING: Calories **276** · Total Fat **22.5g** · Total Carbohydrate **18.8g** · Dietary Fiber **10g** · Protein **6.4g**

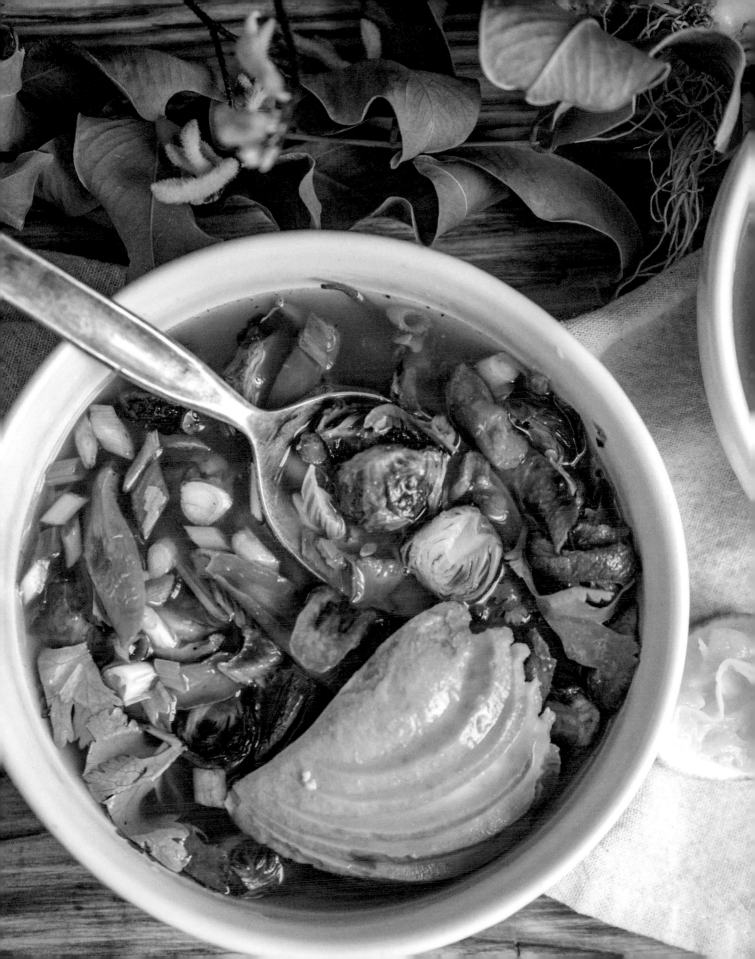

feel-good soup

This soup has a simple yet powerful combination of ingredients that provides the nutrition you need to get back on your feet, along with a delicious and comforting flavor that will make you feel good! I made this soup on a whim when I was in a rut and shared it on my blog, and it quickly became a reader favorite, made hundreds of times during the fall of 2017. Now I share it here, so this feel-good soup can continue to nourish bodies and lift spirits!

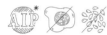

1 tablespoon ghee or coconut oil

2 cups sliced cremini mushrooms

6 cloves garlic, sliced

3 sprigs fresh thyme

1 teaspoon fine Himalayan salt

1 teaspoon ground black pepper

Pinch of ground nutmeg

2 tablespoons coconut vinegar

1 cup bone broth (page 100)

¼ cup coconut cream (see Note, page 144)

1 cup riced cauliflower (see Note)

3 cups baby spinach

3 tablespoons collagen peptides

2 tablespoons nutritional yeast

Makes 2 servings
PREP TIME: 10 minutes   COOK TIME: 20 minutes

○ Heat the ghee in a medium-sized pot over medium heat. When it begins to brown, add the mushrooms, garlic, thyme sprigs, salt, pepper, and nutmeg. Sauté, stirring often, until aromatic and tender, about 8 minutes.

○ Add the vinegar and deglaze the pot, scraping up any goodness that's stuck to the bottom. Add the broth and coconut cream and bring to a simmer.

○ Stir in the riced cauliflower and spinach and cook for 5 minutes, or until the cauliflower is tender. Stir in the collagen peptides and nutritional yeast until dissolved.

○ Serve, sip, enjoy, and feel good! Store leftovers in an airtight container in the fridge for up to 5 days or in the freezer for up to 30 days.

VARIATIONS: If you want to beef up this soup, add ½ pound ground beef, pork, or turkey once the mushrooms and garlic are cooked and brown, before deglazing the pan. Then continue with the recipe as written.

SUBSTITUTIONS: To make this soup AIP-compliant, omit the black pepper and nutmeg and use coconut oil instead of ghee.

CHEF'S NOTE: You can buy riced cauliflower at the grocery store, but it's easy to make it yourself at home. To rice cauliflower, roughly chop a large head of cauliflower (florets plus stem), place it in a food processor, and pulse it into rice-sized pieces. You can also use a box grater instead of a food processor. You'll get about 3 cups of riced cauliflower from 1 large head. Make a bunch at one time and store in the freezer—you'll use it all the time.

PER SERVING: Calories **305** · Fat **16.2g** · Total Carbohydrate **6.8g** · Dietary Fiber **6.9g** · Protein **24.6g**

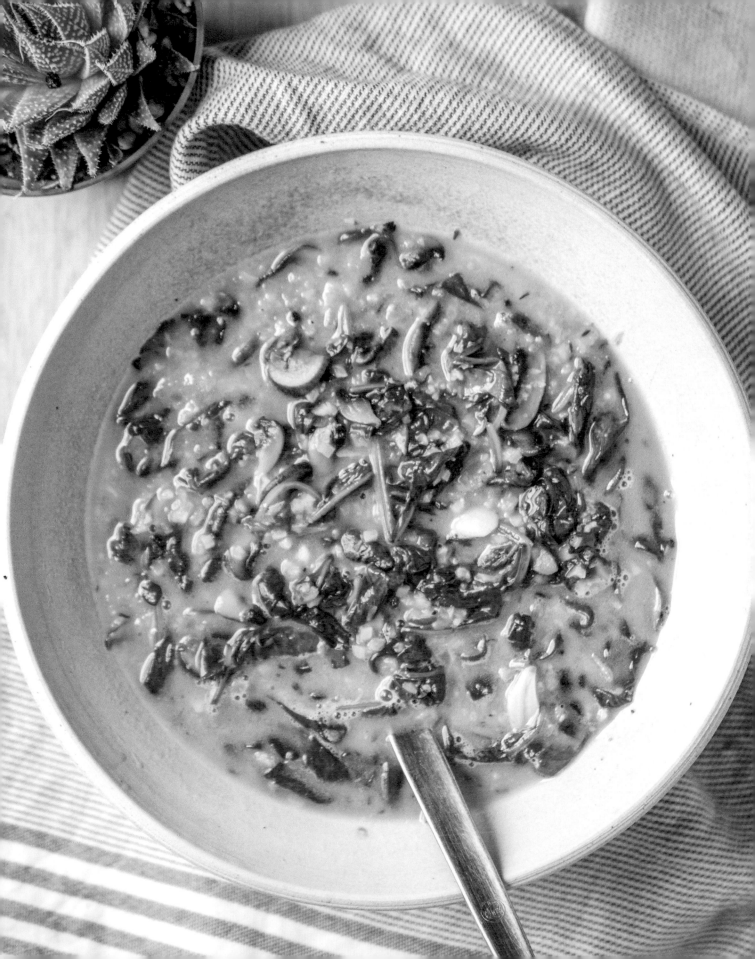

"corn" chowder

I haven't eaten actual corn in at least three years. The last time I ate it was during San Diego Restaurant Week, when we ordered the tasting menu at one of those hipster restaurants in Hillcrest. My favorite dish that day was the corn chowder. It was light and silky, with small little corn kernels floating around. The sweetness of the corn was perfectly emphasized by the slightest bit of spice. This soup re-creates those subtle flavors without the carby corn, using lots of caramelized onion for sweetness, cauliflower pearls for texture, and coconut cream for a thick, creamy feel. This easy soup is the perfect start to any meal.

Makes 4 servings
PREP TIME: 10 minutes   COOK TIME: 50 minutes

3 tablespoons avocado oil

2 cups diced onions

3 cups bone broth (page 100)

2 cups cauliflower pearls
(see Note)

¾ cup coconut cream (see Note,
page 144)

2 teaspoons ground black pepper

1 teaspoon fine Himalayan salt

½ teaspoon ground cumin

½ teaspoon ground nutmeg

2 tablespoons nutritional yeast

Leaves from fresh thyme sprig,
for garnish

2 tablespoons Garlic Confit
(page 76), for garnish

○ Place a medium-sized pot over medium heat. When it's hot, pour in the avocado oil and add the diced onions. Lower the heat to medium-low and cover. Cook for 20 minutes, stirring once halfway through. The onions should be browned but not crispy—they need to be soft and sweet.

○ Add the broth, cauliflower, coconut cream, and seasonings. Stir well and bring to a simmer. Simmer for 20 to 30 minutes, stirring occasionally. When the soup has reduced by one-third and the chunks of onion and cauliflower protrude through the broth, it's time to make it creamy.

○ Pour half of the soup into a blender. Make sure you're not just pouring out broth; you want to get plenty of cauliflower and onion into the blender, too. Blend until silky smooth, then pour the puree back into the pot and stir to combine it all, creating a creamy soup studded with tender pearls of cauliflower and sweet onion.

○ Garnish with the thyme and garlic confit before serving. Store leftovers in an airtight container in the fridge for up to 5 days or in the freezer for up to 30 days. To reheat, bring to a simmer on the stovetop.

CHEF'S NOTE: While bags of cauliflower pearls are available in the grocery store, I like to make my own. Cauliflower pearls are a little bigger than the run-of-the-mill cauliflower rice, and you can easily make them by pulsing cauliflower florets in a blender or food processor until they're the size of corn kernels.

SUBSTITUTIONS: To make this AIP-compliant, omit the black pepper and cumin and add a teaspoon of dried oregano, and replace the nutmeg with a pinch of ground cloves.

PER SERVING: Calories **202** · Fat **12.6g** · Total Carbohydrate **14.3g** · Dietary Fiber **5.6g** · Protein **12g**

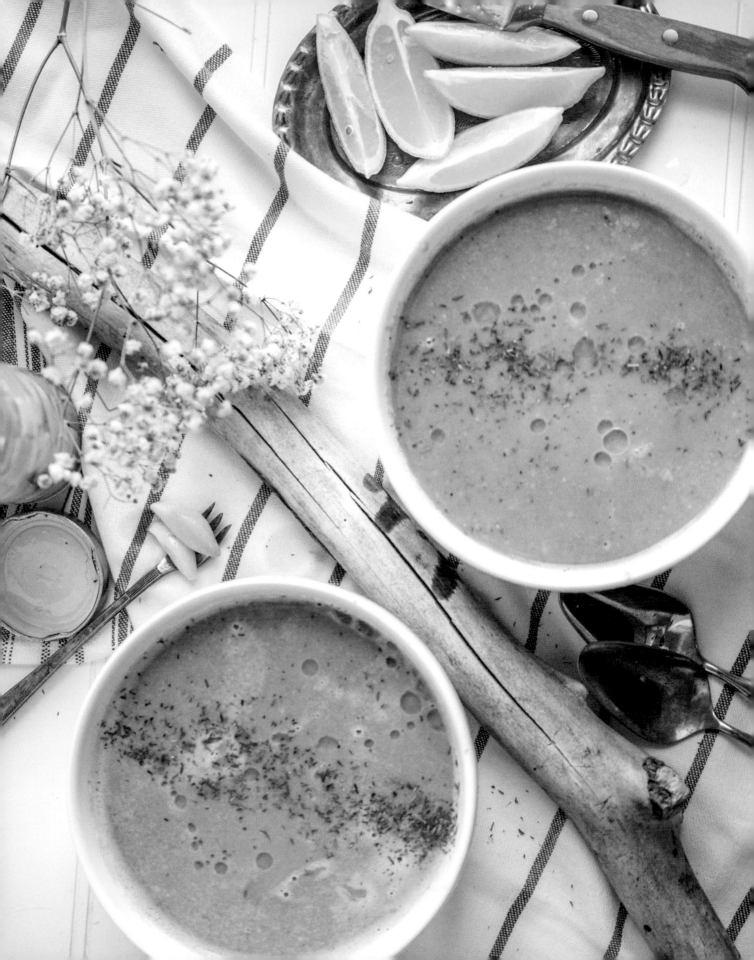

creamy broccoli soup

Creamy, silky, and savory, this soup can be made in a pressure cooker or on the stovetop—the only difference is the simmering time. The deciding factors in the incredible flavor it delivers happen in the early phases of this recipe: the bacon and the browning. I love to pile avocado on top of this soup and serve Everything Flaxseed Meal Crackers (page 326) on the side.

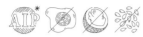

6 slices bacon, chopped

4 heaping cups broccoli florets

5 cloves garlic, peeled

¼ cup nutritional yeast

1 teaspoon dried dill weed

1 teaspoon fine Himalayan salt

1 teaspoon onion powder

½ teaspoon ground black pepper

3 cups bone broth (page 100)

3 tablespoons Homemade Mayo (page 82) or coconut cream (see Note)

Makes 4 servings
PREP TIME: 10 minutes   COOK TIME: 35 minutes

○ Heat a large pot over medium heat. Add the bacon and cook until crispy, stirring occasionally. Remove half of the crispy bacon with a slotted spoon and set aside—it will be used later as a garnish. Leave the rendered bacon fat and the other half of the bacon at the bottom of the pot.

○ Add the broccoli and garlic. Sauté for about 10 minutes, until the garlic becomes aromatic and the broccoli is bright green, then mix in all of the seasonings and pour in the broth.

○ Bring to a simmer, stir well, and cook for 15 minutes. Remove from the heat and carefully transfer the mix to a blender.

○ Add the mayo or coconut cream and blend to your desired consistency. I like mine silky smooth.

○ Ladle the soup into four small bowls and garnish with the reserved crispy bacon. Store leftovers in an airtight container in the fridge for up to 5 days or in the freezer for up to 30 days. To reheat, bring to a simmer on the stovetop.

CHEF'S NOTE: You can buy canned unsweetened coconut cream at the store, or make it at home from a can of full-fat coconut milk: chill the coconut milk in the refrigerator overnight and then skim off the separated cream, which will make up about half of the can of full-fat coconut milk.

SUBSTITUTIONS: To make this AIP-compliant, omit the black pepper and use coconut cream instead of mayo. If you are avoiding yeast, omit the nutritional yeast and use 1 tablespoon fish sauce instead.

VARIATIONS: To make this soup richer and sweeter, use ⅓ cup Garlic Confit (page 76) instead of fresh garlic cloves.

PER SERVING: Calories **214** · Fat **18.9g** · Total Carbohydrate **9.6g** · Dietary Fiber **7.3g** · Protein **9.6g**

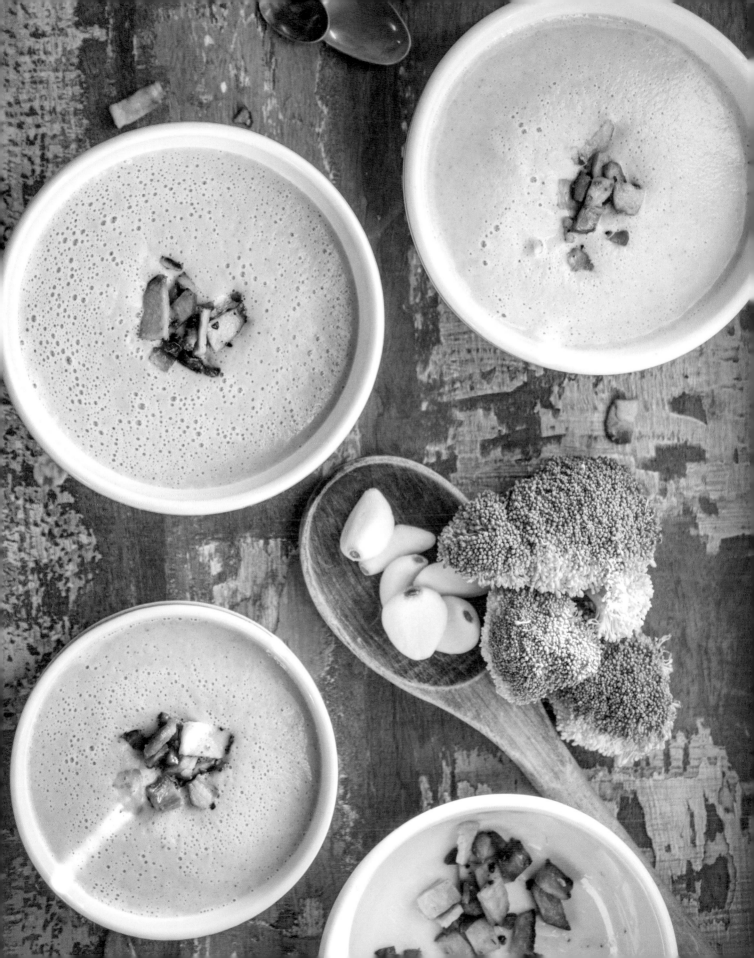

egg drop soup

If you've got broth and a few eggs on hand, you've got egg drop soup. The rest of the ingredients just jazz up the flavor a bit. I often have this for lunch after a good workout; it's so satisfying without being heavy. Such a feel-good soup, and it's easy as pie. Just kidding—it's easier. (Who ever said pie was easy to make?)

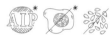

Makes 4 servings
PREP TIME: 5 minutes   COOK TIME: 25 minutes

2 tablespoons toasted sesame oil

1 (2-inch) piece fresh ginger, peeled

4 cloves garlic, peeled

4 cups bone broth (page 100)

1 tablespoon coconut aminos

1 tablespoon fish sauce

Pinch of fine Himalayan salt

4 large eggs, whisked

2 green onions, sliced, for garnish

4 sprigs fresh cilantro, minced, for garnish

○ In a 6- or 8-quart pot, heat the sesame oil over medium heat. Add the ginger and garlic and stir until lightly browned.

○ Add the broth, coconut aminos, fish sauce, and salt. Bring to a low simmer, reduce the heat to low, cover, and cook for 20 minutes.

○ Slowly drizzle in the eggs while stirring the soup so the eggs cook instantly in ribbons as they hit the broth.

○ Garnish with the green onions and cilantro and serve hot. Store leftovers in an airtight container in the fridge for up to 5 days. I don't recommend freezing this soup.

VARIATIONS: I love to add shredded chicken to this soup and make a meal out of it. Other killer additions are Crispy Kalua Pork (page 282) and Carne Molida (page 244)!

SUBSTITUTIONS: You can't really have egg drop soup without eggs, but if you're on AIP, the flavored broth is divine! Use coconut oil instead of sesame oil, skip the eggs, add 2 tablespoons of coconut butter for texture, and add shredded cooked chicken. You still get one heck of a soup.

PER SERVING: Calories **185** · Fat **12g** · Total Carbohydrate **4.2g** · Dietary Fiber **0.1g** · Protein **15.8g**

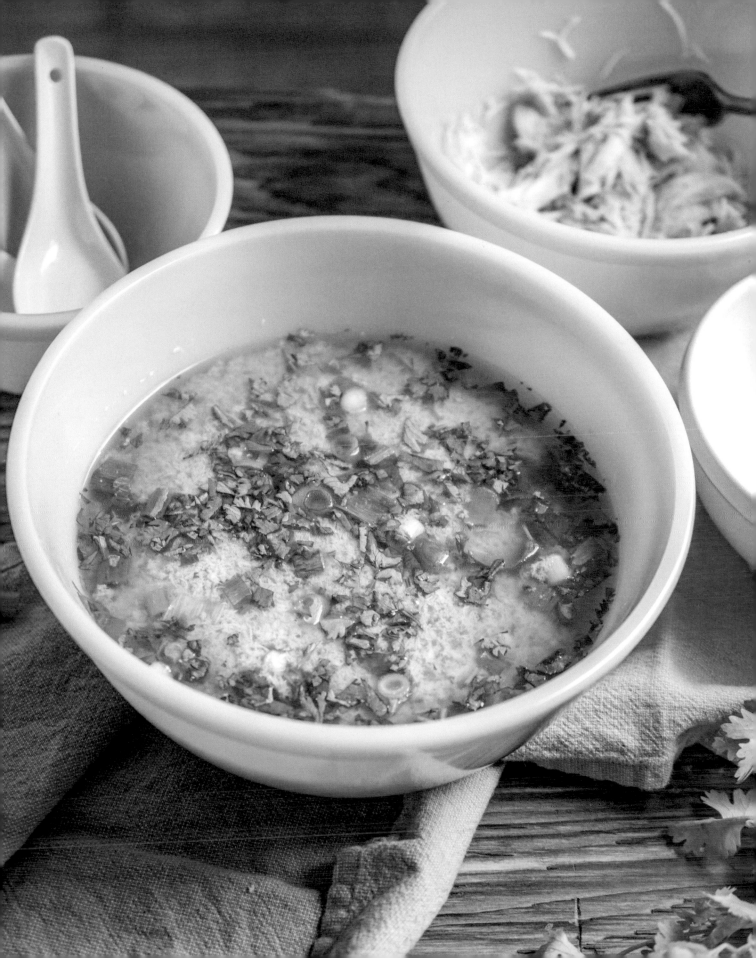

thai coconut soup

I could eat this every day (at least, I could if it weren't so hot all the time in Hawaii). This soup is bursting with flavor; it's satisfying and nourishing without feeling heavy. I think the combination of digestion-aiding lemongrass and ginger really cuts the sometimes-heavy coconut milk for a soup that packs plenty of good fats but goes down light. You can enjoy this soup vegetarian-style with only mushrooms and aromatics, or add your protein of choice! I like to use baby bella mushrooms, but you can use shiitake, cremini, or chanterelles—whatever you can source in your area.

Makes 6 to 8 servings
PREP TIME: 15 minutes   COOK TIME: 25 minutes

1 tablespoon avocado oil

2 tablespoons peeled and minced fresh ginger

2 tablespoons minced garlic

2 stalks lemongrass, cut into large pieces

3 cups sliced baby bella mushrooms

2 tablespoons coconut aminos

2 tablespoons fish sauce

4 cups bone broth (page 100)

2 (13.5-ounce) cans full-fat coconut milk

1 teaspoon fine Himalayan salt

¼ cup minced fresh cilantro, for garnish

3 to 4 sprigs basil, for garnish

2 limes, cut into wedges, for serving

◦ Heat a large pot over medium heat. When it's hot, pour in the avocado oil. Then add the ginger, garlic, and lemongrass. Sauté, stirring often, for 2 to 3 minutes, until the garlic is lightly browned and aromatic.

◦ Add the mushrooms and sauté, stirring often, for 5 to 6 minutes, until they have softened. Stir in the coconut aminos and fish sauce, mixing well and scraping up any bits of garlic or ginger that are stuck to the bottom of the pot. Pour in the broth and bring to a simmer.

◦ Stir in the coconut milk and salt. Simmer for 10 minutes, then remove from the heat. Fish out the pieces of lemongrass.

◦ Garnish with the minced cilantro and basil sprigs and serve with lime wedges on the side. Store leftovers in an airtight container in the fridge for up to 5 days. To reheat, bring to a simmer on the stovetop.

CHEF'S NOTE: A scoop of warm cauliflower rice would go nicely with this soup. Top with a scoop of Crispy Kalua Pork (page 282) or shredded cooked chicken to make it a complete meal.

VARIATIONS: If you want to add shrimp to the soup, add up to 1 pound peeled, deveined, thawed shrimp when the soup is simmering (after adding the bone broth) and cook until the shrimp are no longer translucent, then continue with the recipe as written.

PER SERVING (8 servings): Calories **217** · Fat **19.3g** · Total Carbohydrate **4.4g** · Dietary Fiber **3.1g** · Protein **3.6g**

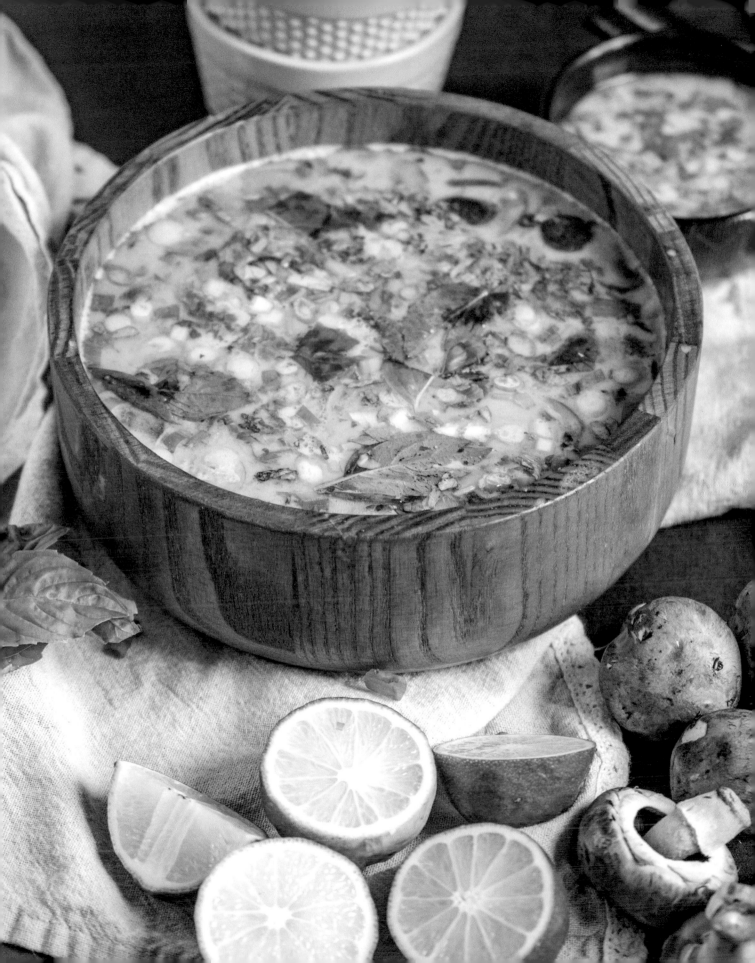

pumpkin chili

Autumn in a bowl. This soup combines the natural sweetness of pumpkin with warm spices, ground beef, and creamy mayo to create a rich soup that will fill you up and warm you up!

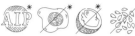

1 tablespoon unsalted butter, ghee, or avocado oil

1 medium onion, diced

3 radishes, diced

2 cloves garlic, minced

4 ribs celery, diced

1 teaspoon dry mustard

1 teaspoon fine Himalayan salt

1 teaspoon garam masala

1 teaspoon ground black pepper

1 pound ground beef (85% lean)

½ cup canned unsweetened pumpkin puree

2 cups bone broth (page 100)

¼ cup Homemade Mayo (page 82)

2 tablespoons coconut cream (see Note, page 144), for garnish

¼ cup minced fresh cilantro, for garnish

Makes 4 servings
PREP TIME: 5 minutes   COOK TIME: 40 minutes

◦ Heat a large pot over medium-high heat. Melt the butter in the pot, then add the onions, radishes, garlic, and celery. Sauté, stirring often, until the onions are translucent and aromatic, about 8 minutes.

◦ Add the seasonings, mix well, and cook until they become fragrant, about 2 minutes.

◦ Add the ground beef, crumbling it up as you go. Use a whisk to make sure it breaks apart well.

◦ Cook, stirring often, until all of the ground beef is browned and crumbly, about 8 minutes.

◦ Add the pumpkin puree and the broth and bring to a simmer. Reduce the heat to low and simmer for 10 to 15 minutes.

◦ Stir in the mayo until well dissolved and remove from the heat. Swirl in the coconut cream and sprinkle with the cilantro. Enjoy!

◦ Store in an airtight container in the fridge for up to 5 days or in the freezer for up to 30 days. To reheat, bring to a simmer on the stovetop.

SUBSTITUTIONS: Make this soup AIP-compliant by omitting the seasonings listed; instead, use 1 teaspoon each of dried thyme leaves, ginger powder, turmeric powder, and ground cinnamon. In addition, omit the mayo and use ¼ cup more coconut cream instead.

Alternatively, if you can't have coconut, garnish with avocado or add more mayo instead.

PER SERVING: Calories **502** · Fat **34.5g** · Total Carbohydrate **7.8g** · Dietary Fiber **1.6g** · Protein **41.3g**

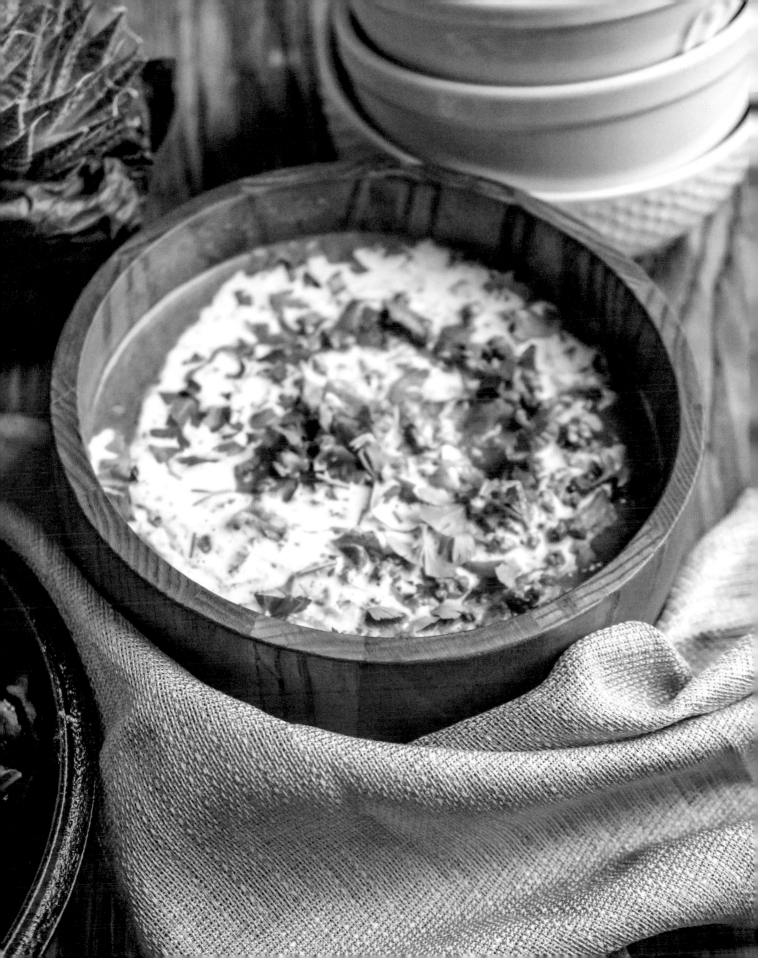

chicken + dumpling soup

Hearty and chock-full of comforting goodness, this easy-peasy soup is the perfect dinner for a winter evening. The dumplings are based on the pie crust dough from page 92, formed into balls and dropped into the soup. They cook quickly into delicate and fluffy dumplings that you can cut into with a spoon and slurp up with some broth.

2 tablespoons avocado oil

1 medium onion, diced

3 ribs celery, diced

3 small radishes, diced

1 small carrot, sliced

4 cloves garlic, minced

1 pound boneless, skinless chicken thighs

1 bay leaf

3 sprigs fresh oregano

4 cups bone broth (page 100)

1 teaspoon fine Himalayan salt

1 teaspoon ground black pepper

FOR THE DUMPLINGS:

2 large eggs

2 tablespoons coconut oil or melted unsalted butter

3 tablespoons coconut flour

Pinch of fine Himalayan salt

Pinch of ground nutmeg

Fresh parsley, for garnish (optional)

Makes 4 servings
PREP TIME: 10 minutes   COOK TIME: 40 minutes

◦ Heat a 5-quart pot over medium heat. Pour in the avocado oil and add the onions, celery, radishes, carrots, and garlic. Sauté, stirring often, for 8 minutes, until the onions are aromatic and translucent.

◦ Push the sofrito to the side and place the chicken thighs flat on the bottom of the pot with the bay leaf and the oregano sprigs on top. Brown for 3 minutes on each side, then mix the chicken thighs well with the sofrito and pour in the broth. Stir in the salt and pepper. Bring the soup to a boil and cook for 20 minutes.

◦ While the soup cooks, make the dumplings: In a medium-sized bowl, whisk together the eggs and coconut oil. Add the coconut flour, salt, and nutmeg and mix until a dry dough forms. Shape into eight equal-sized balls.

◦ Reduce the heat to low and stir the soup, bringing it down to a simmer. Use tongs to gently tear apart the chicken thighs.

◦ Carefully add the dumplings to the soup one at a time. Simmer for about 5 minutes, turning them over with tongs once. They're done when they begin to puff up a little—do not let them swell too much.

◦ Remove the soup from the heat, garnish with fresh parsley if desired, and serve right away. I like to give each serving two dumplings, but you can hoard them if you like.

◦ I do not recommend storing this soup with the dumplings; the longer they sit in the soup, the more they will disintegrate. We like to eat up all the dumplings on first go-round and enjoy the lighter chicken soup, sans dumplings, for leftovers. Store the soup in an airtight container in the refrigerator for up to 6 days. To reheat, bring to a simmer on the stovetop.

CHEF'S NOTE: Sofrito is the combination of sautéed vegetables, seasonings, and bay leaves that are cooked down until tender to give soups and other meals a depth of flavor. Traditionally, in a Cuban sofrito, there are bell peppers and onions, but I like to omit the peppers and use radishes or celery instead.

SUBSTITUTIONS: To make this soup AIP-compliant, leave out the dumplings and the black pepper.

TIME-SAVING TIP: Make this soup in an electric pressure cooker: Make the sofrito (sautéed vegetables) and brown the chicken on sauté mode. Then add the broth, close the cooker, and cook on high for 10 minutes. Open the lid, bring the soup to a simmer on sauté mode, add the dumplings, and cook for 5 minutes.

PER SERVING: Calories **430** · Fat **20g** · Total Carbohydrate **13.1g** · Dietary Fiber **6.2g** · Protein **47.7g**

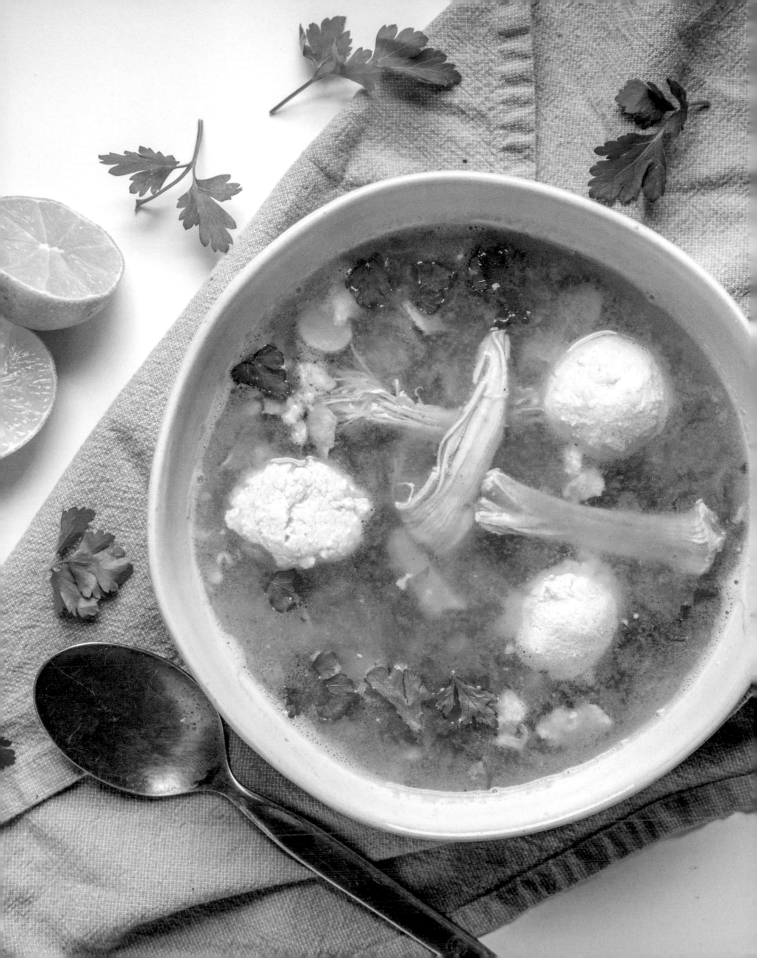

salmon salad avocado boats

No-cook meals don't have to be boring. These delicious avocado boats come together in minutes. Canned wild-caught salmon is a fantastic affordable option that delivers omega-3 fats and protein. I always opt for the boneless, skinless version. Mixed with crunchy and spicy radishes, sweet and juicy blueberries, and creamy homemade mayo, it makes this seafood salad absolutely stunning. So many textures, flavors, and colors packed into one easy meal!

  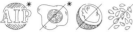

Makes 2 servings
PREP TIME: 10 minutes

1 medium Hass avocado

¼ cup blueberries

¼ cup sliced radishes

2 tablespoons minced fresh parsley

1 (6-ounce) can wild-caught salmon

3 tablespoons Homemade Mayo (page 82)

Pinch of fine Himalayan salt

½ teaspoon ground black pepper

Squeeze of lemon (optional)

¼ cup Pickled Red Onions (page 88), for serving

○ Cut the avocado in half and remove the pit. Cut a ¼-inch grid pattern into each avocado half with a paring knife. Use a spoon to scoop out a few squares of avocado where the pit used to be and surrounding that area. You want to make space for the salad.

○ Place the scooped-out avocado in a small bowl. Add the blueberries, sliced radishes, and parsley. Drain the salmon and use a fork to flake it into the bowl.

○ Add the mayo, salt, and pepper. Mix until well combined. Then spoon half of the mixture into one avocado boat and the rest into the second. Give them a squeeze of lemon (if desired) and serve with pickled onions on the side.

CHEF'S NOTE: I confess, I don't always share this meal. If I've been fasting all day or had an extra-intense workout, I will eat both boats—all 900 calories of goodness—and I don't bat an eye. Because nutrient density, real food, and deliciousness!

SUBSTITUTIONS: If you don't have radishes or just don't like them, cucumber or celery will work well. To make this AIP-compliant, use Toum (page 72) instead of mayo and omit the black pepper.

PER SERVING: Calories **450** · Fat **36.9g** · Total Carbohydrate **13g** · Dietary Fiber **7.5g** · Protein **19.1g**

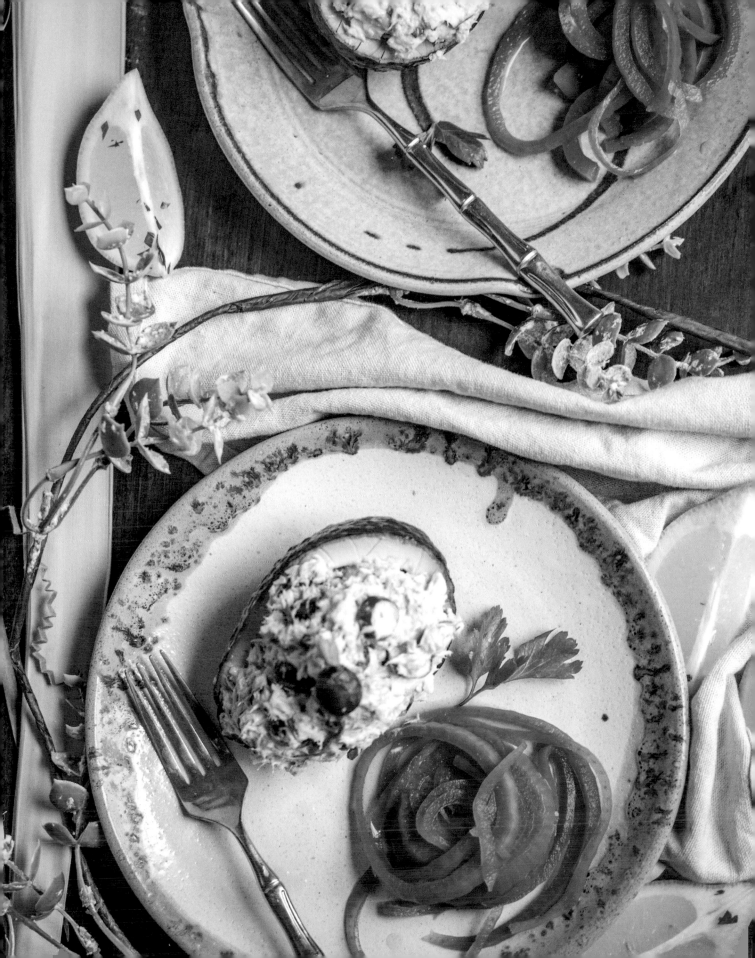

curried crab cake salad

Crab cakes are tasty but usually one of those dishes reserved for eating out. Well, not anymore. Jumbo lump crab meat is preferred for crab cakes because it's white and tender. But it also costs a lot more. Claw meat might not be as pretty, but it works just fine! These curried crab cakes will turn out delicious either way. Served over a super-simple salad with lots of Homemade Mayo (page 82) and fresh lemons, this salad delivers the perfect bistro experience!

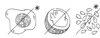

Makes 4 servings
PREP TIME: 15 minutes   COOK TIME: 12 minutes

FOR THE CRAB CAKES:

8 ounces pasteurized blue crab meat

¼ cup minced red onions

2 tablespoons minced celery

2 tablespoons minced fresh parsley

1 tablespoon Dijon mustard

1 teaspoon garam masala

1 teaspoon turmeric powder

1 large egg

2 tablespoons flaxseed meal

½ cup coconut oil or ghee, or more if needed, for frying

FOR THE SALAD:

2 hearts of romaine, shredded

¼ cup crispy bacon crumbles

¼ cup raspberries

¼ cup Pickled Red Onions (page 88)

FOR SERVING (OPTIONAL):

¼ cup Homemade Mayo (page 82)

2 lemons, cut into wedges

° In a large bowl, combine the crab meat, onions, celery, and parsley, using your fingers to break apart the meat. Use a spatula to mix in the Dijon mustard, garam masala, and turmeric, and then add the egg and finally the flaxseed meal.

° Heat a large skillet over medium heat. When it's hot, pour in the coconut oil; it should be ½ inch deep. Line a plate with a paper towel or set out a cooling rack.

° Form the crab meat mixture into eight cakes, using your hands to mold dense, smooth cakes. Add half of the cakes to the skillet with the coconut oil. Brown for 3 minutes, then gently flip, using a thin spatula and a spoon so they don't break. Fry on the other side for another 3 minutes, or until golden brown and crispy. Remove from the pan and set on the lined plate or cooling rack to drain. Repeat with the remaining half of the crab cakes.

° Make the salad: Divide the shredded lettuce among four plates and top with the bacon crumbles, raspberries, and pickled onions.

° Serve the crab cakes with a squirt of mayo, with the salad and lemon wedges on the side.

° Store leftover crab cakes and salad in separate airtight containers in the fridge for up to 4 days. To reheat the crab cakes, bake in a preheated 400°F oven for 5 minutes.

SUBSTITUTIONS: If you can't have flaxseed meal, use 1 tablespoon coconut flour instead. For an egg-free option, lose the cakes and sauté the curried crabmeat mix until toasty. Still delicious! Serve with Toum (page 72) or Green Goddess Dressing (page 106) instead of mayo.

VARIATION: If you don't like crab, try making the cakes with canned tuna or salmon!

PER SERVING: Calories **470** · Fat **44g** · Total Carbohydrate **5.6g** · Dietary Fiber **3g** · Protein **17g**

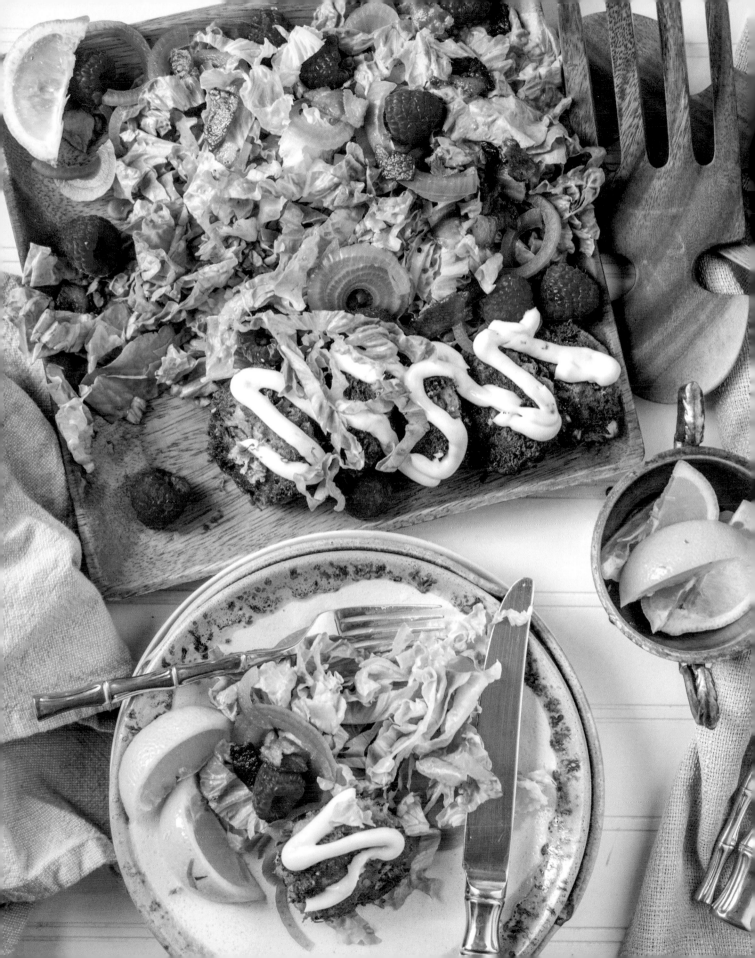

broiled salmon salad

Colorful and flavorful, this big salad is a favorite lunch of mine. The lime zest on the salmon adds freshness to this bouquet of satiating fats over a bed of greens. With Everything Bacon (page 84) and Raspberry Vinaigrette (page 104) on hand, this meal comes together in twenty minutes!

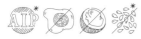

FOR THE SALMON:

1 tablespoon cooking fat (see page 53)

2 (3-ounce) salmon steaks

1 teaspoon fine Himalayan salt

Grated zest of 1 lime

FOR THE SALAD:

2 cups fresh arugula

1 medium Hass avocado, peeled, pitted, and sliced

1 green onion, sliced

6 slices Everything Bacon (page 84), chopped

FOR SERVING:

¼ cup Raspberry Vinaigrette (page 104) or other dressing

Lime wedges

Makes 2 servings
PREP TIME: 10 minutes   COOK TIME: 10 minutes

○ Turn on the broiler and set the oven rack 3 to 5 inches from the heat source.

○ Spread half of the cooking fat on a sheet pan and place the salmon steaks on it skin side down. Sprinkle the salt and lime zest evenly over the salmon steaks and then add the rest of the cooking fat to the tops of the salmon steaks.

○ Broil for 6 minutes, or longer if the steaks are very thick. The salmon will be ready when you can flake the thickest part of it easily with a fork. After 6 minutes, check for doneness in 1-minute intervals.

○ While the salmon cooks, make the salad: Place the arugula, avocado, green onion, and bacon in a large bowl. Gently toss to combine, then divide evenly between two plates.

○ When the salmon is ready, remove it from the oven and use a spatula to gently separate the salmon fillet from the skin. You should be able to do this quite easily just by running the spatula under the meat.

○ Place a salmon steak on each salad and drizzle with 2 tablespoons of dressing. Serve with lime wedges on the side.

○ If you're preparing this to eat later, store the salad base, dressing, and salmon in separate airtight containers in the fridge for up to 3 days. Toss all together to eat.

CHEF'S NOTE: If you're a salmon-skin eater—and you should be; it's very good for you—after you've assembled the salmon salads, scrape the skins off of the sheet pan and flip them over. Broil for another 5 minutes or until crispy, sprinkle with salt, and eat them like chips!

PER SERVING: Calories **419** · Fat **29.5g** · Total Carbohydrate **8.4g** · Dietary Fiber **8.9g** · Protein **20.9g**

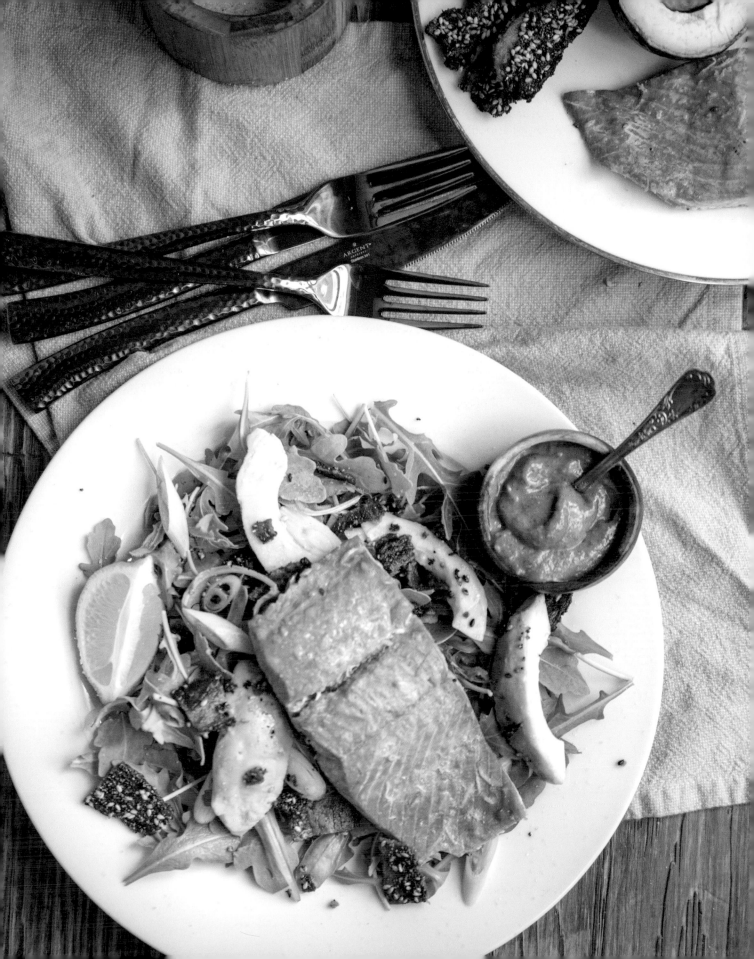

chicken caesar lettuce cups

Chicken Caesar salad just got keto-fied. Toasted cubes of Nut-Free Keto Bread (page 324), succulent chicken thighs, and finger-licking-good creamy dressing, all piled into crisp romaine lettuce cups—I don't think Caesar Cardini, the Italian American chef who invented the Caesar salad in the 1920s, would mind. We've done his salad justice with this fun and delicious combination.

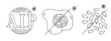

4 boneless, skinless chicken thighs

1 tablespoon avocado oil

1 teaspoon fine Himalayan salt

1 teaspoon ground black pepper

½ teaspoon liquid smoke

1 tablespoon nutritional yeast

¼ cup Ranch Dressing (page 94)

3 slices Nut-Free Keto Bread (page 324)

6 large romaine lettuce leaves

Makes 6 lettuce cups (3 per serving)
PREP TIME: 5 minutes   COOK TIME: 20 minutes

○ Preheat the oven to 425°F.

○ Score the bottom of each chicken thigh with shallow cuts in a crisscross pattern. Place them on a sheet pan, drizzle with the avocado oil, sprinkle with the salt and pepper, and add the liquid smoke. Toss to combine, then lay them flat, scored side down, and spread out. Place in the oven and roast for 20 minutes.

○ While the chicken cooks, stir the nutritional yeast into the ranch dressing, then set aside. Toast the slices of bread for 5 to 6 minutes, until well toasted and hard. Cut them into cubes and set aside.

○ When the chicken is done, dice it and distribute it evenly among the romaine leaves on a serving plate. Do the same with the croutons. Drizzle the dressing over the cups and serve!

○ This salad stores best unassembled. Store the diced chicken in one container and the dressing in another, and wrap the leaves in clean kitchen towels. Keep these in the fridge for up to 5 days. Store the toasted bread in an airtight container at room temperature for up to 3 days.

TIME-SAVING TIP: Use leftover chicken or, really, any protein you have on hand. If you have the bread and dressing ready, this meal can be thrown together in minutes. A great leftover-meal idea!

CHEF'S NOTE: This peppery and slightly smoky chicken is divine. Double the batch and you'll have extra on hand to throw over other salads or to quickly make more Chicken Caesar Lettuce Cups.

SUBSTITUTIONS: To make these egg-free, omit the croutons. To make them AIP-compliant, omit the black pepper, use Toum (page 72) instead of ranch dressing, and replace the croutons with chunks of avocado or pork rinds.

PER SERVING: Calories **751** · Fat **48.8g** · Total Carbohydrate **14.6g** · Dietary Fiber **8g** · Protein **64.1g**

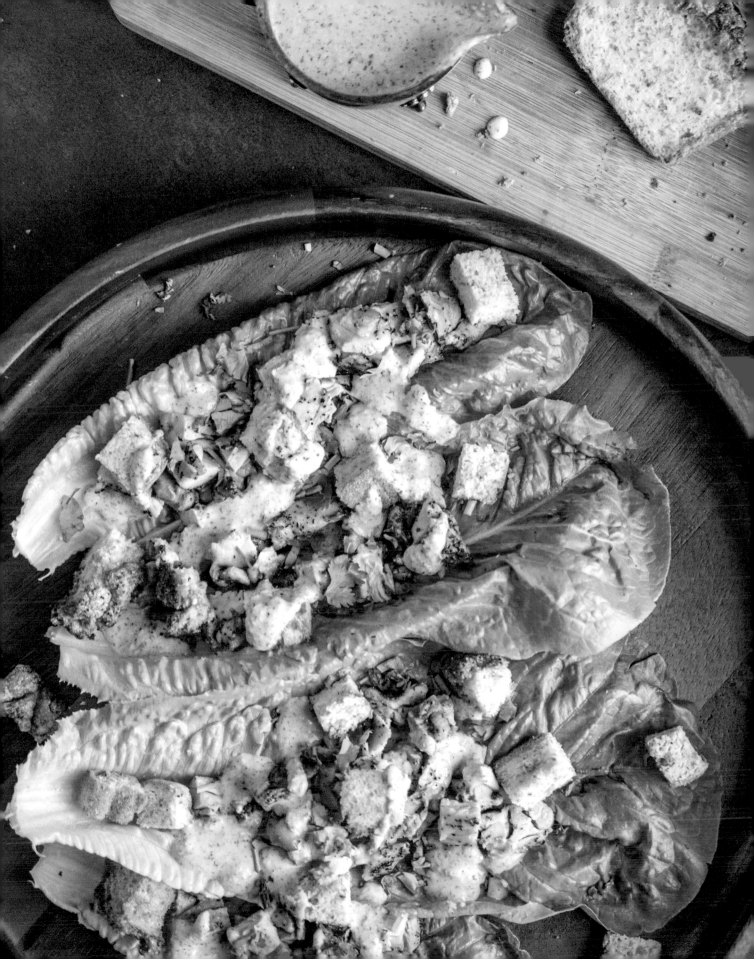

taco salad

This salad is always on repeat in my house. The best thing about it is that you can make it as simple or as complex as you like. If you have Carne Molida (page 244), an avocado, and romaine lettuce, you can make a taco salad—just start with that and build from there.

Makes 4 servings
PREP TIME: 15 minutes

4 hearts of romaine, shredded

2 cups chopped baby spinach

1 recipe Carne Molida (page 244)

2 tablespoons avocado oil

½ red onion, sliced, or ¼ cup Pickled Red Onions (page 88)

¼ cup nutritional yeast

2 cups Fiesta Guacamole (page 90)

½ cup pitted black olives

2 limes, halved, for serving

○ Divide the shredded romaine and spinach among four bowls. Spoon the carne molida over each bowl of greens. Drizzle 1½ teaspoons of avocado oil over each salad.

○ Add a few slices of red onion and a tablespoon of nutritional yeast to each salad.

○ Pile ½ cup of guacamole on each salad. Add a few olives to each bowl and serve with half a lime.

○ Serve, share, enjoy, and get your taco on! This salad is best stored unassembled. Store all the components in separate airtight containers in the fridge for up to 5 days.

VARIATIONS: While I love the combination of guacamole and carne molida here, there are many ways to taco! Leftover Beef Carnitas (page 246) or Chicken Katsu (page 220) will work, too. If you don't have guacamole ready to go, sliced avocado will do just fine. If you have pickled red onions on hand, definitely use those!

PER SERVING: Calories **474** · Fat **37.6g** · Total Carbohydrate **9.8g** · Dietary Fiber **15.1g** · Protein **23.2g**

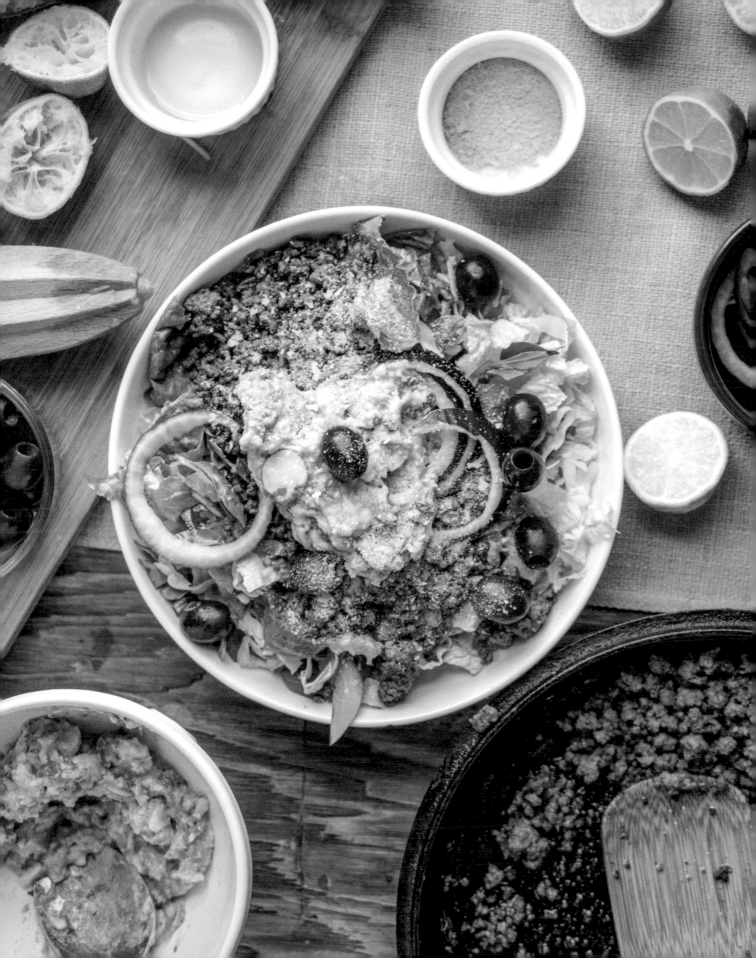

castaway chicken salad

I love chopped salads! Each bite has the potential to be that perfect bite that has a little piece of each ingredient. This crunchy, saucy, slightly sweet combination is inspired by the classic Waldorf salad. It's perfect for making ahead—keep a tub of it in the fridge for lunch all week. Eat it as is or spoon it into lettuce wraps for the perfect finger-food meal!

Makes 6 servings
PREP TIME: 15 minutes

4 cooked chicken cutlets, diced (about 4 cups)

10 slices crispy bacon, chopped

4 green onions, sliced

2 cups diced celery

2 cups halved strawberries

½ cup Homemade Mayo (page 82)

¼ cup Garlic Confit (page 76; optional)

2 tablespoons Dijon mustard

1 teaspoon fine Himalayan salt

1 large head butter lettuce, for serving (optional)

○ Place all of the ingredients except the lettuce in a large bowl and mix until well combined.

○ Spoon the chicken salad onto the lettuce leaves for wraps, or enjoy as is!

○ Store leftovers in an airtight container in the fridge for up to 5 days.

CHEF'S NOTE: If you have a batch of Everything Bacon (page 84) ready to go, chop it up and use it here; it will add lots of extra flavor and texture. I like to use leftover roasted chicken or rotisserie chicken to make short work of this salad.

SUBSTITUTIONS: To make this recipe AIP-compliant, use Toum (page 72) instead of mayo and omit the mustard.

PER SERVING: Calories **375** · Fat **22.9g** · Total Carbohydrate **6g** · Dietary Fiber **2.3g** · Protein **32.8g**

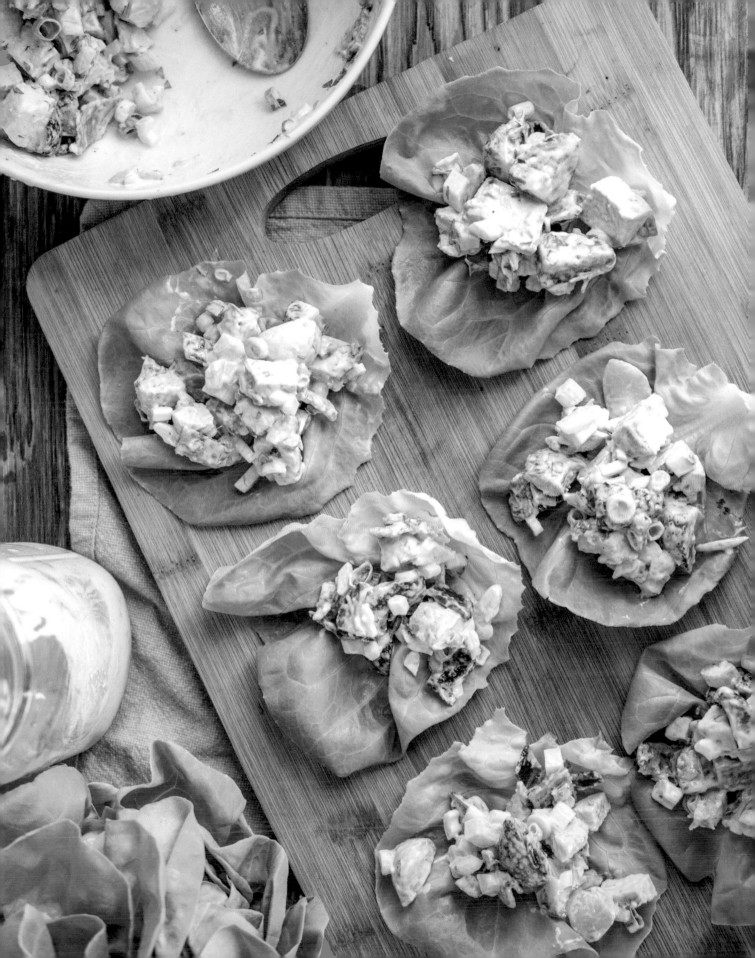

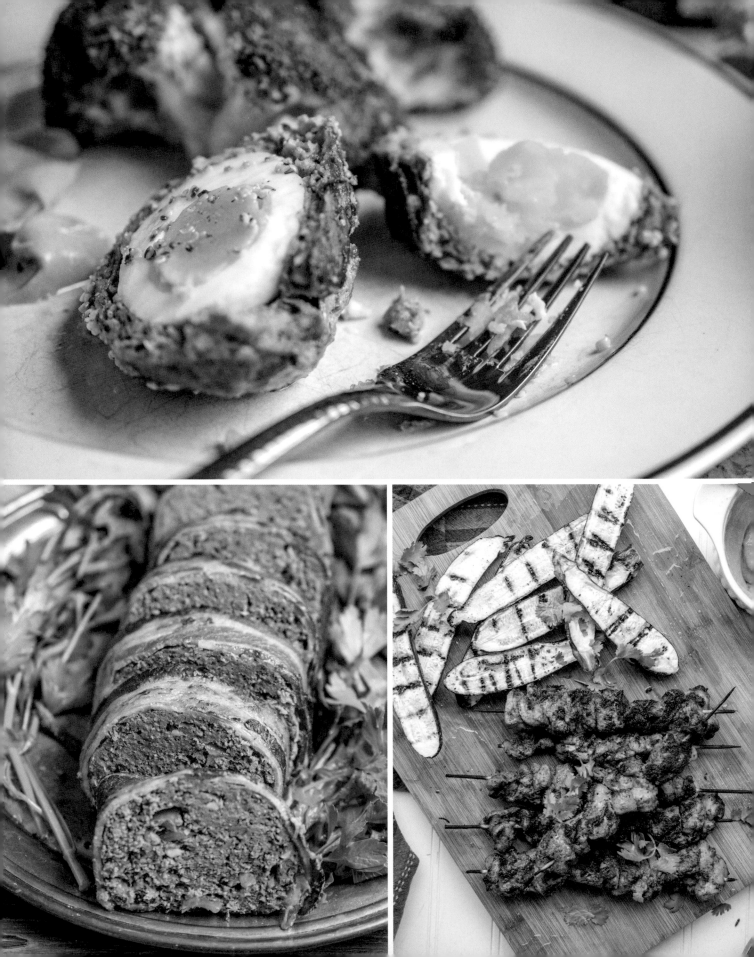

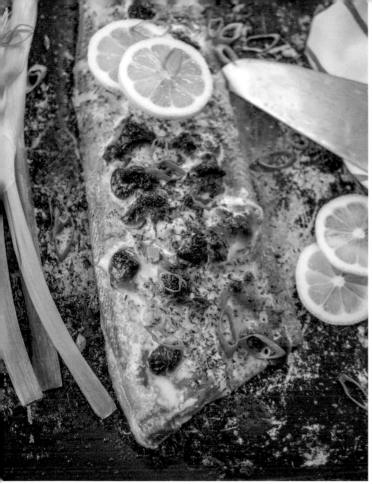

MAINS

Here we go! The main events. These dishes range from holiday table–worthy to weeknight rescues. They bring flavors from all around the world right to your kitchen. I want you to have fun with these recipes—enjoy the process and make them your own. In creating these recipes, I have become healthier, happier, and stronger than ever before. I truly hope that these meals make you feel Made Whole!

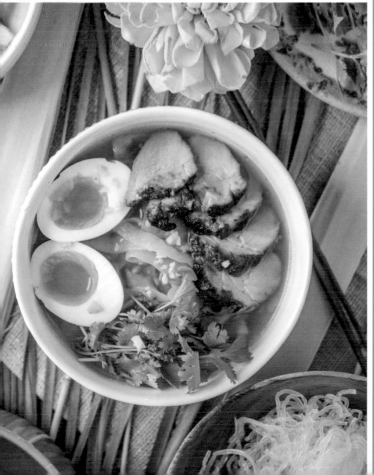

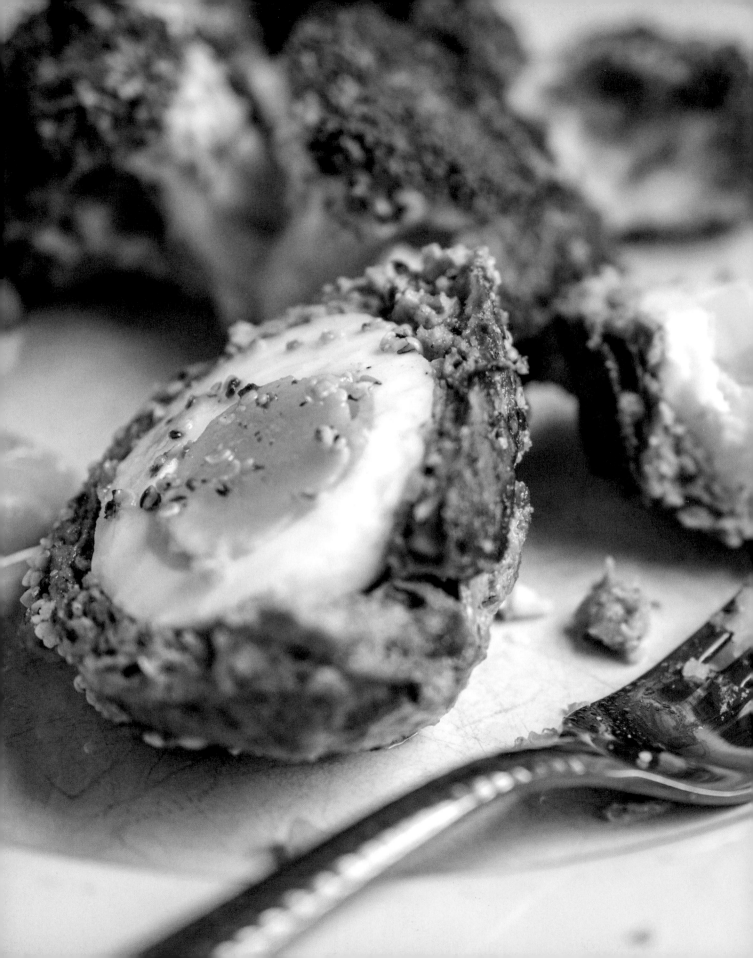

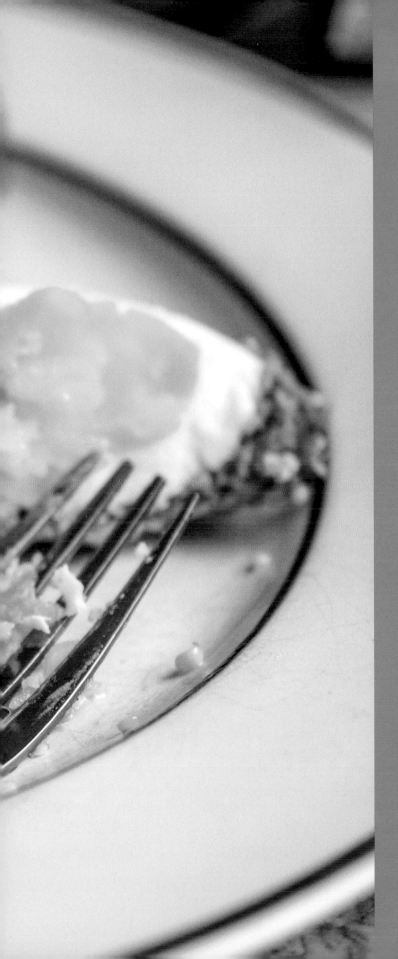

EGGS

Not strictly about morning meals, eggs are welcome any time of day! These eggscellent options include brunch-worthy dishes and meals that are ready in minutes. Eggs are an amazing source of nutrition, containing all essential amino acids. Large eggs contain 5 grams of good fats, 6 grams of protein, and zero carbs, making them an optimal keto food!

kailua breakfast bowl

Eating out can sometimes be difficult when you're trying to be vigilant about what goes into your body. (Will I ever be able to indulge in a chef's tasting menu again?) So when a place opens up in my neighborhood with made-from-scratch lactose-free yogurt, thoughtfully sourced ingredients, and a spotless open kitchen, I am all over it. This dish is an ode to Over Easy in Kailua, the best breakfast spot on the island. The perfect brunch dish is now available in your kitchen.

1 large egg

1 tablespoon avocado oil

5 or 6 leaves curly or dinosaur kale, chopped (about 1 cup)

¼ teaspoon fine Himalayan salt

2 tablespoons Coconut Yogurt (page 96)

¼ cup Carne Molida (page 244)

2 tablespoons Pickled Red Onions (page 88)

Makes 1 serving
PREP TIME: 5 minutes   COOK TIME: 7 minutes

○ Bring a small pot of water to a rapid boil over high heat. In the meantime, heat a large skillet over medium heat.

○ When the water begins to boil, gently add the egg and set a timer for 6 minutes.

○ While the egg cooks, pour the avocado oil into the skillet and add the kale. Sprinkle with the salt. Sauté, stirring often, until the kale wilts and begins to brown, about 6 minutes. Remove from the heat and transfer the kale to a serving plate.

○ After 6 minutes, remove the pot with the egg from the heat and drain the water, leaving the egg in the pot. Fill the pot with cool water and ice, enough to cover the egg. Let the egg sit in the ice bath for 2 minutes while you prepare the rest of the dish.

○ Smear the yogurt on the plate across from the kale. Spoon the carne molida between the kale and the yogurt and top with the pickled onions.

○ Tap the egg on the counter to crack the shell and then submerge it under the water to peel it.

○ Place the egg on the yogurt and use a paring knife to make a vertical slit in it, letting the yolk spill out over the yogurt.

○ Serve right away and dig in! The best way to store this dish is by storing the different components in separate airtight containers in the fridge for up to 5 days.

VARIATIONS: Instead of carne molida, use whatever protein you have ready—Everything Bacon (page 84), Crispy Kalua Pork (page 282), ham . . . whatever makes this super fast and easy! Same goes for the greens: if you don't have kale on hand, spinach, collards, or other leafy greens will work.

PER SERVING: Calories **478** · Fat **31.3g** · Total Carbohydrate **12.5g** · Dietary Fiber **2.3g** · Protein **33.6g**

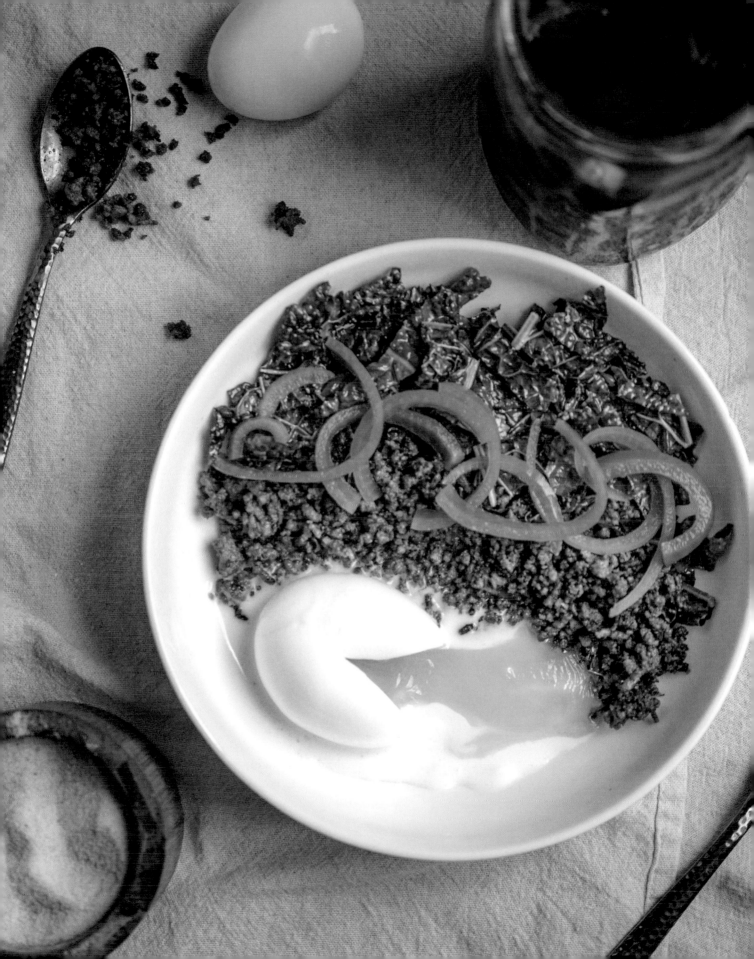

mini quiche muffins

Egg muffins aren't a new idea. I've definitely made my share, but I always get bored of eating them before the batch is gone. Something is missing: a buttery crust! So, I fixed that. A tiny, totally legit quiche that delivers bacon and colorful vegetables? Yes, please! These muffins are simple to make; the crust is no-fail easy. And they're so good that even my four-year-old eats them, and that's saying something!

Makes 12 muffins (1 per serving)
PREP TIME: 15 minutes   COOK TIME: 35 minutes

FOR THE FILLING:

4 slices bacon, diced

2 cups rainbow slaw (see Note)

1 teaspoon fine Himalayan salt, divided

5 large eggs

½ teaspoon ground black pepper

½ teaspoon dried Italian herb blend

½ cup full-fat coconut milk

¼ cup nutritional yeast

FOR THE CRUST:

¼ cup coconut flour

4 to 5 tablespoons flaxseed meal

¼ cup lard, unsalted butter, or ghee, softened

1 to 3 tablespoons ice-cold water

CHEF'S NOTE: You can buy premade rainbow slaw at the grocery store or make it yourself at home. It's simply a mix of a variety of vegetables that are shredded or cut into matchsticks. I like to include broccoli stems, cauliflower stems, cabbage, and carrots. Broccoli slaw, coleslaw, or any shredded cruciferous vegetable blend will work as a substitute in any recipe that calls for rainbow slaw.

○ Preheat the oven to 400°F. Line a standard-size 12-cup muffin tin with baking cups and lightly grease them with coconut oil or avocado oil.

○ In a large skillet, cook the bacon over medium-high heat until crispy, stirring occasionally. Remove the bacon from the skillet and set it on a plate to cool, leaving the fat in the skillet. Add the rainbow slaw and ½ teaspoon of the salt to the skillet. Cover and cook for about 10 minutes, stirring occasionally.

○ While the slaw cooks, make the crust: Mix together the coconut flour and flaxseed meal in a small bowl. Add the lard and use your fingertips to break it up until a crumbly dough forms. Add the water a tablespoon at a time, until the dough comes together and you can form it into a large ball. Cover the bowl and place it in the fridge.

○ The slaw should be done by now. Remove the skillet from the heat and transfer the slaw to the plate with the bacon to cool.

○ In a large bowl, whisk together the eggs, the remaining ½ teaspoon of salt, the seasonings, and the coconut milk. Add the nutritional yeast and whisk until well combined but not too frothy.

○ Grab the dough from the fridge. Break off ½-inch pieces and press them down into the bottoms of the baking cups, creating little crusts. Par-bake the crusts for 5 minutes.

○ While the crusts par-bake, mix the cooled slaw and bacon into the egg mixture.

○ Remove the crusts from the oven and ladle the egg-and-slaw mixture into the muffin cups, filling them three-quarters full. Bake for 15 minutes, or until the centers are set and the muffins are fluffy and golden. Let cool for 5 minutes before serving.

○ Store in an airtight container in the fridge for up to 1 week. To reheat, toast in a preheated 350°F oven for 8 minutes or microwave on high for 1 minute.

PER SERVING: Calories **155** · Fat **12.5g** · Total Carbohydrate **4.6g** · Dietary Fiber **2.3g** · Protein **6.6g**

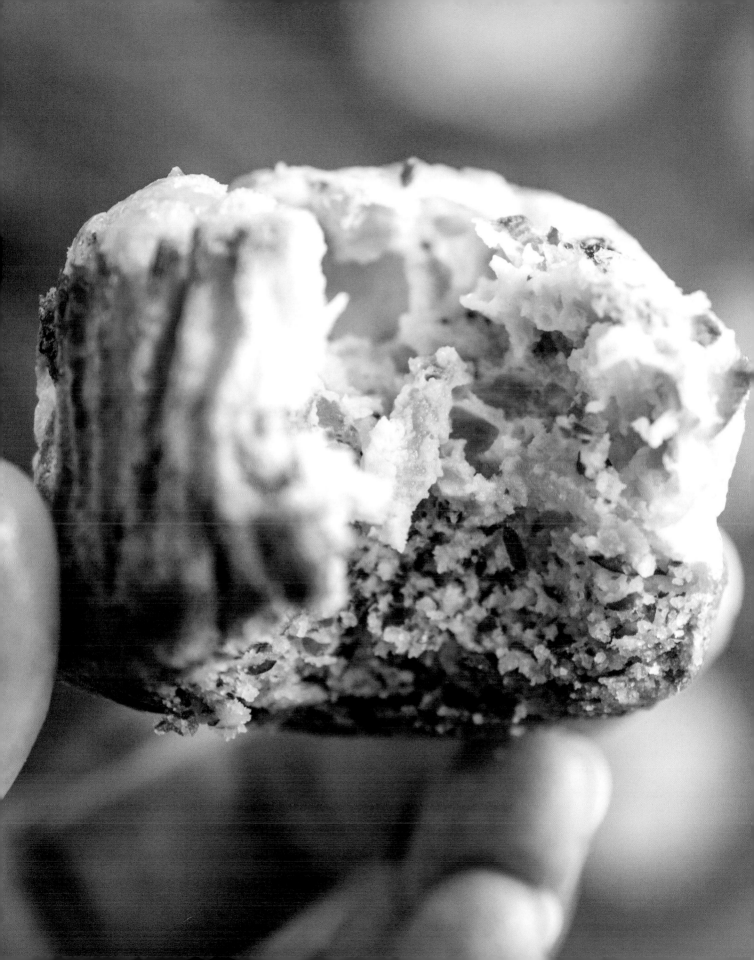

crispy eggs + cabbage

This is the kind of meal I make for myself when I come home from the gym, super ready to break my fast. A one-skillet, five-ingredient meal that takes less than fifteen minutes to make! I like to drizzle some Chimichurri (page 80) on my eggs or pile on some Pickled Red Onions (page 88).

1 tablespoon coconut oil or avocado oil

½ medium head cabbage, sliced (about 2 cups)

2 slices prosciutto, ham, or bacon

2 large eggs

½ teaspoon fine Himalayan salt

Makes 1 serving
PREP TIME: 5 minutes   COOK TIME: 10 minutes

○ Heat an 8-inch skillet or griddle over medium heat. When it's hot, melt the oil in the skillet, swirling it around to grease the entire surface.

○ Add the cabbage, distributing it evenly over the whole skillet in one even layer. Let it cook undisturbed for about 5 minutes, until the bottom of the cabbage browns. Move the cabbage to one side of the skillet, forming a little mound.

○ Put the prosciutto slices on the other side of the skillet and cook for 2 to 3 minutes, until crispy, flipping once. Then push the prosciutto to the side, snuggled up against the cabbage.

○ Crack the eggs into the remaining space in the skillet and sprinkle everything with the salt. Let the eggs cook for 2 to 3 minutes, until the whites are no longer translucent and the edges are crispy. If the eggs look done except for little pools of raw white near the yolk, use a spatula to gently distribute the loose egg white over the cooked egg parts until they too are cooked.

○ Serve right away. You can even eat it right out of the skillet! If you have leftovers, store them covered in the fridge for up to 3 days.

VARIATIONS: This cooking method works with any green veggie. Use broccoli florets, shredded Brussels sprouts, spinach, kale, collard greens, or Swiss chard! The possibilities are endless with this classic.

PER SERVING: Calories **437** · Fat **33.6g** · Total Carbohydrate **8.7g** · Dietary Fiber **3.5g** · Protein **30.4g**

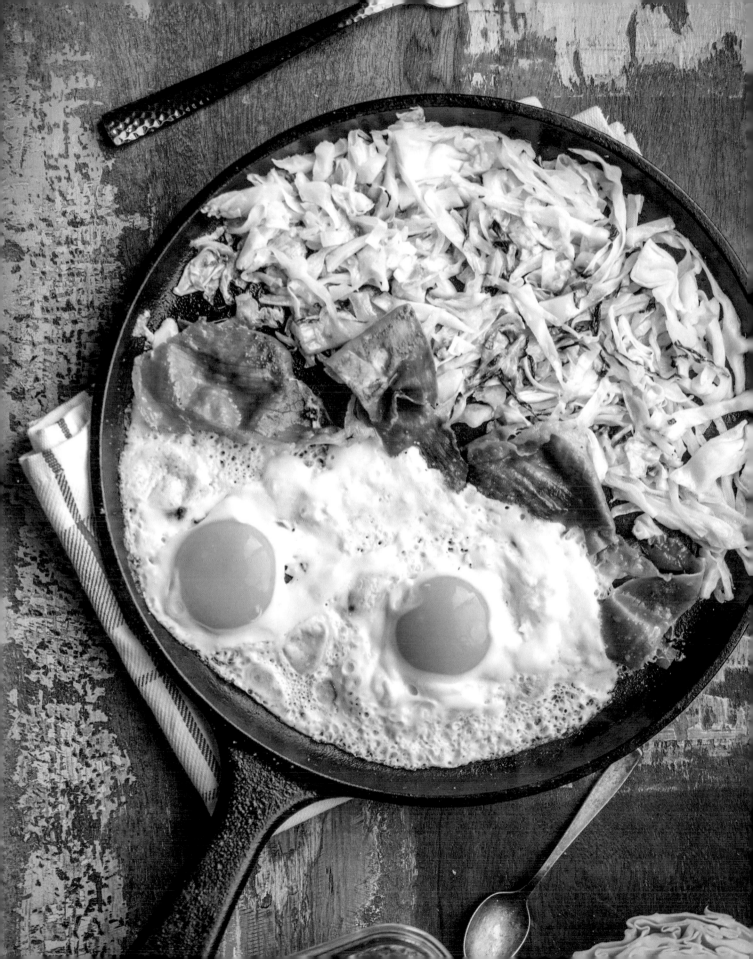

eggs benny

My favorite weekend brunch or breakfast-for-dinner meal, this dish is ultimately satisfying, rich, and flavorful. Use this no-fail poached-egg method and become a brunch pro yourself!

Makes 4 servings
PREP TIME: 10 minutes   COOK TIME: 15 minutes

8 slices bacon

12 spears asparagus, trimmed

4 cups water

1 tablespoon white vinegar

4 large eggs

4 Savory Flax Waffles (page 328), for serving

¼ to ½ cup Hollandaise (page 196), for serving

CHEF'S NOTE: To reheat the hollandaise, microwave it in 10-second increments until warm, not hot, stirring after each increment.

VARIATIONS: Use toasted slices of Nut-Free Keto Bread (page 324) or Mini Pumpkin Waffles (page 330)! Want to skip the waffle altogether? Use Spiced Pork Tenderloin (page 292) as the base and "beef" up this dish!

○ Place the bacon slices on a sheet pan, spaced about 1 inch apart. Distribute the asparagus around the bacon. Place the sheet pan in the oven and set it to 400°F. Cook until the oven comes to temperature, then for 10 to 15 more minutes.

○ Once the asparagus tips are lightly browned and the bacon is toasty on the edges, turn off the oven and crack the door a bit so everything stays warm. I like to put my waffles in there, too.

○ Begin poaching the eggs: Line a plate with paper towels. Heat the water in a small saucepan over medium heat. Add the vinegar and bring to a steady simmer. Crack each of the eggs into its own small ramekin.

○ With a slotted spoon, stir the water in the saucepan to create a whirlpool, then slowly add an egg to the center of the whirlpool. Gently stir the water around the edge of the pot for another 10 seconds, until the swirling motion of the water wraps the egg white around the yolk to create a neat poached egg. Cook undisturbed for 3 minutes, until the white is opaque and the egg looks like a teardrop or a little ghost in the water.

○ Remove the egg from the water with a slotted spoon and place on the lined plate. Repeat with the remaining eggs.

○ Assemble the eggs bennys like so: a waffle on the bottom, a layer of asparagus, 2 slices of bacon, a poached egg, and then 1 to 2 tablespoons of hollandaise.

○ I don't recommend saving leftover poached eggs, as reheating them will cause them to overcook. However, you can store the rest of the meal by packing each component separately in an airtight container. They will keep in the fridge for up to 5 days.

PER SERVING (without the hollandaise): Calories **410** · Fat **30.1g** · Total Carbohydrate **11.7g** · Dietary Fiber **9.7g** · Protein **23.3g**
PER 2 TABLESPOONS of hollandaise: Calories **112** · Fat **11.8g** · Total Carbohydrate **0.7g** · Dietary Fiber **0g** · Protein **0.5g**

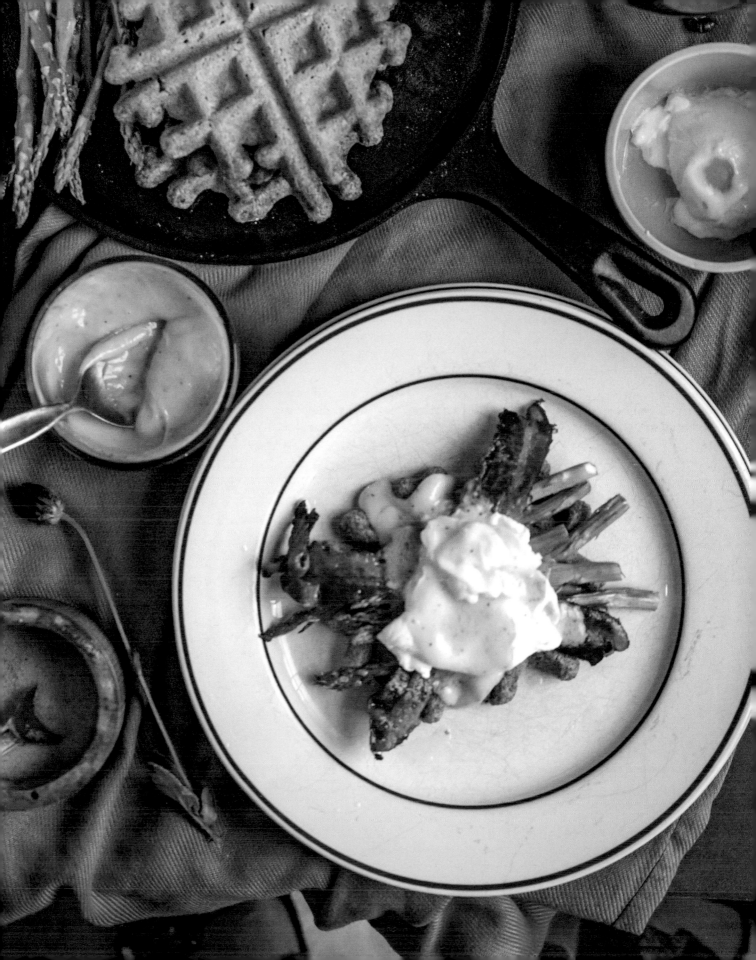

baked scotch eggs

If you haven't had Scotch eggs before, you're in for a treat! I gave this pub-food staple—normally made by wrapping a hard-boiled egg in sausage, then breading and deep-frying it—a makeover. I wrap soft-boiled eggs in homemade Pork Sausage (page 280), sprinkle on some shelled hemp seeds, and bake them to crispy perfection while leaving the yolks moist and jammy. This hearty concoction is a meal in and of itself, but it also pairs nicely with some leftover veggies. Take these to your next potluck or pack them for lunch. I promise, they will not disappoint.

6 cups water

8 large eggs

1 recipe Pork Sausage (page 280), uncooked

2 tablespoons avocado oil

2 tablespoons shelled hemp seeds (aka hemp hearts) (optional)

1 teaspoon fine Himalayan salt

CHEF'S NOTE: Let me let you in on a little secret, especially if the idea of making eight Scotch eggs terrifies you: you don't have to make everything all at once. You can keep a dozen soft-boiled eggs in the fridge for up to a week.

TIME-SAVING TIP: Kill two meal-prep birds with one stone: make a batch of the sausage, cook up half of it, and save the rest of the raw mix for a half batch of these Scotch eggs. When the time comes to make the eggs, it won't be such a production—you'll have it all done in about 30 minutes.

Makes 8 eggs (1 per serving)
PREP TIME: 10 minutes   COOK TIME: 35 minutes

○ Preheat the oven to 400°F.

○ Bring the water to a rapid boil in a large pot. Gently place the eggs in the water and cook for 8 minutes.

○ Meanwhile, form the sausage mix into eight ¼-inch-thick, 4-inch-diameter patties. Place them on a sheet of parchment paper or a cutting board and set aside.

○ When the eggs are done, drain the hot water from the pot, leaving the eggs in it, then fill the pot with cold water and ice. Let the eggs chill in the ice bath for 2 minutes, then immediately peel them under the cold water.

○ Wrap the eggs: Place a pork patty in one hand. Using your other hand, place an egg in the center of the patty. Close your hand holding the pork around the egg and use your other hand to pinch the sausage closed. Gently shape the Scotch egg with both hands until it's smooth and even. Place the egg on a sheet pan, seam side down. Repeat with the remaining eggs and pork patties.

○ Brush or spray the eggs with the oil. Sprinkle with the hemp seeds (if using) and salt. Bake for 25 minutes.

○ Remove from the oven and dig in! Or you can let the eggs cool and store in an airtight container in the refrigerator for up to 5 days. I eat the leftovers cold, with a smear of Homemade Mayo (page 82) on top.

PER SERVING: Calories **260** · Fat **20.2g** · Total Carbohydrate **1.4g** · Dietary Fiber **1.9g** · Protein **17.1g**

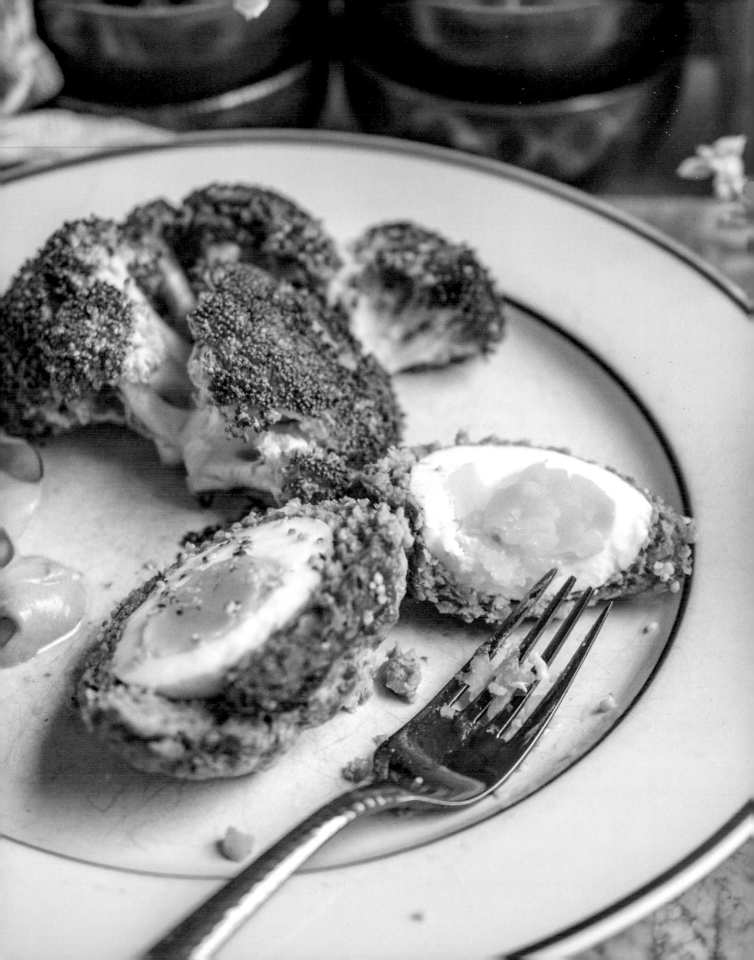

brussels + bacon frittata

Frittata is like quiche's casual cousin: much simpler, crustless, yet just as delicious. Frittatas are perfect to make on the weekend for grab-and-go meals all week. Delicious cold or warm, always welcome at potlucks and in brunch spreads ... If you're not acquainted with frittatas, now's the time! If you don't like Brussels sprouts or don't have them, shredded cabbage or broccoli florets work here, too! You know, we keep things flexible around here.

5 slices bacon, chopped into 1-inch pieces

12 large eggs

¼ cup full-fat coconut milk

1½ teaspoons fine Himalayan salt, divided

1 teaspoon ground black pepper

1 teaspoon dried dill weed

½ onion, sliced

2 cups shredded Brussels sprouts (see Note)

1 tablespoon Dijon mustard

1 tablespoon avocado oil

SUBSTITUTIONS: You may omit the coconut milk; instead, use ¼ cup cold water or your preferred milk.

CHEF'S NOTE: I like to shred Brussels sprouts by carefully holding them at the base and using a sharp knife to thinly slice, starting at the top. Like mini cabbages, they slice into thin shreds. If you're not comfortable with your knife skills, you can also use the slicer or grater attachment of your food processor to get this done.

Makes one 9-inch frittata (8 servings)
PREP TIME: 10 minutes   COOK TIME: 35 minutes

○ Preheat the oven to 350°F.

○ Heat a 9-inch oven-safe skillet over medium heat. Add the bacon pieces and cook, stirring occasionally, for 10 minutes, or until the bacon begins to crisp up.

○ In the meantime, in a large mixing bowl, whisk together the eggs, coconut milk, 1 teaspoon of the salt, the pepper, and the dill until light yellow, smooth, and frothy. Set aside.

○ When the bacon is done, add the onions and Brussels sprouts to the skillet. Mix well, cover, and cook for 3 minutes. Stir in the mustard, oil, and remaining ½ teaspoon of salt until well combined.

○ Pour in the egg mixture and cook undisturbed for about 5 minutes, until the edges begin to look cooked and dry and are separating from the skillet.

○ Carefully transfer the skillet to the middle rack of the oven. Bake for 15 minutes, then check for doneness. When the center is set, meaning it does not jiggle when the skillet is moved, the frittata is done. After 15 minutes, check every 2 minutes until it is set.

○ Remove the skillet from the oven and let the frittata cool for a few minutes.

○ Run a spatula around the edge of the frittata and a little under it to make sure it has not stuck to the skillet. To flip it out of the skillet, put a plate or cutting board over the top of the skillet and, in one swift motion, quickly flip it over. Cut the frittata into eight equal slices.

○ Store leftovers in an airtight container in the fridge for up to 1 week. Enjoy cold or reheat in a preheated 350°F oven for 8 minutes.

PER SERVING: Calories **358** · Fat **26g** · Total Carbohydrate **6g** · Dietary Fiber **1.2g** · Protein **14g**

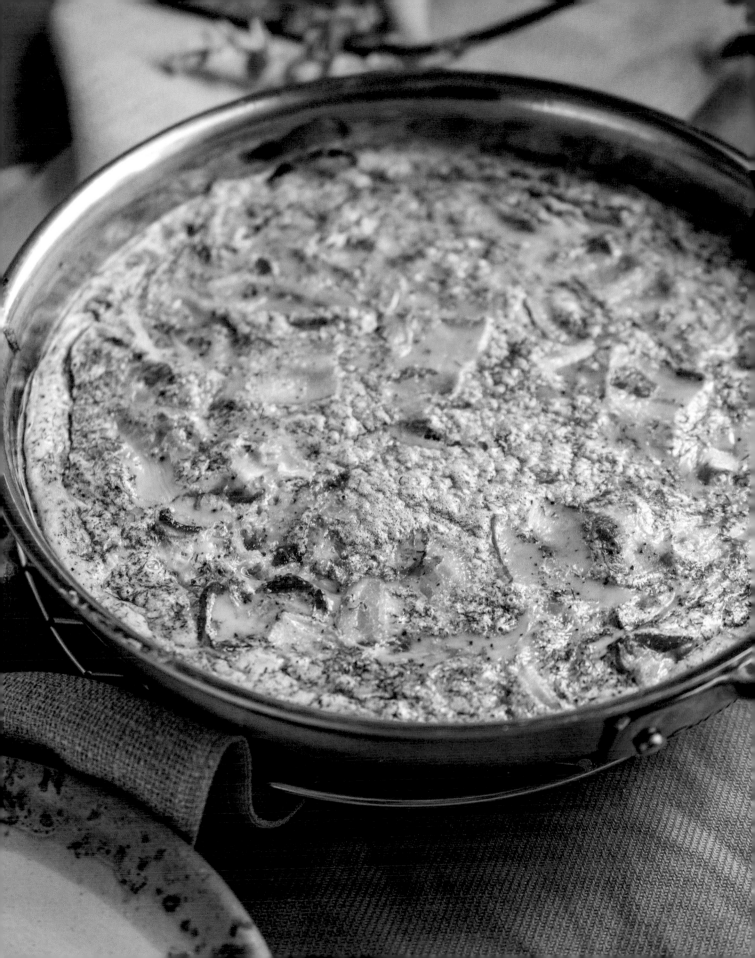

egg tart

Inspired by khachapuri, a Georgian cheese bread, this breakfast tart combines Cheesy Yellow Sauce (page 68) or Cauliflower Alfredo (page 86) and Pie Crust (page 92) with salty prosciutto and a few eggs for a creamy showstopping dish. This beauty reheats well, so feel free to bake it ahead of time and reheat to serve. A handful of arugula or fresh herbs also goes really well atop or alongside a slice of this tart.

1 cup Cheesy Yellow Sauce (page 68) or Cauliflower Alfredo (page 86)

1 baked Pie Crust (page 92)

4 large eggs

¼ teaspoon fine Himalayan salt

¼ teaspoon ground black pepper

4 slices prosciutto di Parma

Makes one 8-inch pie (4 servings)
PREP TIME: 20 minutes   COOK TIME: 20 minutes

◦ Spread the sauce evenly on the bottom of the baked pie crust. Crack the eggs over the sauce and sprinkle with the salt and pepper. Distribute the prosciutto slices around the eggs. Wrap the edges of the crust in aluminum foil so they do not burn.

◦ Bake for 20 minutes, or until the egg whites are completely set. You can test this by gently shaking the pie to watch for a jiggle—when it doesn't move, it's done.

◦ Remove from the oven and serve hot, or let cool and store in the refrigerator, covered, for up to 3 days. To reheat, cut into four large slices, cover each slice with foil, and bake in a preheated 300°F oven for 10 minutes.

CHEF'S NOTE: The eggs can be slightly beaten before adding for a smooth yellow tart, and you can always use regular-cut bacon instead of prosciutto.

PER SERVING: Calories **471** · Fat **40.6g** · Total Carbohydrate **9.2g** · Dietary Fiber **6.3g** · Protein **19.1g**

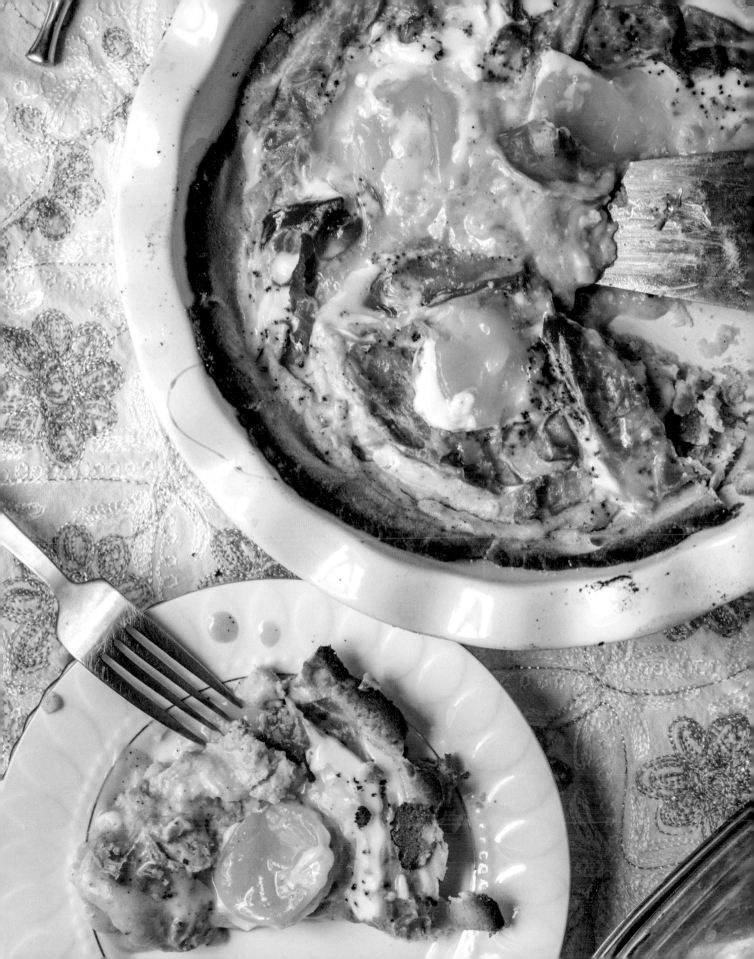

smoky shrimp omelet

Cloves of tender Garlic Confit (page 76) with sautéed shrimp cooked into fluffy eggs. Slightly spicy from the black pepper, with a hint of smoky flavor, this omelet is a combination of tortilla española and Cajun omelets. The mash-up of flavors comes together for a surprising dish that is perfect for brunch, holiday spreads, or breakfast-for-dinner!

6 large eggs

1½ teaspoons fine Himalayan salt, divided

1 teaspoon ground black pepper

1 teaspoon liquid smoke

¼ cup Garlic Confit (page 76), with oil

¾ to 1 pound large shrimp (about 12), peeled and deveined

2 teaspoons avocado oil, divided

1 cup arugula

Makes 2 servings
PREP TIME: 15 minutes   COOK TIME: 15 minutes

○ Place the eggs, ½ teaspoon of the salt, the pepper, and the liquid smoke in a large mixing bowl. Whisk until frothy, then set aside.

○ Heat a 6-inch skillet over medium heat. When it's hot, place the confit in the skillet, quickly followed by the shrimp. Add the remaining teaspoon of salt and sauté for 2 to 3 minutes, until the shrimp are pink and beginning to coil. Then transfer everything from the skillet to a plate. Don't clean the pan.

○ In the same skillet, quickly add 1 teaspoon of the avocado oil, swirl it around, and pour in half of the whisked eggs. Once the bottom is no longer translucent, add 6 shrimp and half of the garlic. Cover the skillet with a tight-fitting lid and cook for 4 to 5 minutes.

○ Remove the lid and pick up the skillet to swirl the contents around for 30 seconds. There will be a thin layer of egg still fluid on the top, and moving it around like this will spread that layer out over the top of the omelet so it will finish cooking while leaving the omelet slightly moist. (If you like a dry omelet, you can pop it under the broiler for 1 to 2 minutes.)

○ Run a spatula along the edge of the omelet and slide it onto a plate. Put the skillet back on the stove and use the remaining ingredients to make the second omelet in the same way, starting with adding the remaining teaspoon of avocado oil.

○ Top each omelet with ½ cup arugula and serve right away. (I do not recommend making this to serve later as reheating will brown the eggs and overcook the shrimp.)

SUBSTITUTIONS: The garlic-infused oil of the confit is just divine in this dish, but if you don't have confit already made, you can mince and quickly sauté some garlic in avocado oil before adding it to the shrimp. You'll get the same flavor, but you'll miss out on the potato-like texture of the confit.

If you don't have liquid smoke or can't find a quality brand, just omit it from the recipe. You might use smoked salt instead of Himalayan salt.

TIME-SAVING TIP: You can use precooked shrimp or langostinos for this and skip the first step of sautéing the shrimp with the garlic confit.

PER SERVING: Calories **403** · Fat **20.5g** · Total Carbohydrate **4.9g** · Dietary Fiber **0.3g** · Protein **42g**

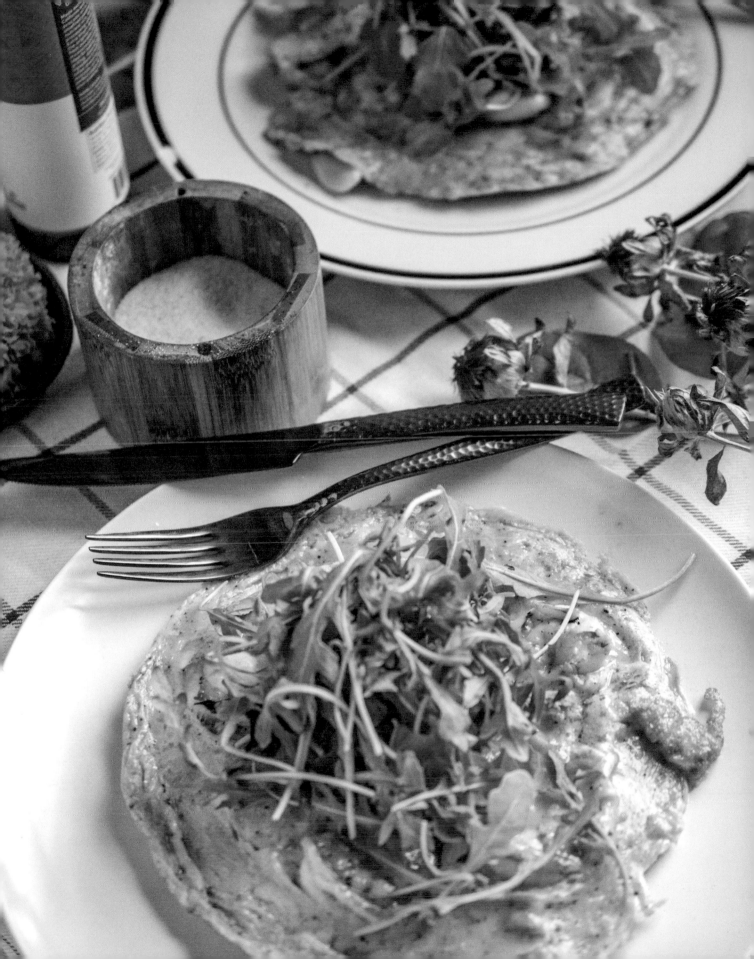

egg roll-ups

Bloggers like to help each other out; we even have groups that comment on and promote each other's recipes. Sharing is caring, right? It was during my participation in this that I found Irena of Eat Drink Paleo's egg roll-ups with ham and carrots and leeks. It was a mind-blown moment. So I messed around a few variations and made my own version, and it broke the internet. Here I have simplified it a bit because variety is the spice of life and sometimes less is more. The perfect make-ahead, grab-and-go breakfast!

4 slices bacon

8 large eggs

¼ cup full-fat coconut milk

½ teaspoon fine Himalayan salt

½ teaspoon ground black pepper

2 cups baby spinach

3 tablespoons Pistou (page 74)

VARIATIONS: In place of the pistou, you could use Homemade Mayo (page 82), Toum (page 72), Roasted Beet Marinara (page 78), or any sauce you wish.

SUBSTITUTIONS: If you can't have coconut milk, you can use any kind of milk you wish instead, in the same amount.

Makes 6 roll-ups (2 per serving)
PREP TIME: 10 minutes   COOK TIME: 30 minutes

○ Lay the bacon slices flat on a 13 by 18-inch sheet pan, put it in the oven on the middle rack, and set the oven to 375°F. Cook the bacon until the oven comes to temperature and then for up to 10 minutes more. When it's crispy, remove it from the oven. Use a spatula to scrape it off the pan and set aside. Drain some of the bacon grease off (into a receptacle to save it, of course). Line the greasy sheet pan with parchment paper.

○ Place the eggs, coconut milk, salt, and pepper in a blender. Blend on high for 45 seconds.

○ Pour the egg mixture into the prepared sheet pan. Distribute the baby spinach evenly over the egg mixture. Carefully place the sheet pan in the oven, using smooth and slow movements.

○ Bake for 10 minutes, or until the edges of the omelet begin to lift from the pan and the center is set.

○ Holding the edges of the parchment paper, lift the giant omelet off of the pan and transfer it to a cutting board or countertop. Let it cool for a few minutes, until you can handle it without burning your fingers. While it cools, chop the bacon into small pieces. Then gently lift the omelet away from the parchment paper. Place it on a flat surface, like a large cutting board.

○ Spread the pistou on the center of the omelet from top to bottom in a 3-inch-wide column. Then sprinkle the bacon over the pistou.

○ Starting from the left side, roll the omelet until you have what looks like a giant egg roll.

○ Cut the roll into six pieces, serve, and enjoy! Store leftovers in an airtight container in the refrigerator for up to 5 days. Enjoy them cold or gently reheat in the microwave on high for 30 seconds or in a 300°F oven for 5 minutes.

PER SERVING: Calories **432** · Fat **35.1g** · Total Carbohydrate **4.2g** · Dietary Fiber **1.6g** · Protein **26g**

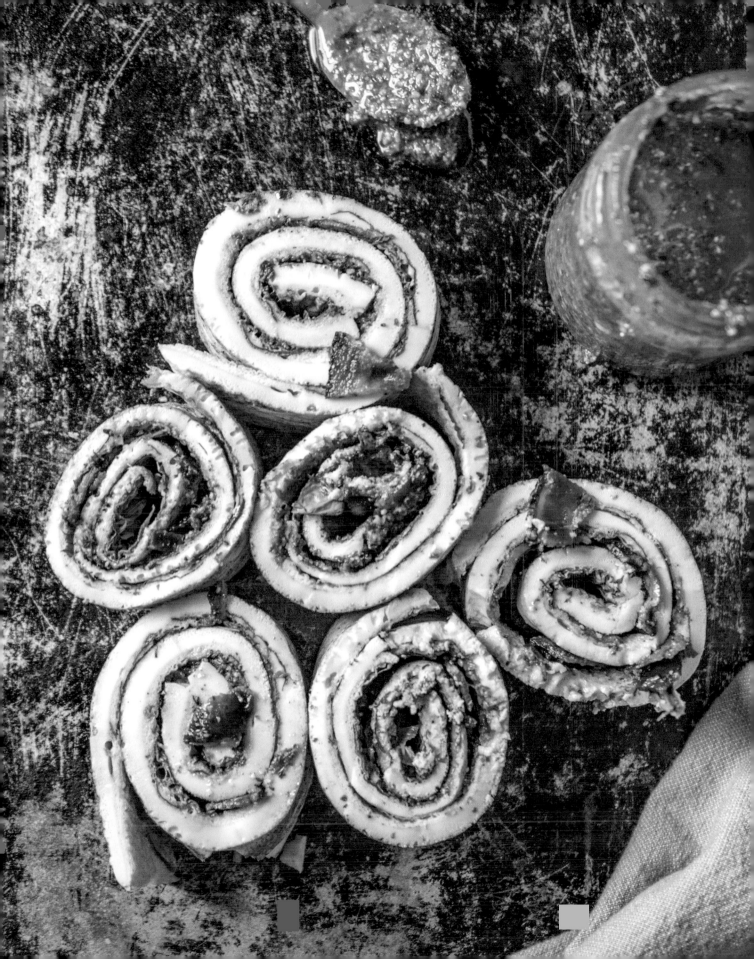

persian herb frittata

This is a clean-out-the-fridge kind of recipe. Personally, I think the parsley is a must, but the rest of the herbs can be swapped out for what you have on hand, even some wilting kale or spinach. My favorite thing about this recipe, other than its deliciousness, is that it delivers some awesome nutrients. Parsley usually isn't consumed in such large doses, but this famous garnish is a powerful little herb with antioxidant, anti-inflammatory, antifungal, and antibacterial properties. Feeling bloated or have some swelling that's lingering? Make one of these bad boys, feast, and feel better. Serve with a generous dollop of Homemade Mayo (page 82)!

Makes one 8-inch frittata (4 servings)
PREP TIME: 10 minutes   COOK TIME: 20 minutes

4 tablespoons avocado oil or olive oil, divided

1 large onion, diced

2 cloves garlic, minced

1 green onion, white part only, minced

6 large eggs

1 teaspoon baking powder (see Note)

1 teaspoon dried dill weed

1 teaspoon turmeric powder

½ teaspoon fine Himalayan salt

½ teaspoon ginger powder

1 cup minced fresh cilantro

1 cup minced fresh parsley

½ cup minced fresh basil

○ Heat an 8-inch skillet over medium or medium-low heat. If your stove runs hot, adjust the temperature; you don't want the bottom of the frittata to burn. When the skillet is hot, pour in 2 tablespoons of the avocado oil. Add the onions, garlic, and green onions and cook, stirring often, for 8 minutes, or until tender, translucent, and aromatic. Remove the onion mix from the skillet and set aside to cool. Put the skillet back on the stove over medium heat.

○ In a large bowl, whisk together the eggs, baking powder, seasonings, and fresh herbs. Add the cooled onion mix.

○ Turn on the broiler and set an oven rack just below it.

○ Drizzle the remaining 2 tablespoons of avocado oil into the skillet and pour in the egg mixture. Cover with a tight-fitting lid. Cook for 7 minutes, or until the edges of the frittata begin to separate from the skillet and the frittata is almost set but still wet in the center. Then remove the lid and place the skillet under the broiler for 1 to 2 minutes. Watch it carefully; you only need to broil it until the center is just set.

○ Remove the frittata from the oven. Run a spatula around the edge of the frittata and carefully shake it out of the skillet and onto a cutting board. Cut into four pieces, serve, and share.

○ Once the frittata has cooled to room temperature, you can store it in an airtight container in the refrigerator for up to 5 days. Enjoy the leftovers cold or gently warmed up in a 300°F oven for 5 minutes.

CHEF'S NOTE: Finding quality baking powder that is corn-free and aluminum-free can be impossible. I make my own by sifting together equal parts tapioca starch, baking soda, and cream of tartar. Store in a jar in a cool dry place for up to 30 days.

PER SERVING: Calories **265** · Fat **22g** · Total Carbohydrate **8g** · Dietary Fiber **2g** · Protein **11g**

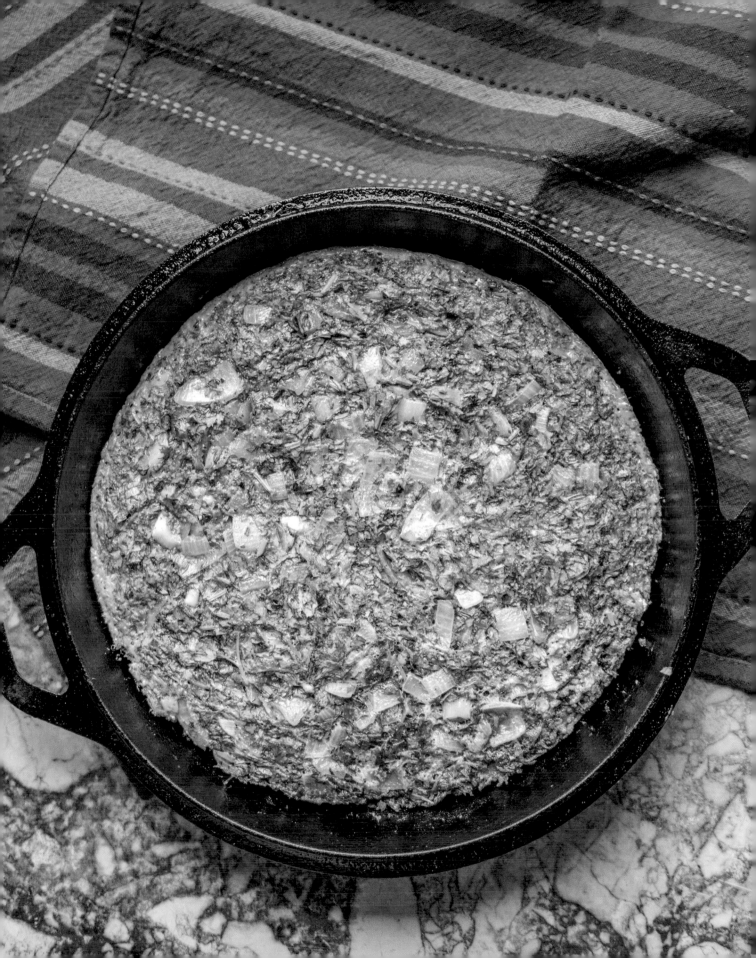

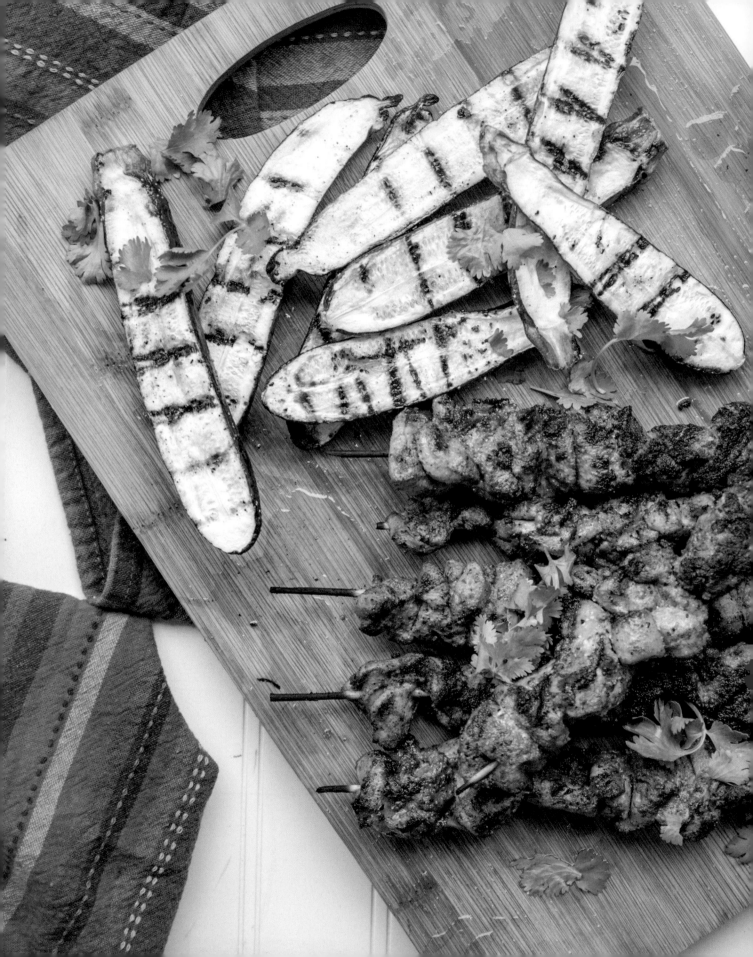

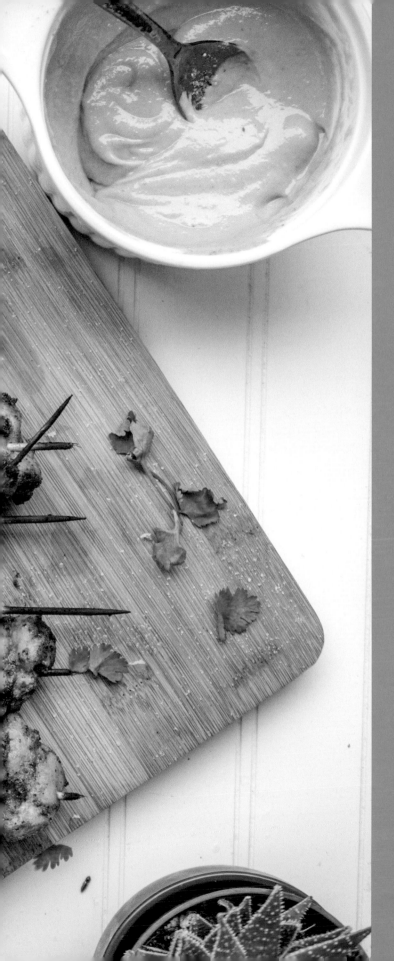

POULTRY

Growing up, I was a strictly white-meat girl. Oh, how I was missing out! There's so much more, from whole birds to crispy cutlets to my current favorite, boneless, skinless chicken thighs. This section gives you all the reasons to enjoy this versatile, reasonably priced protein. Bland chicken is a thing of the past—these recipes will have you praising poultry!

sheet pan dinner: pad thai

While I have a fierce zeal for igniting a passion for cooking in other people, I'm also a realist. Sometimes we just need to get dinner on the table in a hurry! But fast doesn't have to mean boring, and this meal is proof. Chicken cutlets marinated in a thick, seedy sauce that bakes up almost breaded and served over crispy rainbow slaw, this hands-off oven meal goes from prep to table in forty minutes. All your favorite flavors of pad Thai over noodle-like veggies! Double the amount of chicken and do some meal prep while you're at it.

1 pound boneless, skinless chicken breasts

2 tablespoons coconut aminos

2 tablespoons Dijon mustard

2 tablespoons sunflower seed butter

2 teaspoons ginger powder

2 teaspoons fine Himalayan salt, divided

2 tablespoons unsweetened shredded coconut

4 cups rainbow slaw (see Note, page 172)

3 tablespoons avocado oil or olive oil

1 teaspoon garlic powder

SUBSTITUTIONS: If you don't have rainbow slaw or can't find it at your store, bags of coleslaw mix work just fine for this, too. And you can leave out the shredded coconut if you don't like it!

To make this AIP-compliant, use coconut butter in place of the sunflower seed butter and omit the mustard from the marinade.

Makes 4 servings
PREP TIME: 5 minutes   COOK TIME: 40 minutes

○ Preheat the oven to 400°F.

○ Cut each chicken breast into two thin cutlets: Lay the chicken breast flat on a cutting board, place one hand flat on top of it, and gently press down. Then, run the knife straight through the middle horizontally. Be careful not to cut your fingers.

○ Place the coconut aminos, mustard, sunflower seed butter, ginger powder, and 1 teaspoon of the salt in a large bowl. Add the chicken and mix until well combined and the chicken is well coated.

○ Lay the cutlets flat on a sheet pan without overlapping. Sprinkle with the shredded coconut. Put the sheet pan on the middle rack in the oven and cook for 20 minutes.

○ Spread the rainbow slaw evenly on a second sheet pan. Drizzle the avocado oil over it and sprinkle with the remaining teaspoon of salt. Toss to combine and spread evenly over the sheet pan again.

○ When the chicken has been in the oven for 20 minutes, add the second sheet pan to the oven on the bottom rack. Roast for another 10 to 15 minutes. The chicken will be golden with toasty bits and the rainbow slaw will be tender.

○ Remove the chicken from the oven and turn on the broiler. Move the veggies to the middle rack and toast under the broiler for 1 to 3 minutes. Remove the veggies from the oven and serve alongside the chicken. Enjoy!

○ Store leftovers in an airtight container in the fridge for up to 4 days. To reheat, bake in a preheated 350°F oven for 5 to 8 minutes.

PER SERVING: Calories **349** · Fat **18.5g** · Total Carbohydrate **16.1g** · Dietary Fiber **3.4g** · Protein **32g**

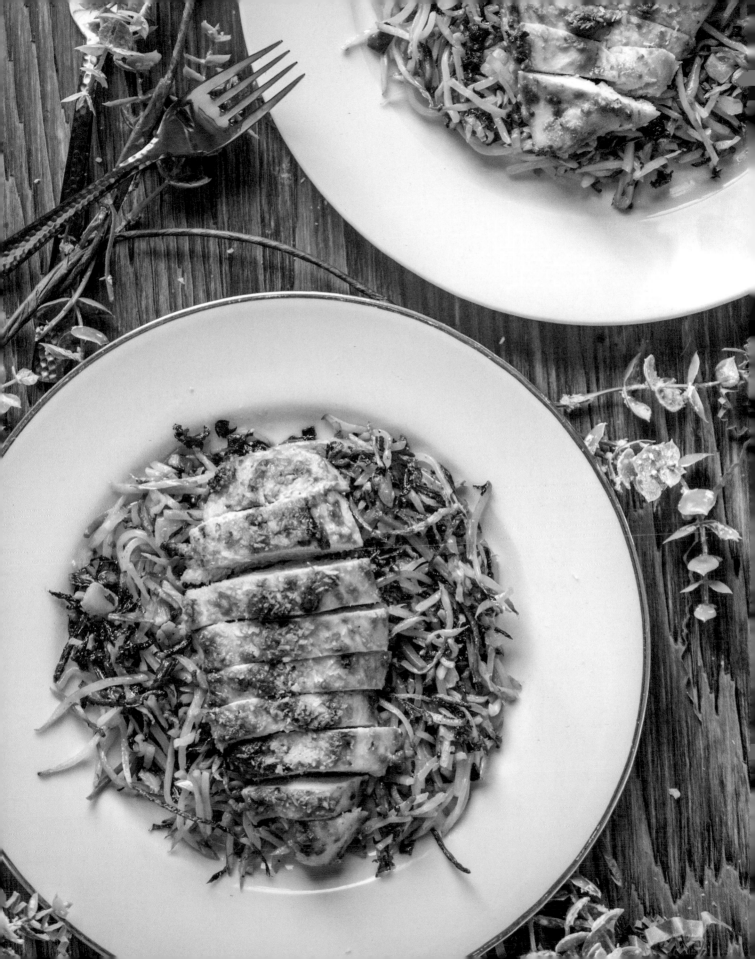

spinach alfredo chicken bake

This is the kind of family meal that is so effortless, it's almost not fair how delicious it is. It's made with the Cauliflower Alfredo on page 86, chicken breasts, and plenty of baby spinach. Pop this bad boy in the oven and be a dinner hero! It's great on its own or served over zoodles.

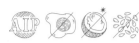

2 pounds boneless, skinless chicken breasts

1 tablespoon avocado oil

1 teaspoon fine Himalayan salt

½ teaspoon ground black pepper

3 cloves garlic, sliced

4 cups baby spinach

2 cups Cauliflower Alfredo (page 86)

Chopped fresh parsley or 2 tablespoons nutritional yeast, for garnish

Makes 6 servings
PREP TIME: 5 minutes   COOK TIME: 45 minutes

◦ Preheat the oven to 400°F.

◦ Cut each chicken breast into two thin cutlets: Lay the chicken breast flat on a cutting board, place one hand flat on top of it, and gently press down. Then, run the knife straight through the middle horizontally. Be careful not to cut your fingers.

◦ Drizzle half of the avocado oil on the bottom of a 9 by 13-inch casserole dish, then place the chicken cutlets in one flat layer on the bottom and drizzle with the remaining oil. Sprinkle evenly with the salt and pepper. Distribute the garlic evenly over the chicken cutlets.

◦ Place the casserole dish in the oven and bake for 15 minutes, or until the chicken is white all the way through and the garlic slices are golden.

◦ Add the spinach on top of the chicken and pour the Alfredo sauce over everything. Use a spatula to spread it out evenly.

◦ Place the casserole dish back in the oven and bake for 30 minutes. The Alfredo will be slightly browned and bubbling.

◦ Place the chicken cutlets on serving plates and spoon copious amounts of bubbling sauce and wilted spinach over them. Garnish with fresh parsley or nutritional yeast.

◦ Store leftovers in an airtight container in the fridge for up to 5 days. Heat by microwaving on high for 2 minutes, or heat the chicken in the Alfredo sauce in a skillet over medium heat for 10 minutes.

VARIATIONS: This template works with any sauce. Try it with Cheesy Yellow Sauce (page 68) or Roasted Beet Marinara (page 78)!

PER SERVING: Calories **367** · Fat **22.2g** · Total Carbohydrate **10.2g** · Dietary Fiber **2.8g** · Protein **35g**

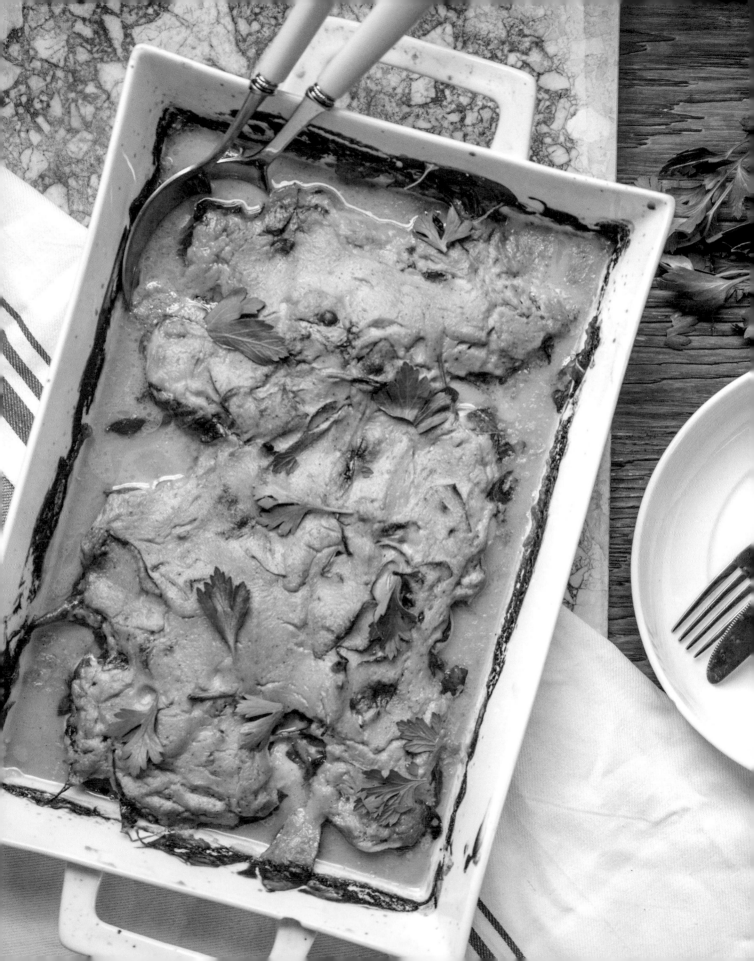

crispy chicken milanese with hollandaise

This dish is inspired by the milanesa my stepfather loves so much. Fernando is from Argentina, and when he joined our family, so did the many delicious foods from his country. Aside from chimichurri (see page 80), this dish of thin cuts of meat, breaded and fried to crispy perfection, is my favorite. Chicken cutlets work best. Dredged in coconut flour and lightly seasoned, these crispy cutlets are the perfect pairing for this Julia Child–worthy hollandaise. I love this rich hollandaise, and it turns out exceptionally well with the ghee for a lactose-free sauce. Serve it all over shaved zucchini ribbons, made easily with a vegetable peeler, and you have a restaurant-worthy meal the whole family will love!

FOR THE CHICKEN:

2 boneless, skinless chicken breasts (about 1 pound)

1 teaspoon fine Himalayan salt

½ cup coconut flour

3 large egg whites

½ cup avocado oil or coconut oil, divided, for frying

FOR THE HOLLANDAISE:

3 large egg yolks (separated from the egg whites above)

Juice of 1 lemon

⅛ teaspoon fine Himalayan salt

1 cup ghee, unsalted butter, or duck fat, divided

½ teaspoon ground black pepper

2 medium zucchini

Chopped fresh parsley, for garnish

Makes 4 servings
PREP TIME: 15 minutes   COOK TIME: 15 minutes

∘ Put the chicken breasts on a cutting board. Place one hand flat on top of a breast and, with a sharp knife, cut into the side horizontally. Open the breast like a book. Repeat with the other chicken breast.

∘ Place a piece of plastic wrap over the chicken breasts and gently pound them with the smooth side of a mallet until they are about ¼ inch thick. Cut the chicken into eight equal-sized pieces and sprinkle with the salt.

∘ Heat an 8- or 10-inch skillet over medium heat.

∘ Put the coconut flour in a shallow bowl. Crack the eggs into a medium-sized bowl. Carefully remove the egg yolks and set them aside for the hollandaise. Whisk the egg whites.

∘ When the skillet is hot, pour ¼ cup of the avocado oil into the skillet.

∘ Dredge one chicken piece in the coconut flour, then dip it in the egg whites and then back in the coconut flour. Shake off any excess flour and place the piece in the skillet. Repeat with three more pieces of chicken. Cook for 6 to 8 minutes, until the chicken is crispy and golden brown, turning over halfway through. Remove the chicken from the skillet and set on a cooling rack to drain.

∘ Add the remaining ¼ cup of avocado oil to the skillet and cook the last four pieces of chicken in the same fashion.

∘ While the last of the chicken cooks, make the hollandaise: Whisk the egg yolks in a small saucepan for 1 minute, or until they become light yellow. Add the lemon juice, salt, and 1 tablespoon of the ghee.

∘ Heat the remaining ghee in the microwave for 30 to 40 seconds, until liquid and warm.

PER SERVING (without the hollandaise): Calories **312** · Fat **18.2g** · Total Carbohydrate **10.8g** · Dietary Fiber **10g** · Protein **27.8g**

PER 2 TABLESPOONS of hollandaise: Calories **112** · Fat **11.8g** · Total Carbohydrate **0.7g** · Dietary Fiber **0g** · Protein **0.5g**

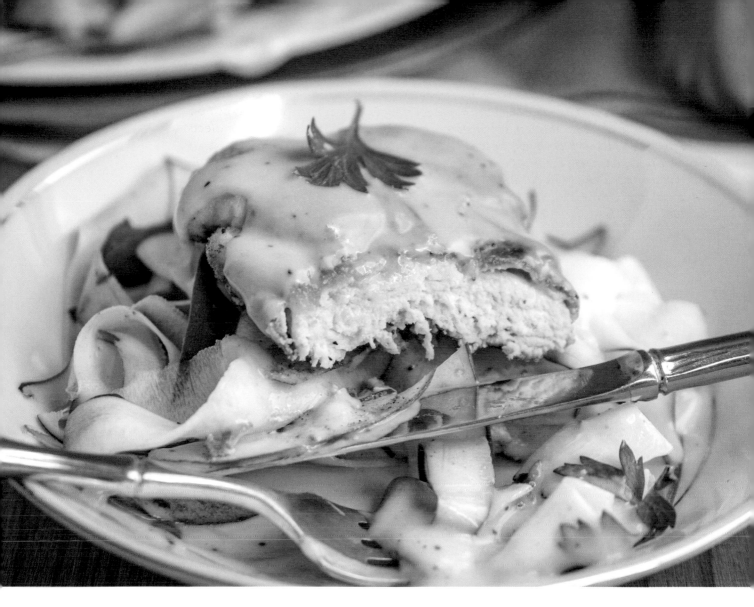

VARIATIONS: You can make this dish with veal or beef cutlets, too!

CHEF'S NOTE: If you have leftover hollandaise, as I always do, save it for Eggs Benny (page 176).

SUBSTITUTION: If you can't tolerate ghee, don't be afraid to use duck fat to make hollandaise—it turns out rich and delicious!

◦ Set the saucepan over medium-low heat. (I like to put it on the burner next to the chicken so I can flip it when I need to.) Keep whisking the hollandaise at a moderate speed until the sauce thickens and you can see the bottom of the pot in streaks between stirs.

◦ Lower the heat to low. Add the melted ghee a tablespoon at a time, mixing it in completely before adding in the next spoonful, until thick and creamy. Stir in the pepper. Remove from the heat.

◦ By now the last of the chicken should be done. Remove the chicken pieces from the skillet and set them on the cooling rack.

◦ With a vegetable peeler, shave the zucchini into ribbons. Divide the ribbons among four plates.

◦ Place two pieces of chicken on each plate and spoon hollandaise liberally over them. Garnish with fresh parsley.

orange chicken skewers

I made these skewers for an impromptu barbecue with some friends from Jack's school. The minute we all bit into them, I knew this recipe was a keeper. They're bursting with flavor, tangy and sweet, with perfectly charred bits. The orange and cumin–marinated skewers only need a drop of sweetness to really set off the flavor. I like to marinate them overnight, but two hours will do. Throw some romaine hearts or sliced zucchini on the grill with these skewers for a quick dinner that won't wreck your kitchen.

  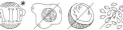

2 pounds boneless, skinless chicken thighs (about 8 thighs)

1 navel orange, halved

1 lemon, halved

1 large onion, quartered

3 tablespoons coconut aminos or 20 drops liquid stevia

1 tablespoon olive oil or avocado oil

2 teaspoons fine Himalayan salt

2 teaspoons ground cumin

1 teaspoon Dijon mustard

1 teaspoon dried thyme leaves

1 teaspoon ground black pepper

Special equipment:

Bamboo, wooden, or metal skewers

Makes 4 skewers (1 per serving)
PREP TIME: 20 minutes, plus 2 hours to marinate   COOK TIME: 20 minutes

○ Cut the chicken thighs in half lengthwise and put them in a large bowl. Squeeze the orange halves into the bowl and throw them in; do the same thing with the lemon halves. Add the rest of the ingredients and mix thoroughly. Cover the bowl with plastic wrap and place it in the refrigerator to marinate for at least 2 hours.

○ Set the chicken out about 30 minutes before you thread it on the skewers; otherwise it will be uncomfortably cold to handle. If you're using bamboo or wooden skewers, use this time to soak the skewers in water.

○ Give the chicken mix a toss and remove the orange and lemon halves. Thread four pieces of chicken and one piece of onion onto each skewer.

○ Spray or brush the grill with cooking fat. Heat the grill to medium-high heat (between 350°F and 400°F). Place the skewers on the hottest part of the grill. Cook for 20 minutes, turning every 5 minutes.

○ Remove the skewers from the grill and serve right away! If you're making extra, let the skewers cool to room temperature, use a fork to remove the pieces from the skewers, and store them in an airtight container for up to 5 days in the refrigerator.

CHEF'S NOTE: I highly suggest doubling the recipe; these make fantastic leftovers. And they're great with anything. Use leftovers in Collard Chicken Wraps (page 204) or in Chicken Caesar Lettuce Cups (page 160) to spice things up a bit. Serve with grilled veggies, Spinach Salad (page 348), or Curried Vegetable Salad (page 338)!

SUBSTITUTIONS: Omit the cumin, mustard, and pepper to make these AIP-compliant. Add 1 teaspoon ginger powder instead. If you don't have stevia or coconut aminos, you can use 2 tablespoons to ¼ cup of your preferred sweetener in this recipe.

PER SERVING: Calories **456** · Fat **23.7g** · Total Carbohydrate **5.1g** · Dietary Fiber **1.5g** · Protein **54.3g**

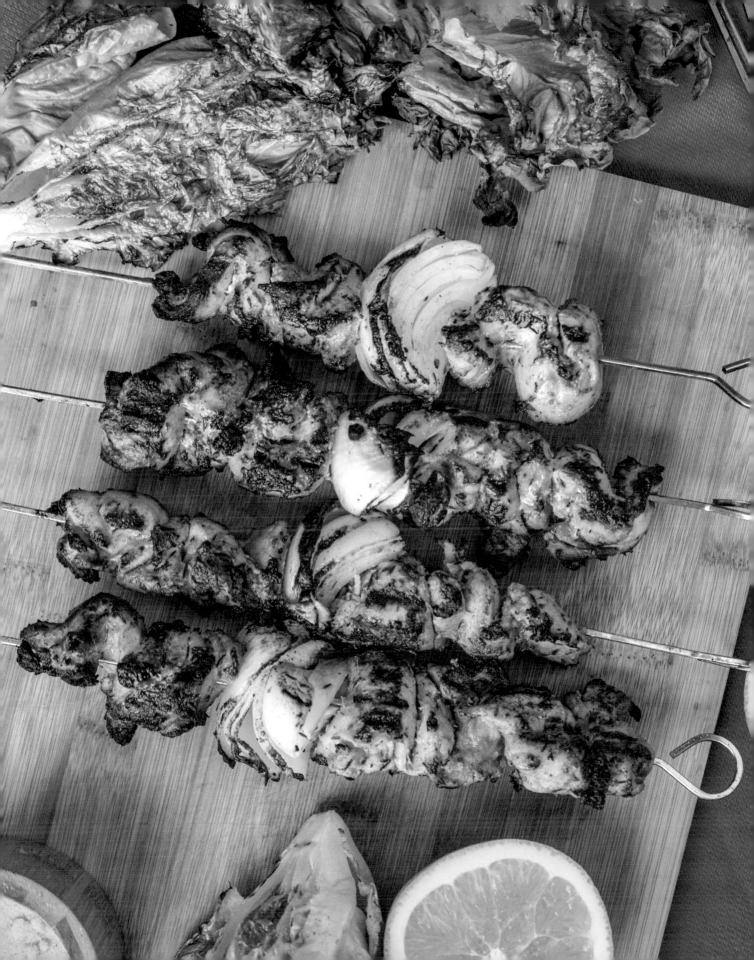

fricase de pollo

This is a soupy sauté of chicken and vegetables that simmers in a fragrant sauce until the encuentros de pollo (chicken thighs) are tender and the whole neighborhood has gathered at your door to see where the aroma is coming from. I wasn't sure how to tackle this staple from my childhood without tomatoes (a nightshade), but then I saw the recipe for ropa vieja by Aleana Haber of Grazed and Enthused, and it all clicked for me. The basis of flavor for this, and for all Cuban recipes, is sofrito, the sautéed aromatics that breathe life into dishes. Its smell will always remind me of home, and this anti-inflammatory rendition of a Cuban classic would make Mama proud. This is perfect over cauliflower rice or served with Street Taco Tortillas (page 332).

 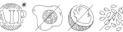

Makes 3 servings
PREP TIME: 10 minutes   COOK TIME: 35 minutes

4 tablespoons avocado oil, ghee, or lard, divided

2 large carrots, diced

4 ribs celery, diced

1 large onion, diced

2 cloves garlic, minced

2 bay leaves

2 pounds boneless, skinless chicken thighs, cut into 3-inch strips

2 teaspoons fine Himalayan salt

1 teaspoon ground black pepper

1 teaspoon ground cumin

2 sprigs fresh oregano

½ cup bone broth (page 100)

2 green onions, sliced, for garnish

○ Heat 2 tablespoons of the avocado oil in a large pot or skillet over medium heat. Add the carrots, celery, onions, garlic, and bay leaves. Sauté over medium heat for 8 to 10 minutes, until the sofrito is very fragrant and the onions have become tender and translucent.

○ Remove the sofrito from the pot and set aside. Heat the remaining 2 tablespoons of avocado oil in the pot and add the chicken strips. Add the salt, pepper, cumin, and oregano sprigs. Stir to combine. Cook until the chicken is browned, about 10 minutes, turning the pieces occasionally.

○ While the chicken browns, place half of the sofrito in a blender with the broth and blend until smooth. Once the chicken is browned, add the rest of the sofrito and the sauce you just blended back to the pot.

○ Stir well, cover the pot with a tight-fitting lid, and simmer for 10 minutes. You will hear bubbling and sizzling from the pot. Remove the lid; if the mixture has a lot of liquid, reduce over high heat for 5 minutes, stirring occasionally. If not, stir well, garnish with green onions, and serve hot!

○ Store leftovers in an airtight container in the fridge for up to 5 days. Sauté over medium heat for 5 minutes to reheat.

TIME-SAVING TIP: After you brown the chicken and blend half of the sofrito, add everything to a pressure cooker or slow cooker and set it to pressure cook on medium pressure for 20 minutes or slow cook on low for 4 hours. Add frozen riced cauliflower to the pot and make it a super-easy one-pot meal!

SUBSTITUTIONS: To make this dish AIP-compliant, omit the cumin and pepper. Use 1 teaspoon turmeric powder and a pinch of celery salt instead.

PER SERVING: Calories **408** · Fat **25.3g** · Total Carbohydrate **7.7g** · Dietary Fiber **4.2g** · Protein **32.7g**

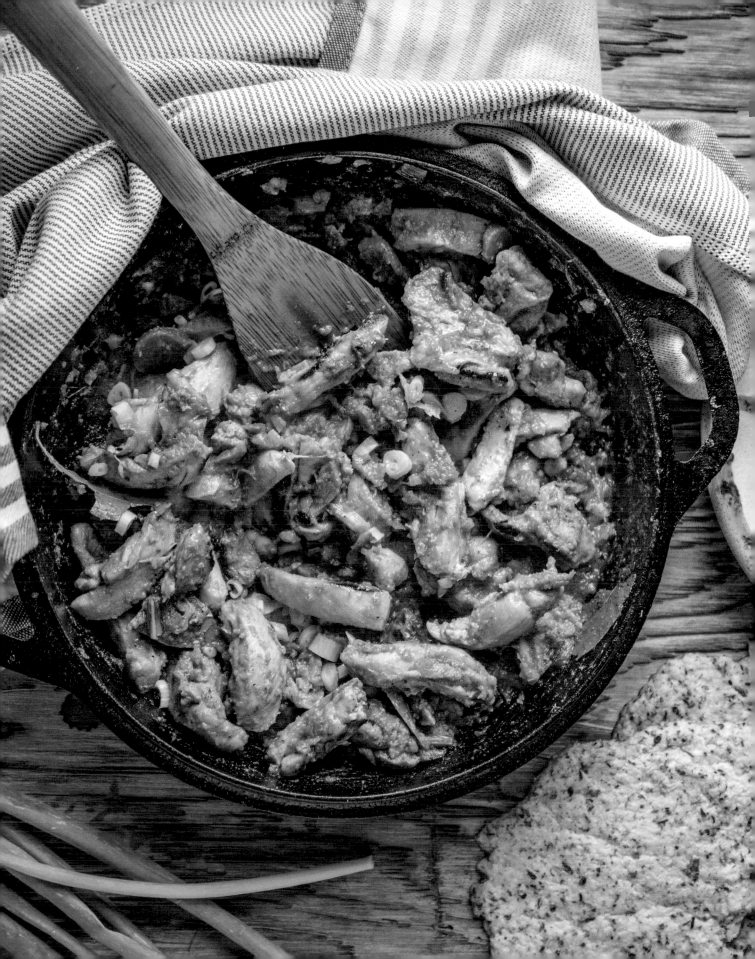

cristina's roast chicken

Everyone needs a solid roast chicken recipe in their arsenal. It's a kitchen staple, the one you use when chickens are on sale and you buy five to batch-cook for weeks of protein. The recipe you bust out when your mother-in-law is coming over and you want to assure her that you're feeding her offspring well. This recipe will always turn out a juicy bird that's bursting with flavor. It's different enough that you won't get tired of it yet easy enough to throw together on a whim. I like to spatchcock the whole chicken—split it in half—so it cooks faster and more of the skin gets crispy. A pair of kitchen shears makes short work of it, so there's no need to be intimidated. Serve with simply prepared vegetables, like steamed asparagus or green salad.

1 (4- to 5-pound) whole chicken

3 tablespoons coconut oil or ghee

2 teaspoons fine Himalayan salt

2 teaspoons ground black pepper

¼ cup minced fresh cilantro

2 tablespoons minced garlic

2 tablespoons peeled and minced fresh ginger

2 tablespoons minced lemongrass

Juice of 2 lemons

2 teaspoons sesame oil (optional)

1 tablespoon coconut aminos

1 tablespoon fish sauce

Makes 4 servings
PREP TIME: 10 minutes, plus 30 minutes to marinate   COOK TIME: 50 minutes

○ Preheat the oven to 375°F.

○ Place the chicken breast side down on a work surface. Hold it firmly with one hand and use kitchen shears to cut up one side of the spine, toward the neck. Then turn the chicken around and cut down the opposite side toward the cavity, trimming any excess skin hanging around the area. Remove the spine. Flip the chicken over and firmly press down on the breast to flatten the bird, cracking the breastbone.

○ Place the chicken breast side up in a large casserole dish. Rub the coconut oil all over the chicken, getting it in every crevice and under the breast skin. Sprinkle the salt and pepper all over.

○ Place the cilantro, garlic, ginger, lemongrass, lemon juice, sesame oil (if using), coconut aminos, and fish sauce in a small bowl. Mix well, then rub this mixture all over the chicken. Turn the chicken over and rub the mixture inside the cavity as well. Leave the chicken breast side down, cover, and allow to marinate for 30 minutes at room temperature.

○ When ready to roast, place the chicken breast side up on a sheet pan or, if it's oven-safe, in the same casserole dish where it marinated. Scrape all of the marinade out of the container and spoon it over the chicken. Roast on the oven's middle rack for 45 minutes, or until juice runs clear from the chicken when you wiggle the leg. Turn on the broiler and broil for 5 minutes from the middle rack. Remove the chicken from the oven and let it rest for 5 minutes before cutting into it.

○ To store leftovers, let the chicken cool to room temperature, then pull all the meat and skin off of the bones and store in an airtight container in the fridge for up to 5 days. Remember to pour off any pan sauce into the container, too!

TIME-SAVING TIP: Prep and marinate the chicken a day in advance; this will save you time and also result in a much more flavorful chicken. Remember to measure out all of the ingredients ahead of time—when handling chicken, it saves time and hand-washing. You don't want to grab a bottle of oil with "chicken hands," but if you have the oil in a small ramekin that you can wash later, it's not a big deal.

SUBSTITUTIONS: Omit the pepper and sesame oil to make this AIP-compliant. Double the fish sauce to amp up the flavor!

PER ¼-POUND SERVING: Calories **436** · Fat **32.7g** · Total Carbohydrate **3.5g** · Dietary Fiber **0.6g** · Protein **30.3g**

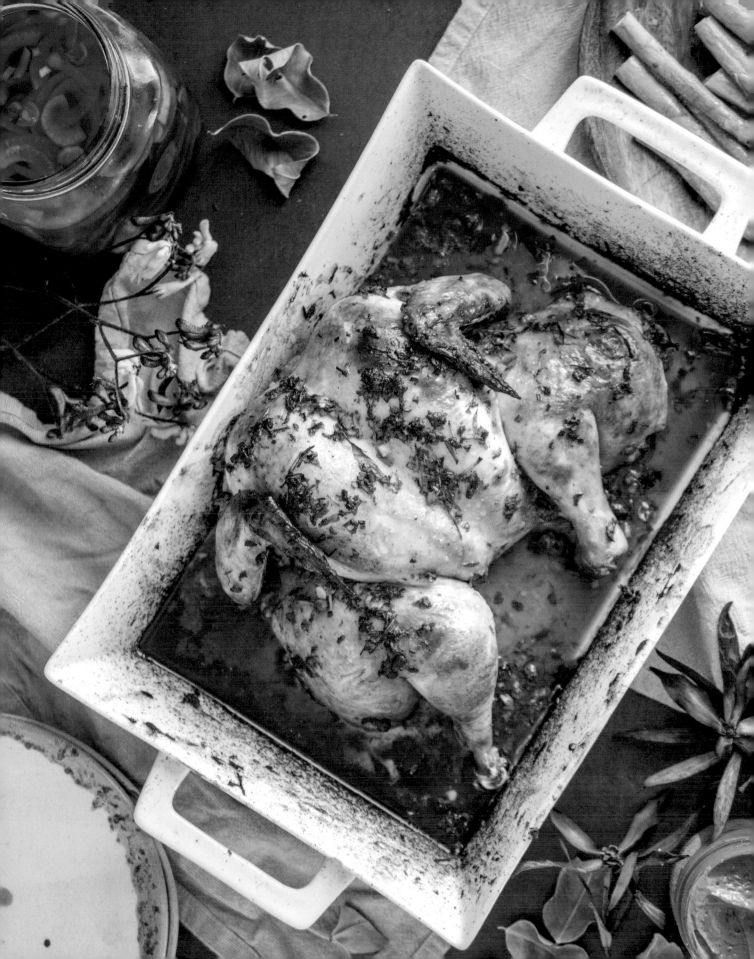

collard chicken wraps

Who doesn't love a good wrap? Blanched collard greens make exceptional low-carb wraps. You can prepare a bunch ahead of time and store them in the fridge layered in kitchen towels or paper towels. They are pliable, have a mild flavor, and hold quite a bit of nutrient goodness! I use leftover chicken, Beet Mayo (page 82), and a few fresh veggies in this ragtag recipe. This is the kind of thing I eat at home all the time. It's not fancy, but it sure is delicious, satisfying, and oh-so-nourishing! Bonus, you can eat it with your hands. Here's a pro tip: wrap it up in parchment paper and eat it burrito-style, peeling away paper as you go. This helps catch leaky sauce and keeps your hands clean. These are great for a quick no-cook meal or as appetizers to feed a crowd.

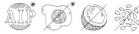

Makes 4 wraps (1 per serving)
PREP TIME: 10 minutes

3 cups water

4 large collard leaves

¼ cup Beet Mayo (page 82)

2 cups shredded cooked chicken

1 medium Hass avocado, peeled, pitted, and sliced

12 spears asparagus, trimmed

Radish sprouts or salad greens

○ Pour the water into a large skillet and bring to a boil. While it heats, trim the collard leaves: Fold them in half lengthwise so the back side of the leaf is on the outside. Use a paring knife to cut in a downward diagonal starting 2 inches above the bottom of the leaf. You want to trim down the vein and cut off the stem in one cut.

○ One at a time, place each leaf in the pot so that it floats on top of the water and cook for 30 seconds. It will turn bright green and pliable when ready. Use tongs to remove the leaf, place it on a kitchen towel, and put it in the fridge to quickly cool. Repeat with all of the leaves, layering them in the fridge until cool to the touch.

○ Lay the collard leaves on a flat surface. Smear 1 tablespoon of the beet mayo lengthwise down the center of each leaf. Make a small mound on the mayo with ½ cup shredded chicken per wrap. Add 2 or 3 slices of avocado and 3 asparagus spears per wrap. Finally, add a few radish sprouts or salad greens over the chicken.

VARIATIONS: I love using leftover roast chicken (page 202) for this, but any protein will do, from cold cuts to Vaca Frita (page 240). Get creative—use Pistou (page 74) or Toum (page 72), add bacon or scrambled eggs. The possibilities are endless!

○ One at a time, take each collard leaf and place it horizontally in front of you. Pick up the side closest to you and fold forward and over the chicken. Then fold in the sides and continue to roll forward to create a burrito-style wrap. Repeat with the rest of the greens.

○ Wrap in parchment paper with the same rolling technique and eat like burritos, or cut in half and serve family-style to share.

○ Do not store assembled wraps as they will fall apart. Rather, store the leaves layered in the paper towels and assemble the wraps when you're ready to eat one.

SUBSTITUTIONS: To make this recipe egg-free and AIP-compliant, replace the beet mayo with Chimichurri (page 80), Toum (page 72), or an AIP-compliant version of Tzatziki (page 98).

PER SERVING: Calories **499** · Fat **32.7g** · Total Carbohydrate **9.7g** · Dietary Fiber **5.1g** · Protein **40.7g**

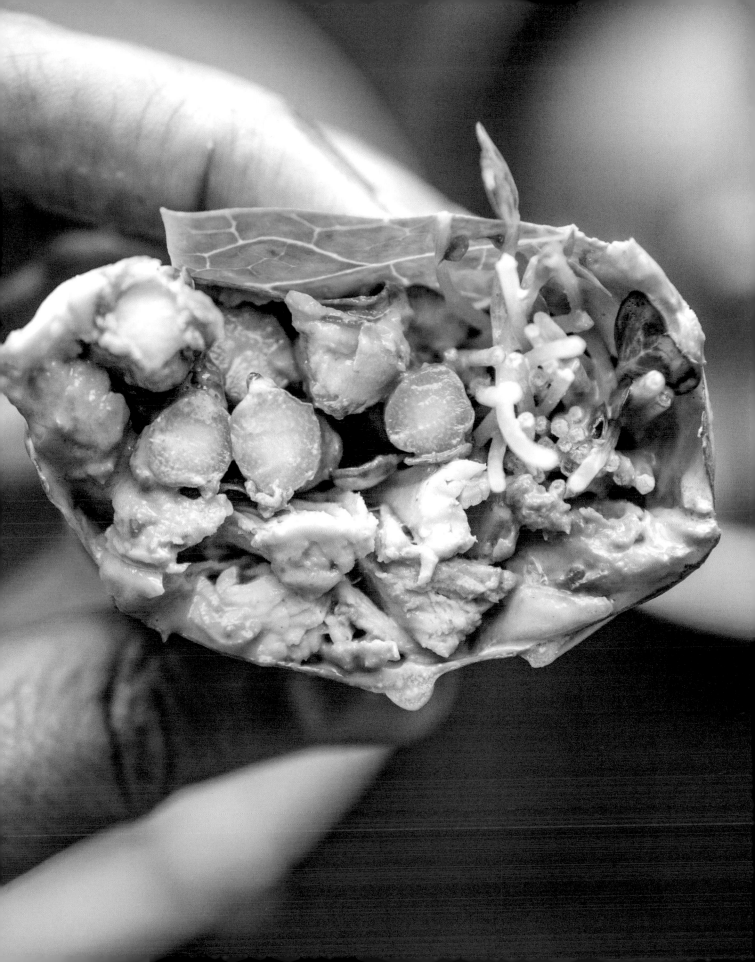

chicken kofta kebabs

Kofta, kafta, kefta… The name for these minced-meat kebabs varies greatly from region to region. I'm partial to the Lebanese variety with parsley, cumin, and yogurt, so we're going to call them kofta kebabs. This simple recipe is made by mixing ground chicken with minced onions, a variety of spices, herbs, and, traditionally, yogurt. If you have Coconut Yogurt (page 96), omit the coconut milk and vinegar from the recipe and use ¼ cup of yogurt instead! I wrote the recipe with the substitutions because I don't want a lack of yogurt to keep you from experiencing these.

2 pounds ground chicken

1 sweet onion, minced

3 tablespoons flaxseed meal

2 tablespoons coconut vinegar

2 tablespoons dried parsley

2 tablespoons full-fat coconut milk

2 teaspoons fine Himalayan salt

1 teaspoon granulated garlic

1 teaspoon ground black pepper

1 teaspoon ground cumin

1 teaspoon turmeric powder

Butter lettuce, for serving

Lemon wedges, for serving

Toum (page 72) or Herb Mayo (page 82), for serving (optional)

Special equipment:

Bamboo, wooden, or metal skewers

Makes 6 skewers (2 per serving)
PREP TIME: 10 minutes   COOK TIME: 20 minutes

○ If you are using bamboo or wooden skewers, soak them in water for 20 minutes. Turn on the broiler and move an oven rack to just under it.

○ Place all of the ingredients in a large bowl and mix until thoroughly combined. Shape the chicken mixture into six large sausages, thread a skewer through each one, and place on a sheet pan.

○ Broil for 15 minutes. Open the oven, use a spatula to carefully unstick each skewer from the pan, and turn them over. Broil for another 5 minutes. The skewers should be nicely browned all over. Remove from the oven and let cool for 5 minutes before serving.

○ Serve with butter lettuce leaves, lemon wedges, and toum or herb mayo for dipping or smearing. I like to remove the kofta from the skewer and eat it in a lettuce wrap with a smear of sauce.

○ Store leftovers in an airtight container in the fridge for up to 5 days. Reheat in a preheated 350°F oven for 10 minutes.

VARIATIONS: You can use any kind of ground protein for this recipe, from lamb to turkey, and it will turn out delicious.

SUBSTITUTIONS: To make this dish AIP-compliant, omit the flaxseed meal, pepper, and cumin and add 1 teaspoon ginger powder and 1 tablespoon coconut flour or unflavored grass-fed beef gelatin.

PER SERVING: Calories **556** · Fat **36.6g** · Total Carbohydrate **8.3g** · Dietary Fiber **5.6g** · Protein **56.8g**

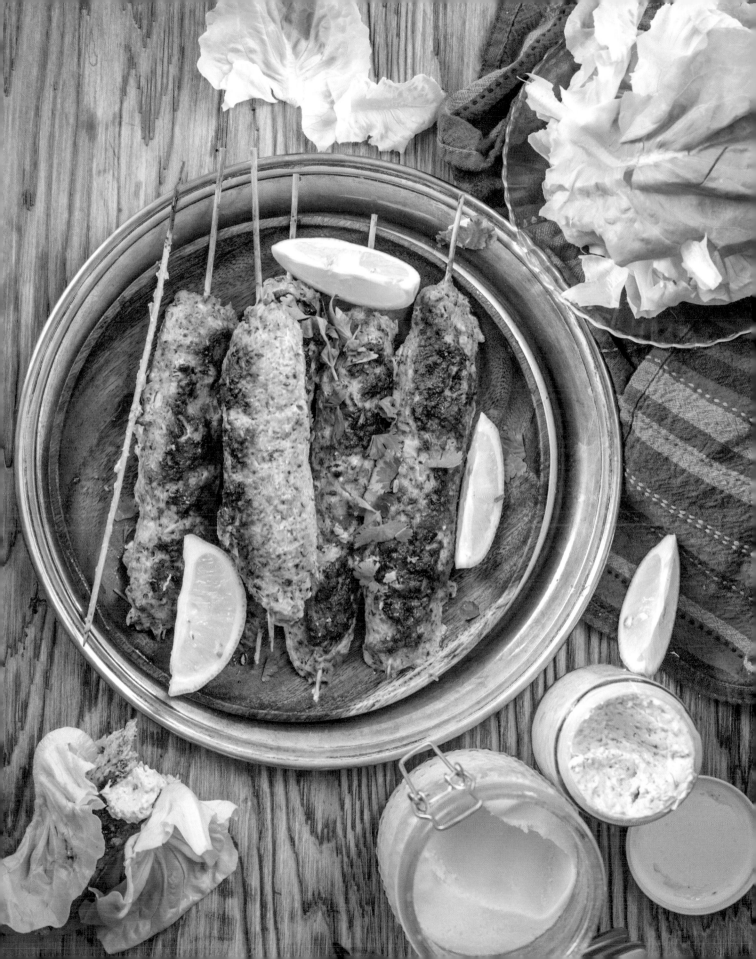

slow cooker arroz con pollo

When I was growing up, our house was always the family hub. My mother loved hosting, cooking, and entertaining, and all holidays and major events, like baptisms, graduations, and birthdays, were celebrated in our home. While all my aunts are talented cooks, each with her own signature dish and area of expertise, my mom always had her own flair, that magic touch. Arroz con pollo risotto-style was one of her specialties. This dish pays tribute to that recipe. Saucier than the classic arroz con pollo, this slow cooker rendition is hands-off and easy, using riced cauliflower and hemp seeds.

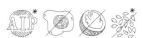

Makes 4 servings
PREP TIME: 10 minutes   COOK TIME: 2½ hours in the slow cooker

½ cup diced carrots

½ cup diced celery

½ cup diced onions

4 cloves garlic, minced

2 tablespoons avocado oil

1 pound boneless, skinless chicken thighs

2 teaspoons minced fresh oregano, or ½ teaspoon dried oregano

1½ teaspoons fine Himalayan salt

1½ teaspoons ground cumin

1 teaspoon ground black pepper

1 cup bone broth (page 100)

½ cup Roasted Beet Marinara (page 78)

2 tablespoons red wine vinegar or coconut vinegar

2 ounces salami, prosciutto, or cooked bacon

2 bay leaves

1½ cups riced cauliflower (see Note, page 140)

½ cup shelled hemp seeds (aka hemp hearts)

8 sprigs fresh cilantro, for garnish

2 green onions, sliced, for garnish

○ Place the carrots, celery, onions, and garlic in the slow cooker and drizzle with the avocado oil. Place the chicken thighs on the vegetables. Sprinkle with the oregano, salt, cumin, and pepper.

○ Add the broth, marinara, vinegar, salami, and bay leaves to the slow cooker. Cook on high for 2 hours.

○ After 2 hours, open the slow cooker and use two forks to shred the chicken into chunks, then mix in the riced cauliflower and hemp seeds. Cook for another 30 minutes on high. Alternatively, if your slow cooker has a simmer or sauté function, you can just bring it to a boil for 10 minutes, stirring occasionally. Serve garnished with fresh cilantro and green onions.

○ This is the kind of meal that tastes better the next day. Store leftovers in an airtight container in the fridge for up to a week. To reheat, bring to a simmer on the stovetop.

TIME-SAVING TIP: I grate my head of cauliflower over the pressure cooker so I have one less dish to wash. You can also use frozen riced cauliflower, of course. If you have a pressure cooker, you can make this by sautéing the carrots, celery, onions, and garlic first, then adding the rest of the ingredients and cooking on high for 30 minutes. Then shred the chicken, stir in the riced cauliflower, and boil for 10 minutes.

SUBSTITUTIONS: To make this dish AIP-compliant, omit the cumin, pepper, and hemp seeds and increase the fresh oregano by ½ teaspoon or the dried oregano by ¼ teaspoon. Also, increase the riced cauliflower by ½ cup. If you do not have roasted beet marinara, you may use ⅓ cup pumpkin puree with 2 tablespoons coconut vinegar instead.

PER SERVING: Calories **552** · Fat **36.9g** · Total Carbohydrate **10.4g** · Dietary Fiber **9.3g** · Protein **45.7g**

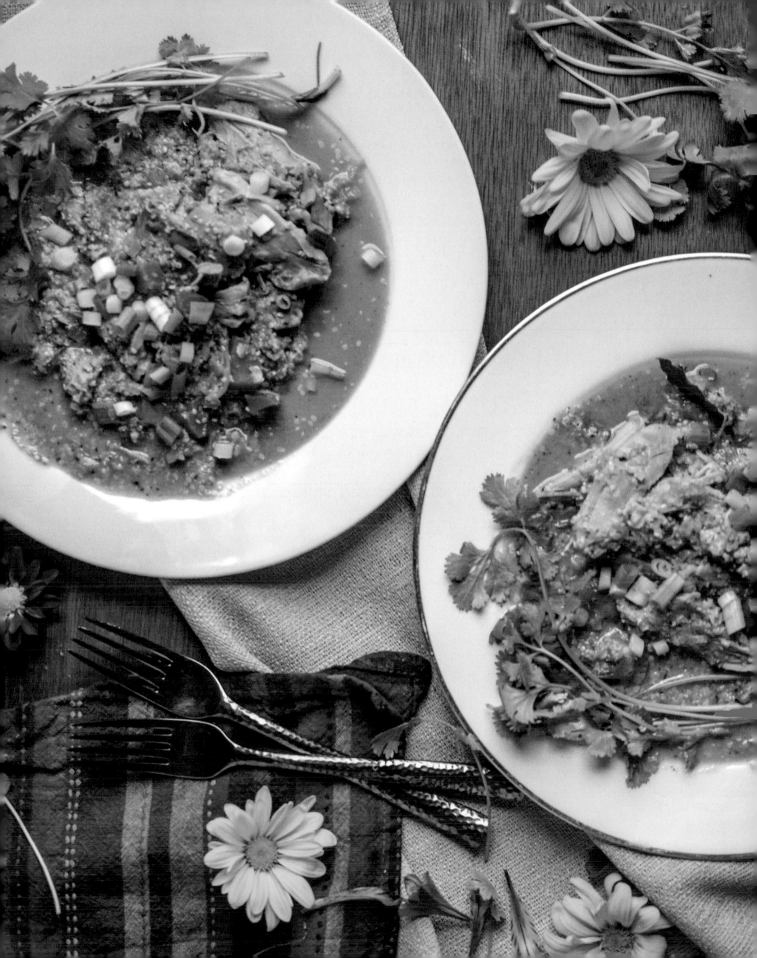

prosciutto-wrapped chicken tenders

This is the kind of meal that everyone loves. It's easy to make, it has a short ingredients list, and everyone will eat it. Yes, it's toddler approved. The mayo makes a delicious coat on the chicken and takes bland, dry chicken breast to another level. Any variation of the mayo recipe on page 82 will work, although I am partial to the one made with garlic confit. This entrée served up with simple salad makes for the ideal weeknight meal.

2 pounds boneless, skinless chicken breasts (about 4 breasts)

¼ cup Homemade Mayo (page 82)

1 teaspoon dried thyme leaves

1 teaspoon fine Himalayan salt

1 teaspoon ground black pepper

8 slices prosciutto di Parma (see Note)

Makes 16 tenders (4 per serving)
PREP TIME: 10 minutes   COOK TIME: 25 minutes

- Preheat the oven to 400°F.

- Cut each chicken breast into 2 thin cutlets: Lay the chicken breast flat on a cutting board, place one hand flat on top of it, and gently press down. Then run the knife straight through the middle horizontally. Be careful not to cut your fingers. Cut each cutlet into two tenders—you should now have sixteen tenders total.

- In a large bowl, combine the mayonnaise, thyme, salt, and pepper. Add the chicken tenders and toss to coat. Make sure that each tender is well coated.

- Tear each slice of prosciutto in half lengthwise; they should come apart quite easily. Wrap one long strip of prosciutto around one tender, starting at one end and working your way to the bottom. It doesn't have to be completely covered. Lay the tender on a sheet pan and repeat with the rest of the tenders and prosciutto.

- Bake for 25 minutes. Remove from the oven and let rest for 5 minutes before serving.

- Store leftovers in an airtight container in the fridge for up to 5 days. To reheat, bake, covered in foil, in a preheated 350°F oven for 10 minutes.

VARIATIONS: You can make these with bacon instead of prosciutto, or leave out the pork altogether.

SUBSTITUTIONS: To make this recipe AIP-compliant, substitute 2 tablespoons avocado oil and 1 tablespoon coconut vinegar for the mayo and omit the pepper.

CHEF'S NOTE: Make sure to read labels on the prosciutto. Real prosciutto contains only pork and salt; avoid brands with lactic starters, spices, or fillers.

PER SERVING: Calories **331** · Fat **24.5g** · Total Carbohydrate **0.5g** · Dietary Fiber **0g** · Protein **30.3g**

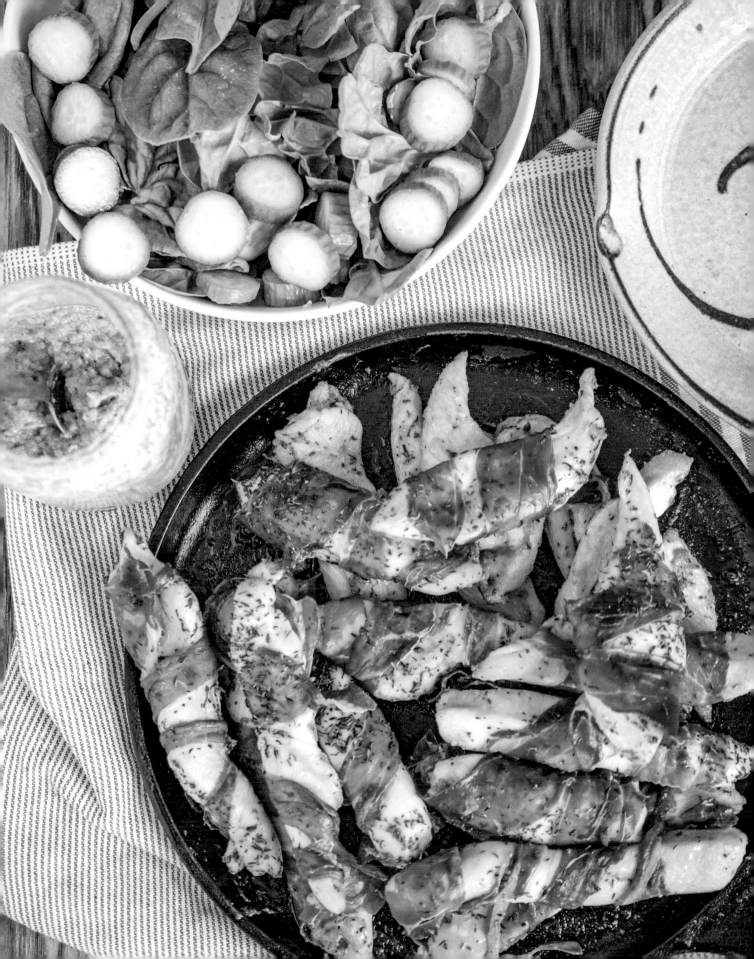

turkey cheeseburgers with crispy rainbow slaw

This fun twist on a classic cheeseburger is easy to make. These stuffed turkey burgers are juicy and filled with gooey melted Hard Cheese (page 70). You'll be amazed at how this dairy-free cheese melts and even toasts in the oven—truly a magic trick. With minimal hands-on time, it's a great option for make-ahead meals, weeknight dinners, or when you're feeding a crowd. Here's a tip: when you buy the rainbow slaw at the grocery store, buy a few bags. When roasted, it's more like crack slaw, and it will go so fast.

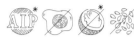

FOR THE CHEESEBURGERS:

2 pounds ground turkey (93% lean)

2 teaspoons dried dill weed

2 teaspoons fine Himalayan salt

1 teaspoon ground black pepper

¼ teaspoon Chinese five-spice powder

2 tablespoons avocado oil, divided

¾ cup grated Hard Cheese (page 70)

FOR THE CRISPY SLAW:

4 cups rainbow slaw (see Note, page 172)

2 tablespoons avocado oil

1 teaspoon garlic powder

½ teaspoon fine Himalayan salt

Salad greens or mashed or sliced avocado, for serving

SUBSTITUTIONS: To make this recipe AIP-compliant, replace the pepper and Chinese five-spice powder in the burgers with 1 teaspoon horseradish or ginger powder.

Makes 6 servings
PREP TIME: 10 minutes   COOK TIME: 30 minutes

○ Preheat the oven to 400°F.

○ Place the ground turkey, dill, salt, pepper, Chinese five-spice powder, and 1 tablespoon of the avocado oil in a large bowl. Mix until well combined.

○ Form the turkey mixture into six large, equal-sized balls. One at a time, flatten the meatball in your hand, place about 2 tablespoons of cheese in the center, and close the meat patty around the cheese, pinching together the meat and smoothing out the seam. Lightly oil your hand with the remaining avocado oil to coat the burger with oil as you shape it. Place it on a sheet pan. Repeat with the remaining meatballs. Cook the turkey burgers in the oven, on the middle rack, for 20 minutes.

○ While the burgers cook, make the crispy slaw: Place the rainbow slaw on a sheet pan, drizzle it with the avocado oil, and sprinkle it with the garlic powder and salt. Toss to combine, then spread the veggies evenly on the sheet pan.

○ At the 20-minute mark, put the sheet pan with the rainbow slaw in the oven on the bottom rack. Roast everything for 10 minutes.

○ Remove the slaw from the oven first; there should be toasted brown bits and colorful bits. Use a spatula to scrape and mix everything together.

○ Remove the turkey burgers from the oven. Some of the cheese may have seeped out of the burgers and browned on the sheet pan; that's okay. Use a spatula to scrape up that goodness and pile it over the burgers.

○ Serve the burgers on salad greens or mashed or sliced avocado, pile on the rainbow slaw, and dig in.

○ Store any leftovers in an airtight container in the fridge for up to 5 days. To reheat, bake in a preheated 350°F oven for 5 minutes or microwave on high for 1 to 2 minutes.

PER SERVING: Calories **353** · Fat **24g** · Total Carbohydrate **9g** · Dietary Fiber **3g** · Protein **37g**

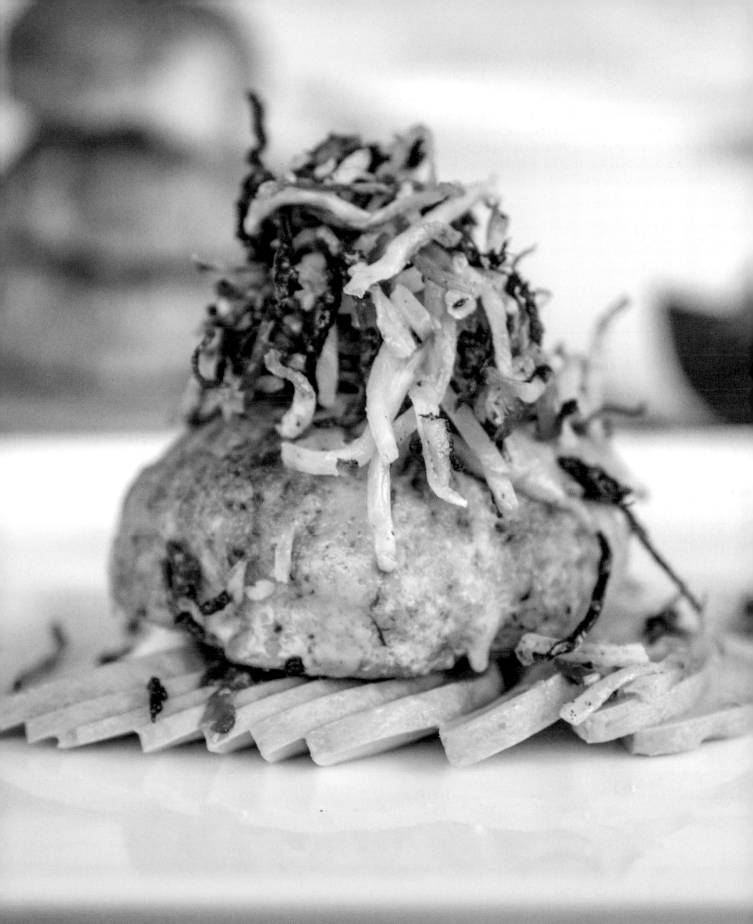

vietnamese crispy chicken

This recipe was inspired by a series of events, something that happens to me more often than not. I went to buy prepared food at a place I assumed would have suitable choices for me, but I found that everything was made with canola oil and/or had some ingredient that's on my not-worth-it list. So I headed home, slightly annoyed, and made my own food. Then something else that often happens to me occurred: my food turned out better than what I would have bought, and all was right in the world. Inspired by Michelle Tam's Cracklin' Chicken and that Vietnamese chicken that I had to pass up at the market, I bring you Vietnamese Crispy Chicken.

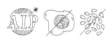

2 tablespoons grated lemongrass

2 teaspoons fine Himalayan salt

2 teaspoons ginger powder

2 teaspoons granulated garlic

2 teaspoons onion powder

1 teaspoon ground black pepper

2 tablespoons coconut aminos

1 tablespoon fish sauce

8 chicken thighs, bone-in, with skin

2 tablespoons avocado oil, divided

CHEF'S NOTE: If you're feeding a crowd, use a sharp knife to slice the chicken thighs into strips. These strips are also perfect on chopped salads or tacos.

SUBSTITUTIONS: To make this dish AIP-compliant, just leave out the pepper. You can double the ginger powder or lemongrass to boost the flavor. If you can't find lemongrass, use 2 tablespoons lemon or lime zest instead.

TIME-SAVING TIP: If you're squeamish about cutting out the bones or you want to save time, ask your butcher to do it for you.

Makes 8 chicken thighs (2 per serving)
PREP TIME: 20 minutes   COOK TIME: 40 minutes

○ Heat a large cast-iron skillet over medium heat.

○ In a small bowl, combine the lemongrass, salt, ginger powder, granulated garlic, onion powder, and pepper. In a separate small bowl or cup, combine the coconut aminos and fish sauce. Set both bowls aside.

○ Prepare a work area with a cutting board, a plate for the chicken, kitchen shears, and a few paper towels. With the shears, cut the bones out of the chicken thighs by cutting along one side of the bone, as close as possible, all the way to the bottom, and then clip the meat right above the tendon. Continue to cut along the other side of the bone and gently pull to release the bone from the thigh.

○ Pat the chicken dry on all sides with a paper towel. Hold one thigh skin side down on one hand and season with a generous pinch of the dry seasoning mix. Gently rub the seasoning in and place the chicken skin side up on the plate. Sprinkle the skin with more seasoning mix and pat it in. Repeat with the rest of the chicken thighs.

○ The skillet should be very hot now. Drizzle 1 tablespoon of the avocado oil into the skillet. Arrange as many chicken thighs as you can in the skillet, skin side down. Make sure they are not crowded or overlapping. Cover the skillet with a splatter guard and cook for 10 minutes. Then use tongs to flip the chicken thighs and pour in half of the coconut amino mix, drizzling a little to the base of each chicken thigh. Cover with the splatter guard again and cook for another 8 minutes. Remove the chicken thighs from the skillet and set on a cooling rack or plate lined with paper towels.

○ Drizzle the remaining tablespoon of the avocado oil into the skillet, add the next batch of chicken to the skillet, and repeat. Let rest for 5 minutes before serving.

○ Store leftovers in an airtight container in the fridge for up to 5 days. To reheat, bake in a preheated 350°F oven for 10 minutes.

PER SERVING: Calories **505** · Fat **38.1g** · Total Carbohydrate **5g** · Dietary Fiber **0.8g** · Protein **37g**

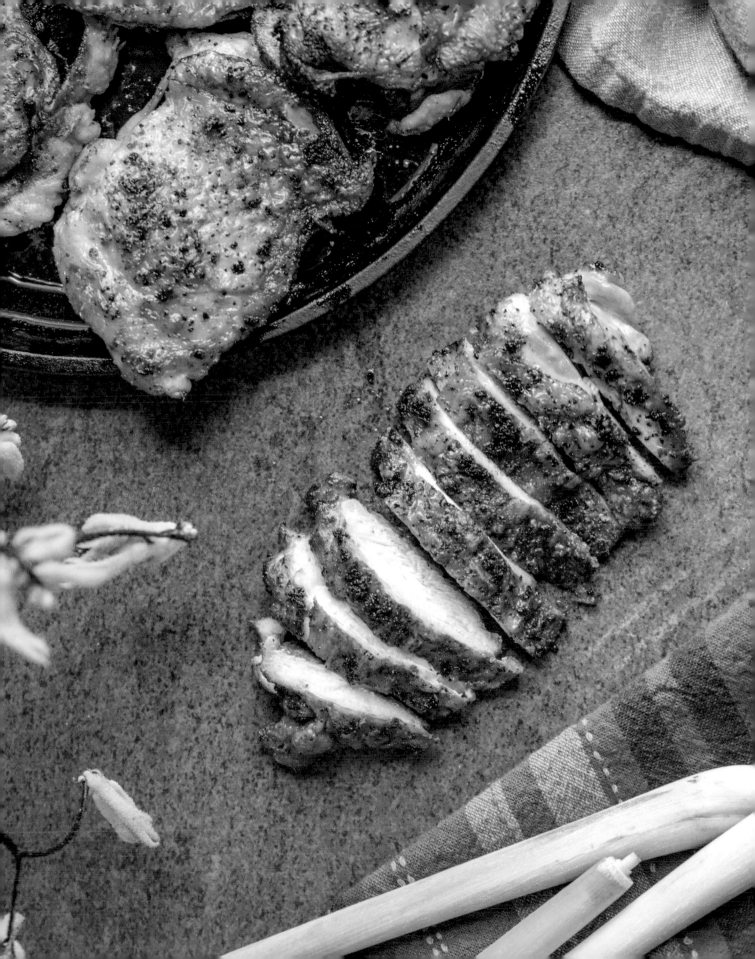

turkey falafel

This is one of those recipes that just popped into my head. There I was, ground turkey in a bowl in front of me, with the usual suspects lined up on the counter—lemon, garlic, herbs, and salt. Then I saw tahini in the fridge, and tahini always reminds me of hummus, which reminds me of chickpeas, which reminds me of falafel. In that moment, standing in my kitchen, fridge door handle in one hand and jar of tahini in the other, I could taste a falafel, just as if I had bitten into it. I decided I would use the tahini to give the turkey the slightly nutty flavor that chickpeas have; aside from the turkey and tahini, the rest would be strictly traditional falafel. I got a little creative with the coating, and hot damn, if these didn't fry up beautifully. So here they are: Paleo protein falafel! Serve them over greens with cucumber slices or Street Taco Tortillas (page 332) for a Mediterranean feast.

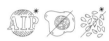

Makes 12 falafel (1 per serving)
PREP TIME: 15 minutes   COOK TIME: 20 minutes

FOR THE FALAFEL:

2 pounds ground turkey (93% lean)

½ cup minced fresh parsley

¼ cup olive oil

2 tablespoons grated lemon zest

Juice of ½ lemon

4 cloves garlic, minced

1 tablespoon tahini

2 teaspoons fine Himalayan salt

2 teaspoons ground cumin

1 teaspoon ground black pepper

⅓ cup coconut oil, or more if needed, for frying

FOR THE COATING:

⅓ cup coconut flour

⅓ cup shelled hemp seeds (aka hemp hearts)

2 teaspoons sesame seeds

1 teaspoon onion powder

2 cups Tzatziki (page 98), for serving

○ Make the falafel: Place all the ingredients for the falafel in a large bowl. Using your hands, mix together thoroughly; set aside.

○ Heat the coconut oil in a Dutch oven or large cast-iron skillet over medium heat until the oil reaches 375°F, or until it sizzles around a wooden spoon handle when it's inserted in the oil. The oil should be approximately 1 inch deep, so the falafel are halfway submerged when frying. (*Note:* As you add the falafel to the oil, the level will rise.)

○ While the oil is heating up, put the ingredients for the coating in a shallow bowl and mix until combined.

○ Shape the falafel mixture into 2-inch balls, then gently flatten them to make thick disks. Coat them in the flour mixture, then toss them between your hands to shake off the excess flour.

○ When the oil is hot, add five or six falafel and fry for 5 minutes, then use tongs or a slotted spoon to turn them over and fry for 5 minutes on the other side. Remove to a cooling rack or paper towel–lined dish. Repeat with the remaining falafel.

○ Spoon the tzatziki liberally over the falafel or serve it on the side. Store extras in an airtight container in the fridge for up to 1 week. Reheat in a preheated 350°F oven for 10 minutes; if you reheat them in the microwave, they will lose their crispiness.

SUBSTITUTIONS: To make these falafel AIP-compliant, omit the tahini, cumin, and pepper from the turkey mixture; add 1 teaspoon turmeric powder and ¼ cup minced fresh parsley or cilantro. In the coating, replace the hemp seeds and sesame seeds with unsweetened shredded coconut, or double the amount of coconut flour.

PER SERVING (without tzatziki): Calories **214** · Fat **14.5g** · Total Carbohydrate **5g** · Dietary Fiber **3.7g** · Protein **17.6g**

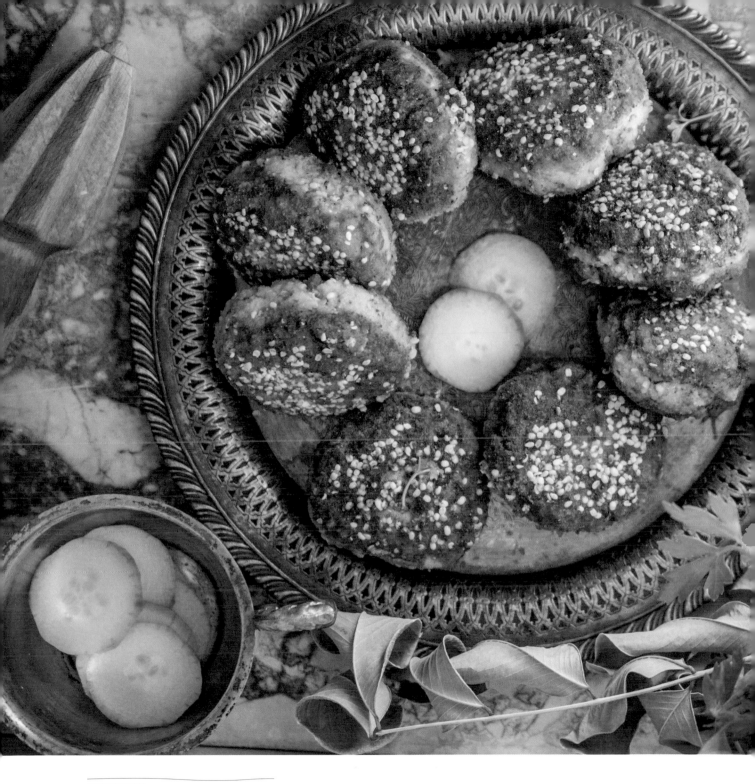

VARIATION: Add 2 tablespoons to ¼ cup minced fresh herbs to the falafel mix and swap out the lemon zest for orange zest to change up the flavor profile! Orange zest is quite delectable in this dish.

shredded jerk chicken

This is a lazy take on a barbecue classic, but what can I say, I love my pressure cooker. Not to worry, I've included stovetop and slow cooker instructions as well. The seasoning here has all the fun without any of the heat, yet this jerk marinade will definitely satisfy. Serve over Creamy Cilantro Rice (page 342) with a wedge of lemon for an epic island-inspired meal.

2 tablespoons avocado oil

2 tablespoons coconut aminos

Juice of 1 lemon

2 teaspoons liquid smoke

2 teaspoons garlic powder

2 teaspoons ground black pepper

1 rounded teaspoon fine Himalayan salt

1 teaspoon Chinese five-spice powder

2 pounds boneless, skinless chicken thighs

3 sprigs fresh thyme

CHEF'S NOTE: If you want to grill the marinated chicken, score the undersides of the thighs in a crisscross pattern before marinating. After marinating, heat a grill to high heat (450°F) and grill the thighs for 5 to 6 minutes per side.

Makes 6 servings
PREP TIME: 15 minutes, plus at least 20 minutes to marinate
COOK TIME: 40 minutes on the stovetop, 20 minutes in a pressure cooker, or 6 hours in a slow cooker

○ Make the marinade: Place the avocado oil, coconut aminos, lemon juice, liquid smoke, garlic powder, pepper, salt, and Chinese five-spice powder in a small bowl and whisk to combine.

○ Place the chicken in a large bowl and add the marinade and thyme sprigs. Mix well to combine. (You can also place the chicken, thyme, and marinade in a freezer bag and shake well to combine.) Cover and place in the fridge to marinate for at least 20 minutes or up to overnight.

○ **Stovetop instructions:** Heat a large pot over medium heat. When it's hot, add the marinated chicken thighs. Reserve the marinade. Brown the chicken, stirring occasionally, for 8 to 10 minutes. Once the chicken is browned, reduce the heat to low and stir in the reserved marinade. Cover with a tight-fitting lid and simmer for 20 to 30 minutes, until the chicken pulls apart easily. Check it halfway through cooking; if all of the liquid has evaporated, add a cup of bone broth (page 100) or water.

○ **Pressure cooker instructions:** Set a pressure cooker to sauté mode. Add the marinated chicken thighs. Reserve the marinade. Brown the chicken, stirring occasionally, for 8 to 10 minutes. Cancel the sauté function, stir in the reserved marinade, and close the lid. Cook on high pressure (or the appliance's poultry setting) for 10 minutes.

○ **Slow cooker instructions:** Heat a large pot over medium heat. When it's hot, add the marinated chicken thighs. Reserve the marinade. Brown the chicken, stirring occasionally, for 8 to 10 minutes. Place the browned chicken and all of the reserved marinade in a slow cooker and cook on high for 4 to 6 hours.

○ When the chicken is done, use two forks or a pair of tongs to shred it. Serve hot, with the cooking liquid spooned over it.

○ Store in an airtight container in the fridge for up to 5 days. To reheat, sauté over medium heat for 10 minutes.

PER SERVING: Calories **223** · Fat **10.8g** · Total Carbohydrate **1.4g** · Dietary Fiber **0.6g** · Protein **32.1g**

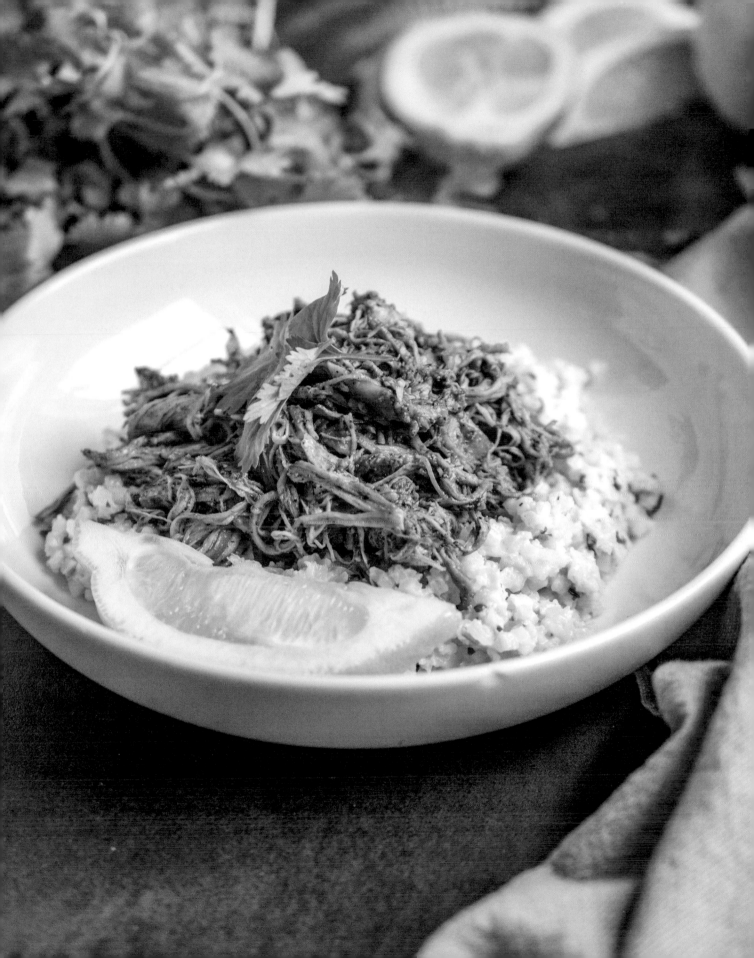

chicken katsu

This Japanese chicken dish is very popular here in Hawaii, and I must say, the crispy strips of chicken at restaurants tempted me many times before I finally took to my own kitchen to create a version that I could eat. Served with thinly shredded cabbage and a mayo-like sauce, chicken katsu is a fried chicken dinner that you can whip up on a weeknight. It's breaded with seasoned coconut flour and shredded coconut, then fried to create a deep golden crust. This breading sticks, it works, it's legit. You won't have soggy cutlets or pieces of breading falling off. Follow me to fried chicken bliss!

2 boneless, skinless chicken breasts

½ cup coconut oil, or more if needed, for frying

½ heaping cup coconut flour

2 teaspoons garlic powder

1 teaspoon fine Himalayan salt

1 teaspoon ground black pepper

3 large eggs

2 tablespoons coconut vinegar

1 cup unsweetened shredded coconut

Makes 4 servings
PREP TIME: 20 minutes   **COOK TIME:** 12 minutes

○ Cut each chicken breast into two thin cutlets, each no more than 2 centimeters thick: Lay the chicken breast flat on the cutting board, place one hand flat on top of it, and gently press down. Then run your knife straight through the middle horizontally. Be careful not to cut your fingers.

○ Pour the coconut oil into a large skillet; it should be about ½ inch deep. Heat the oil over medium heat until it sizzles around the end of a wooden spoon handle when it's inserted into the oil.

○ Set out two shallow dishes and a medium-sized bowl. In one dish, mix together the coconut flour, garlic powder, salt, and pepper. In the bowl, whisk together the eggs and vinegar. Put the shredded coconut in the second dish. In that order, bread the chicken: first, dredge each cutlet in the seasoned coconut flour, then dip it in the eggs, and last, coat it with the shredded coconut. Immediately add the cutlet to the hot oil. Repeat with a second cutlet.

○ Fry two cutlets at a time, making sure they don't touch in the skillet. Fry for 3 minutes, then flip with tongs and fry for another 3 minutes. Use tongs to remove the cutlets from skillet, drain the excess oil from the cutlets, and set them on a cooling rack while you fry the remaining chicken.

○ Place the fried chicken cutlets on a cutting board and cut into strips. Serve hot.

○ Store leftovers in an airtight container in the fridge for up to 5 days. To reheat, bake in a preheated 350°F oven for 10 minutes.

PER SERVING: Calories **597** · Fat **44.4g** · Total Carbohydrate **26.2g** · Dietary Fiber **11.6g** · Protein **23.5g**

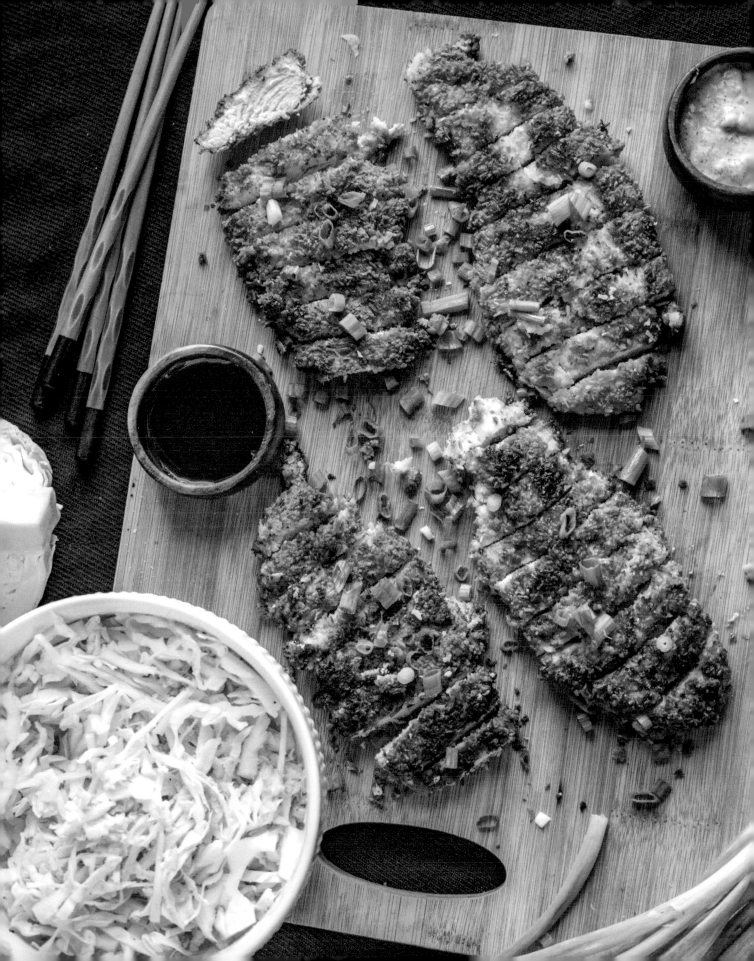

sheet pan dinner: chicken

Sheet pan dinners became one of those Pinterest sensations sometime in 2017, and with good reason—everything cooks together on a sheet pan, and dinner is ready! They're the answer to the weeknight meal. The first key to an excellent sheet pan dinner is pairing foods that have the same cooking needs. If you try to cook a large potato and salmon together, the fish will be burnt to a crisp before the potato softens. When you pair salmon and asparagus, however, both are done at the same time, within minutes. The second component to a killer sheet pan dinner is diversity. You don't want a meal in which everything looks and tastes the same! Here, I've combined chicken thighs and Brussels sprouts, and both cook to crispy perfection. Add a little bacon for extra fat and flavor. Top it off with Ginger Sauce (page 102) to take it to the next level.

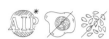

1 pound Brussels sprouts, halved

1 large onion, diced

5 cloves garlic, peeled

3 tablespoons cooking fat (see page 53), divided

2½ teaspoons fine Himalayan salt, divided

1 teaspoon garlic powder

1 teaspoon turmeric powder

2 pounds boneless, skinless chicken thighs

1 teaspoon ground black pepper

1 tablespoon coconut aminos

1 teaspoon fish sauce

4 slices bacon, cut into 1-inch pieces

Ginger Sauce (page 102), for serving (optional)

Makes 4 servings
PREP TIME: 10 minutes   COOK TIME: 40 minutes

○ Preheat the oven to 400°F.

○ On a sheet pan, toss the Brussels sprouts, onions, and garlic with 2 tablespoons of the fat, ½ teaspoon of the salt, the garlic powder, and the turmeric. Use your hands to massage the fat and seasonings into the sprouts, then spread them out in an even layer on the sheet pan—they should take up one-half to three-quarters of the pan.

○ On the empty side of the sheet pan, combine the chicken, the remaining tablespoon of fat, the remaining 2 teaspoons of salt, the pepper, coconut aminos, and fish sauce. Toss to combine and coat the chicken evenly with the seasonings, then lay the chicken thighs flat on the sheet pan. If they don't all fit, you can place the extra chicken in an oven-safe skillet or on a second sheet pan. Distribute the bacon pieces evenly over the sprouts and chicken.

○ Place the sheet pan in the oven and roast for 40 minutes. When it's done, the bacon will be crispy, the Brussels sprouts will be browned on the edges, the chicken thighs will be crispy on the bottom, and everything will smell delicious!

○ If you're using ginger sauce, drizzle it over the chicken before serving.

○ Store leftovers in an airtight container in the fridge for up to 5 days. To reheat, microwave on high for 1 to 2 minutes or place in a skillet over medium heat for 6 minutes.

SUBSTITUTIONS: To make this dish AIP-compliant, use ginger powder in place of the pepper.

VARIATIONS: You can use broccoli or cauliflower florets instead of Brussels sprouts.

CHEF'S NOTE: The seasonings here are really flexible. I love this flavor profile, but you can go with garlic and herbs for a whole different meal.

TIME-SAVING TIP: You can season the chicken and sprouts ahead of time and store them in separate freezer bags in the refrigerator for up to 1 day. When you're ready to cook them, just spread them out on a sheet pan and top with the bacon, and you're good to go.

PER SERVING: Calories **463** · Fat **23.5g** · Total Carbohydrate **15.5g** · Dietary Fiber **5.4g** · Protein **51.3g**

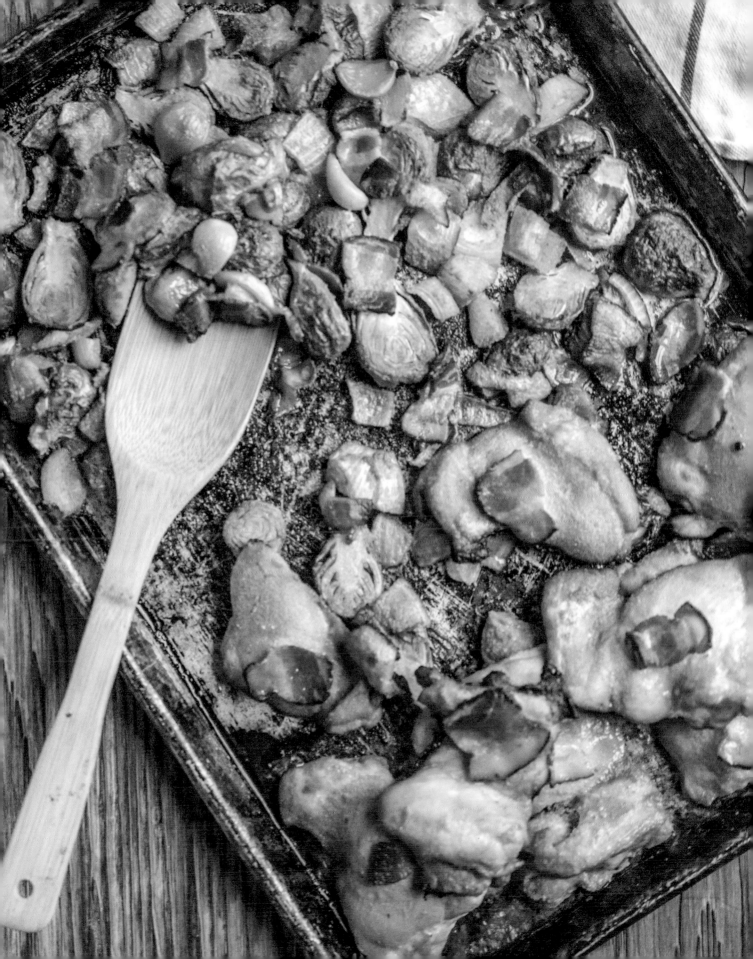

chicken satay + grilled zucchini
with lemon tahini sauce

So many flavors are packed into these easy skewers! Tender chicken thighs are marinated in a combination of warm spices and toasted sesame oil, then cooked on the grill for the perfect satay experience. Since we're grilling, we might as well throw some veggies on there, too, and zucchini is perfect. It grills quickly and beautifully, and it pairs well with the easy tahini sauce. I like to cut up and marinate the chicken as soon as I get home from the market so that when we get a hankering for these—and we always do—it's easy to thread them on skewers, grill, and eat! I love serving this with some fresh cilantro.

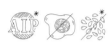

FOR THE SATAY:

1 pound boneless, skinless chicken thighs

1 teaspoon fine Himalayan salt

1 teaspoon ground black pepper

1 teaspoon turmeric powder

½ teaspoon ground toasted cumin seeds or ground cumin

2 tablespoons coconut oil or lard

1 tablespoon coconut vinegar

1 tablespoon toasted sesame oil

FOR THE ZUCCHINI:

3 small zucchini, halved lengthwise

1 tablespoon avocado oil or olive oil

Pinch of fine Himalayan salt

FOR THE TAHINI SAUCE:

Juice of 2 lemons

2 tablespoons tahini

1 tablespoon coconut aminos

½ teaspoon fish sauce

½ teaspoon ginger powder

Special equipment:

Bamboo, wooden, or metal skewers

Makes 3 servings
PREP TIME: 20 minutes, plus 1 hour to marinate   COOK TIME: 10 minutes

○ Cut each chicken thigh lengthwise into two or three strips, then cut the strips in half to make thumb-sized chunks. Place the chicken chunks, salt, pepper, turmeric, cumin, coconut oil, vinegar, and sesame oil in a large bowl. Mix well, cover, and set in the refrigerator to marinate for at least an hour or up to 3 days.

○ If you are using bamboo or wooden skewers, soak them in water for 20 minutes before grilling. Thread four or five pieces of marinated chicken onto each skewer and set aside.

○ Preheat the grill to high heat (450°F).

○ While the grill heats, prepare the zucchini and tahini sauce: Brush the zucchini with the oil and sprinkle with the salt. Place on a tray or cutting board that's large enough to hold everything after cooking.

○ Place all of the sauce ingredients in a small bowl and stir until smooth and well combined. Set aside.

○ When the grill has come to temperature, place the skewers on the hottest part of the grill and close the lid. Cook undisturbed for 3 minutes. Open the lid and turn the skewers over with tongs. Put the zucchini cut side down on the other side of the grill. Close the lid and lower the heat to 400°F. You may have to crack the lid periodically for temperature control. Grill for 5 to 8 minutes, until the chicken has a nice char to it and the internal temperature reaches 175°F. Flip the zucchini once halfway through. Remove the skewers and zucchini from the grill and place everything on the tray or cutting board.

○ Drizzle the tahini sauce over everything or serve on the side for dipping.

○ Store leftover skewers and sauce in separate airtight containers in the fridge for up to 5 days. To reheat the chicken, quickly sear in a hot skillet for 5 minutes.

PER SERVING: Calories **344** · Fat **19.3g** · Total Carbohydrate **5g** · Dietary Fiber **2.8g** · Protein **34.2g**

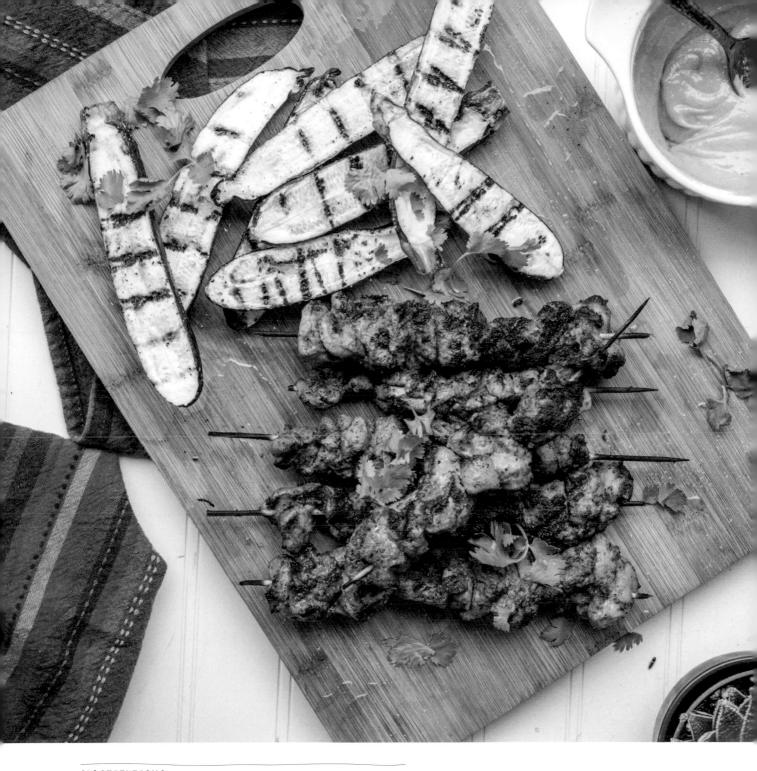

SUBSTITUTIONS: To make this recipe AIP-compliant, omit the pepper and sesame oil from the satay and use Ginger Sauce (page 102) instead of the tahini sauce.

VARIATIONS: In the sauce, use sunflower seed butter instead of tahini for a "peanut sauce" experience. This recipe can also be made with beef; I like to use sirloin steak cut into strips.

coconut-braised curried chicken

This is a slightly unconventional chicken curry method, but it incorporates my two favorite textures, crispy and creamy, so we're going with it. This recipe makes a big batch, perfect for feeding a crowd or when you need to cook once and eat twice. The seasoned chicken is browned to crispy perfection and then braised in coconut milk for pull-apart meat that is bursting with flavor. This dish delivers not only your favorite curry flavor but also lots of good fats to maximize the anti-inflammatory goodness of the turmeric. Serve it with cauliflower rice or a slice of Nut-Free Keto Bread (page 324) to sop up all the sauce.

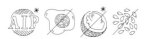

2 pounds boneless, skinless chicken thighs

2 teaspoons fine Himalayan salt

2 teaspoons turmeric powder

1 teaspoon dry mustard

1 teaspoon ginger powder

1 teaspoon ground black pepper

1 teaspoon ground cumin

Pinch of ground cloves

2 tablespoons ghee or lard

3 sprigs fresh thyme

1 cup full-fat coconut milk

2 tablespoons coconut vinegar or red wine vinegar

Fresh cilantro, for garnish (optional)

Makes 6 servings
PREP TIME: 5 minutes   COOK TIME: 35 minutes

○ Heat a large skillet over medium heat. While it heats, place the chicken thighs and seasonings in a large bowl and mix until all the thighs are evenly coated.

○ Place the ghee in the hot skillet and add as many chicken thighs as you can without overcrowding the pan (the thighs shouldn't touch)—you'll probably need to cook the thighs in two batches. Brown for 5 minutes, then flip the chicken over and brown for another 5 minutes. If you're cooking the thighs in batches, remove the first batch, place the second batch in the skillet, and repeat. When all the chicken is browned, return it all to the skillet.

○ Add the thyme sprigs, coconut milk, and vinegar to the skillet. Cover with a tight-fitting lid and let it simmer for 15 minutes.

○ Stir well, scraping the bottom of the skillet to lift any flavorful bits that are stuck to it. Transfer the chicken to a serving platter and pour the pan sauce over it, or serve the sauce on the side. Garnish with fresh cilantro, if desired.

○ Store leftovers in an airtight container in the fridge for up to 5 days. To reheat, sauté over medium heat for 10 minutes.

SUBSTITUTIONS: To make this dish AIP-compliant, omit the pepper and mustard. You can add 1 teaspoon horseradish for some spice. If you can't do coconut milk, use bone broth (page 100) instead.

VARIATIONS: Add cut green beans or frozen riced cauliflower to the skillet after adding the coconut milk. It will cook while the chicken simmers for a quick one-pot dinner!

TIME-SAVING TIP: You can also make this recipe in a pressure cooker. Brown the chicken on sauté mode and then cook it with the sauce on high pressure for 7 minutes instead of simmering on the stovetop for 15.

PER SERVING: Calories **425** · Fat **25.3g** · Total Carbohydrate **3.5g** · Dietary Fiber **1.3g** · Protein **45g**

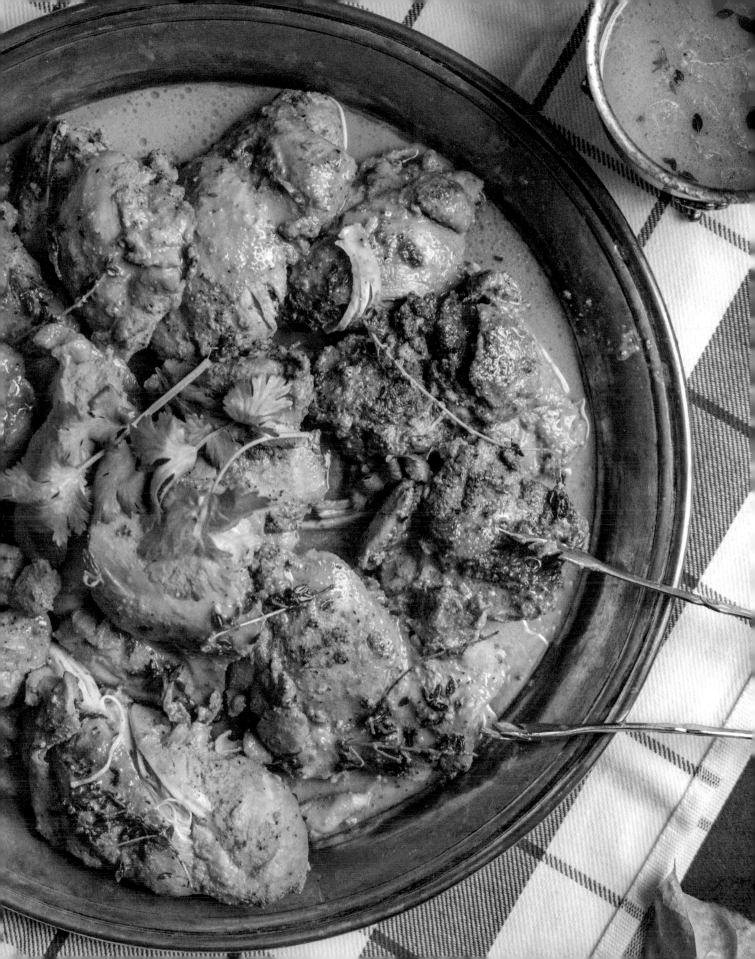

herbed turkey meatballs with lemon caper sauce

These oven meatballs come together in no time. While they bake to juicy perfection, whip up the easy lemon caper sauce. What you get is a restaurant-worthy meal that you can have on the table in under thirty minutes any day of the week. This goes great with Spinach Salad (page 348) and Nut-Free Keto Bread (page 324) or served over Creamy Cauliflower Mash (page 318).

   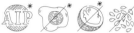

FOR THE MEATBALLS:

2 teaspoons dried rosemary needles

2 teaspoons dried thyme leaves

2 teaspoons fine Himalayan salt

2 teaspoons ground black pepper

Pinch of ground cloves

Pinch of ground nutmeg

2 pounds ground turkey (93% lean)

2 large eggs

2 tablespoons avocado oil, plus more for drizzling

2 tablespoons coconut flour

FOR THE SAUCE:

2 tablespoons salted butter or lard

4 cloves garlic, sliced

2 tablespoons capers, drained

½ teaspoon ground black pepper

Pinch of ground nutmeg

Juice of 1 lemon

¼ cup bone broth (page 100)

1 tablespoon full-fat coconut milk

Lemon slices, for garnish (optional)

Makes 21 meatballs (3 per serving)
PREP TIME: 10 minutes   COOK TIME: 20 minutes

○ Preheat the oven to 350°F. Line a sheet pan with parchment paper.

○ Place the rosemary, thyme, salt, pepper, cloves, and nutmeg in a food processor, coffee grinder, or mortar and pestle. Grind until the herbs, primarily the rosemary, are broken up into pieces the size of grains of sand.

○ Place the ground turkey, seasoning mixture, eggs, avocado oil, and coconut flour in a large bowl. Mix well until the texture is even, without clumps of flour or pools of oil.

○ Use a tablespoon to scoop up the turkey mixture and, with lightly oiled hands, gently shape it into a meatball. One heaping tablespoon per meatball will yield twenty-one meatballs. Line up the meatballs on the sheet pan, spaced ½ inch apart. Spray or drizzle the meatballs with a little extra oil. Bake for 20 minutes.

○ While the meatballs bake, make the sauce: Heat a medium skillet over medium heat. When it's hot, add the butter. Once it has melted, add the garlic, capers, pepper, and nutmeg. Cook, stirring occasionally, for 3 to 4 minutes, until the garlic begins to brown and the butter is frothy.

○ Add the lemon juice and stir, lifting any pieces stuck to the skillet. Add the broth and bring to a simmer. Reduce for 5 minutes. Stir in the coconut milk and remove from the heat.

○ When the meatballs are done, transfer them to a serving dish or bowl. Spoon the sauce over the meatballs or serve it on the side. Garnish with lemon slices, if desired.

○ Store leftovers in an airtight container in the fridge for up to 5 days. Reheat in a small skillet over medium heat.

SUBSTITUTIONS: To make this recipe AIP-compliant, omit the pepper, nutmeg, and eggs from the meatballs; substitute ⅛ teaspoon ground cloves and 2 tablespoons pumpkin puree. For the sauce, use lard or coconut oil instead of butter. To make this dish without coconut, substitute flaxseed meal for the coconut flour and omit the coconut milk from the sauce.

PER SERVING: Calories **300** · Fat **19.3g** · Total Carbohydrate **4.1g** · Dietary Fiber **2g** · Protein **28.4g**

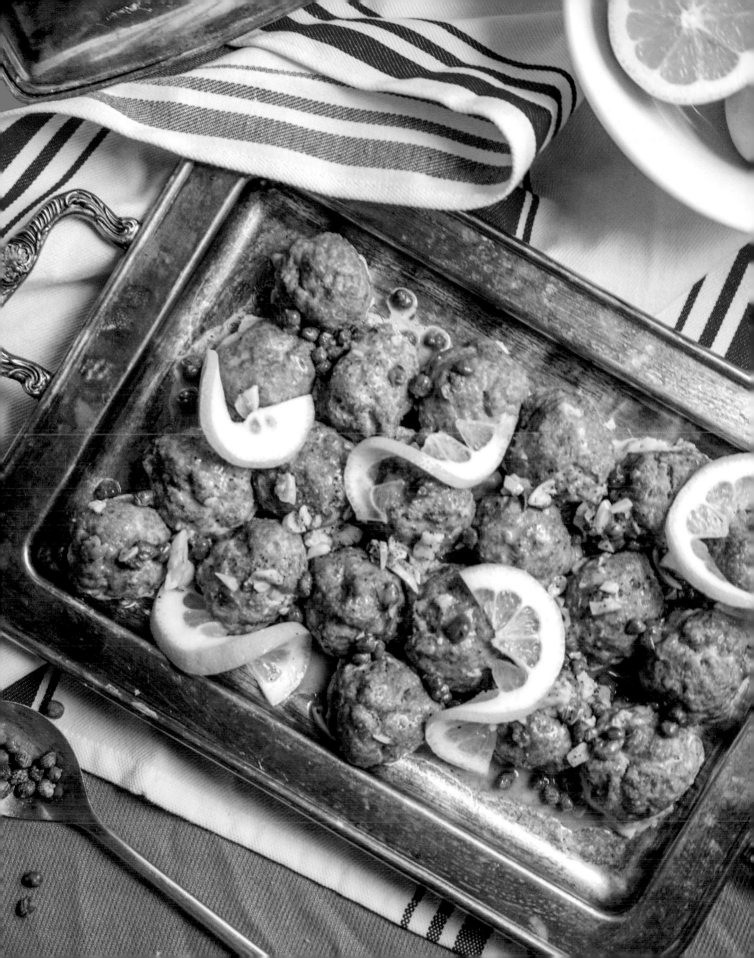

chicken + broccoli bowls

This is the quintessential weeknight dinner—the meal that is so simple, so easy, and so delicious that you can eat it on repeat. This recipe combines my two go-to foods, crispy chicken thighs and crispy broccoli, cooked in the oven simultaneously and deliciously seasoned. Feel free to use the method for chicken thighs always and forever. Same goes for the broccoli; it's my go-to method, and I love broccoli. Bring it all together with some avocado, lemon, and green onion, and voilà! Dinner bowls are done.

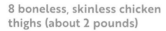

8 boneless, skinless chicken thighs (about 2 pounds)

4 tablespoons avocado oil, divided

3 teaspoons fine Himalayan salt, divided

1 teaspoon dried dill weed

1 teaspoon dried thyme leaves

1 teaspoon ground black pepper

18 ounces broccoli (about 2 crowns), cut into florets

4 cloves garlic, minced

FOR GARNISH (OPTIONAL):

1 medium Hass avocado, sliced

2 green onions, sliced

1 lemon, quartered

Makes 4 servings
PREP TIME: 10 minutes   COOK TIME: 30 minutes

○ Preheat the oven to 425°F.

○ In a large bowl, toss the chicken thighs with 2 tablespoons of the avocado oil, 2 teaspoons of the salt, and the dill, thyme, and pepper. Arrange the chicken thighs on a sheet pan so they are lying flat side by side, not touching.

○ On a second sheet pan, toss the broccoli florets with the remaining 2 tablespoons of avocado oil, the remaining teaspoon of salt, and the minced garlic, massaging the oil into the florets. Then spread them out over the sheet pan so they do not overlap. If there are any large florets, cut them in half.

○ Place the chicken on the middle rack of the oven and the broccoli on the bottom rack and roast for 15 minutes. Switch the chicken to the bottom and the broccoli to the middle and roast for another 15 minutes, or until crispy.

○ Cut up the chicken and divide the broccoli and chicken evenly among four bowls. If you like, garnish each bowl with avocado slices, green onions, and a lemon quarter.

○ Store leftovers in airtight containers in the fridge for up to 5 days. To reheat, sauté over medium heat for 8 minutes.

CHEF'S NOTE: If the chicken thighs are on the plump side, I recommend scoring the undersides. Make shallow cuts with a sharp knife in a crisscross pattern to ensure that they get nice and crispy in 30 minutes.

VARIATIONS: You can easily transform this dish by switching up the seasoning. Toss the chicken with Ginger Sauce (page 102) and toss the broccoli with toasted sesame oil for Asian-inspired bowls. Top with your favorite sauce, Fiesta Guacamole (page 90), or Roasted Beet Marinara (page 78). The possibilities are endless!

SUBSTITUTION: To make this dish AIP-compliant, omit the pepper.

PER SERVING: Calories **426** · Fat **26g** · Total Carbohydrate **4.5g** · Dietary Fiber **2.1g** · Protein **46.1g**

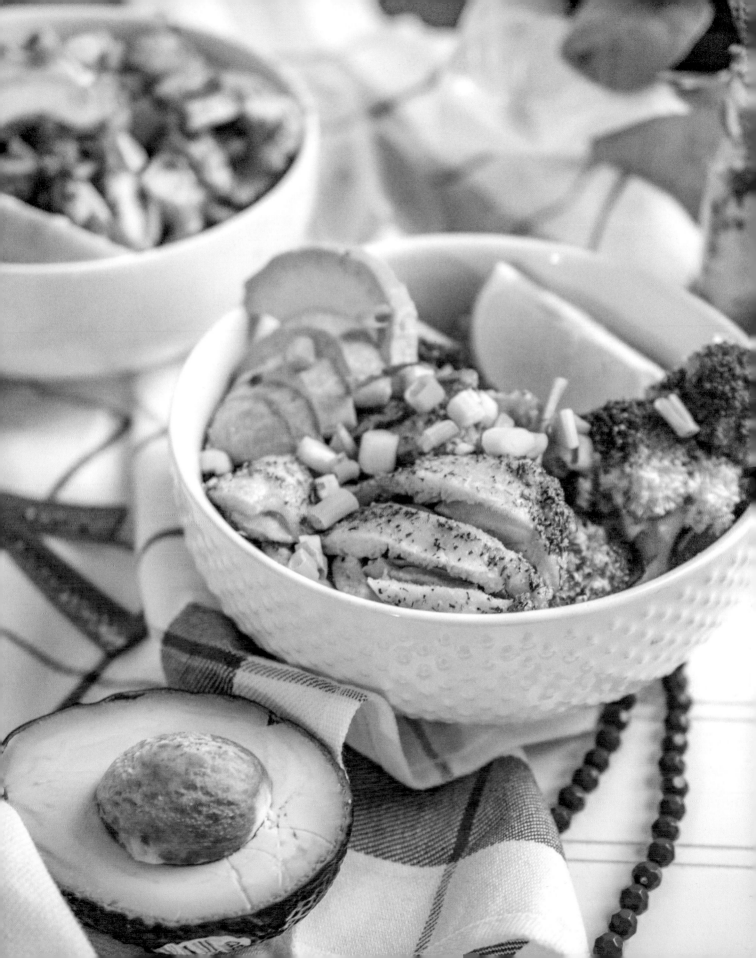

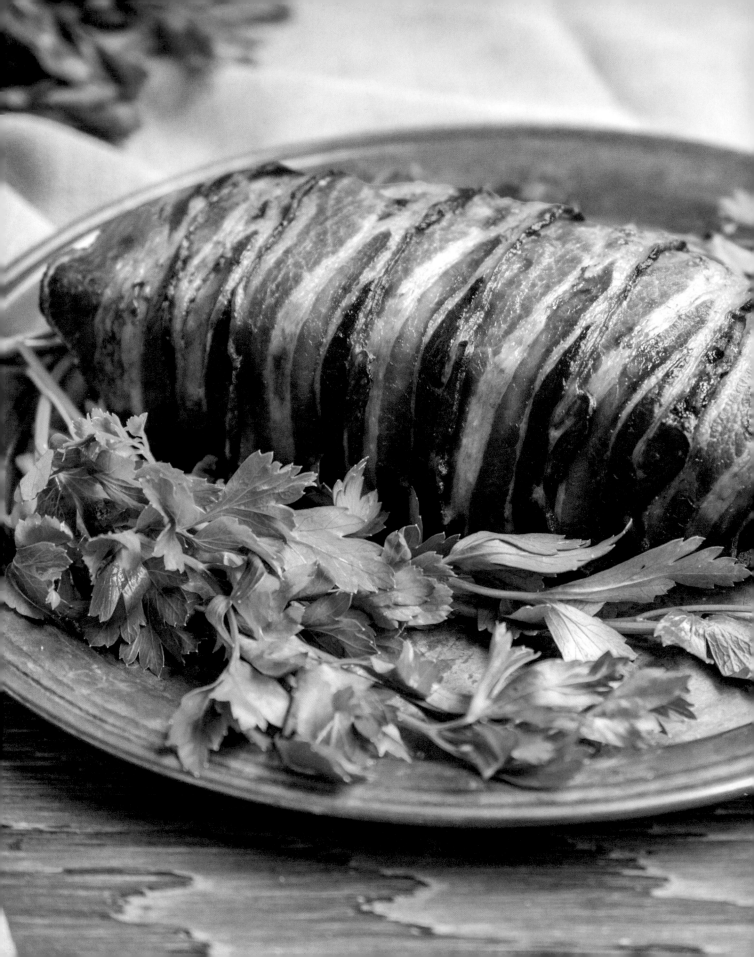

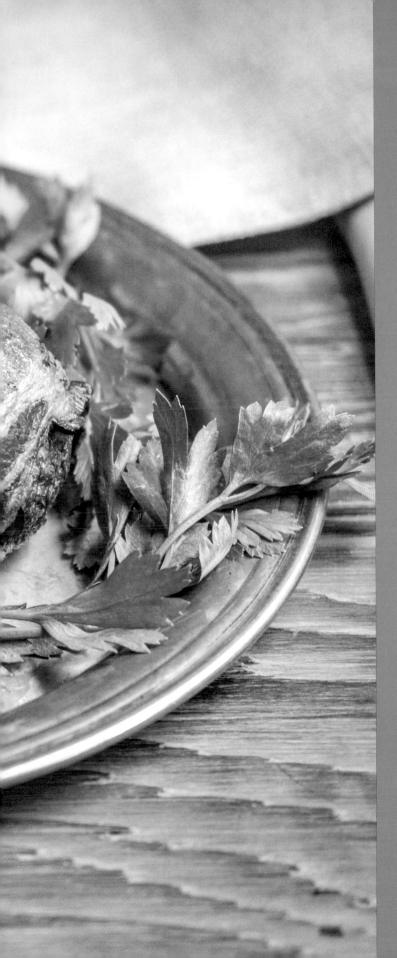

BEEF + LAMB

I have always had an affinity for red meat. (Except for that one time I went vegan—I claim temporary insanity.) I truly enjoy quality meat in my diet. After all, my father is a butcher. Here I've included a variety of red-meat dishes, from the extremely frugal (I am all about the ground beef) to the occasional splurge (hello, rib-eye!). Fire up the grill and heat up those cast-iron skillets!

savory meat pie

This is the kind of recipe for which I like to keep a pie crust in the freezer. It is a great way to stretch leftovers and is perfect for parties and make-ahead meals. Ground beef, shredded veggies, and Cheesy Yellow Sauce (page 68) combine in a low-carb pie crust for an easy meal that makes me nostalgic. I can't put my finger on why; maybe it's because the combination of ground beef and cheese tastes a little like a cheeseburger, taking me back to my childhood days, or at least my pre-grain-free days. This pie stores well in the fridge and reheats like a dream. No need to wait for a special occasion to whip up this bad boy.

1 Pie Crust (page 92), baked in a regular or springform 8-inch pan

1 tablespoon avocado oil

½ small onion, diced

2 cloves garlic, minced

1 pound ground beef (85% lean)

1 teaspoon fine Himalayan salt

1 teaspoon ground black pepper

½ teaspoon ground cumin

½ cup Cheesy Yellow Sauce (page 68), divided

2 cups rainbow slaw (see Note, page 172) or any shredded vegetables

Makes one 8-inch pie (8 servings)
PREP TIME: 5 minutes   COOK TIME: 45 minutes

∘ Preheat the oven to 350°F. Set out the prebaked pie crust. It can be freshly baked or frozen; no need to thaw.

∘ Heat a large skillet over medium heat. When it's hot, add the avocado oil, onions, and garlic. Sauté until tender and aromatic, about 5 minutes.

∘ Add the ground beef, salt, pepper, and cumin. Sauté until browned, breaking up the meat with a whisk or spatula. Stir in ¼ cup of the sauce and quickly use a slotted spoon to transfer the beef mixture to the pie crust. You want to leave behind the pooling liquid in the skillet so the crust doesn't get soggy; let each spoonful drain before transferring it to the crust. Pat the beef down so it's compact in the bottom of the pie crust.

∘ Carefully drain the liquid from the skillet and then put the pan back on the burner. Place the slaw in the skillet and sauté for 5 minutes, or until lightly browned and tender. Mix in the remaining ¼ cup of cheese sauce, then spoon the cheesy slaw over the ground beef in the pie pan. Spread out and pat down.

∘ Bake for 30 minutes. Remove the pie from the oven and let it cool for 5 minutes before cutting it into eight even slices (or unpanning it if you used a springform pan). Enjoy!

∘ You can store slices in an airtight container or cover the entire pie in plastic wrap and store in the refrigerator for up to 6 days. Reheat in a preheated 350°F oven or toaster oven for 10 minutes, or microwave on high for 1 minute.

SUBSTITUTION: To make this pie egg-free, use the crust recipe from Mini Quiche Muffins (page 172): double the recipe and press the dough down into a springform pan, pushing it up the sides to create a 1-inch border.

PER SERVING: Calories **374** · Fat **33g** · Total Carbohydrate **3g** · Dietary Fiber **1g** · Protein **17g**

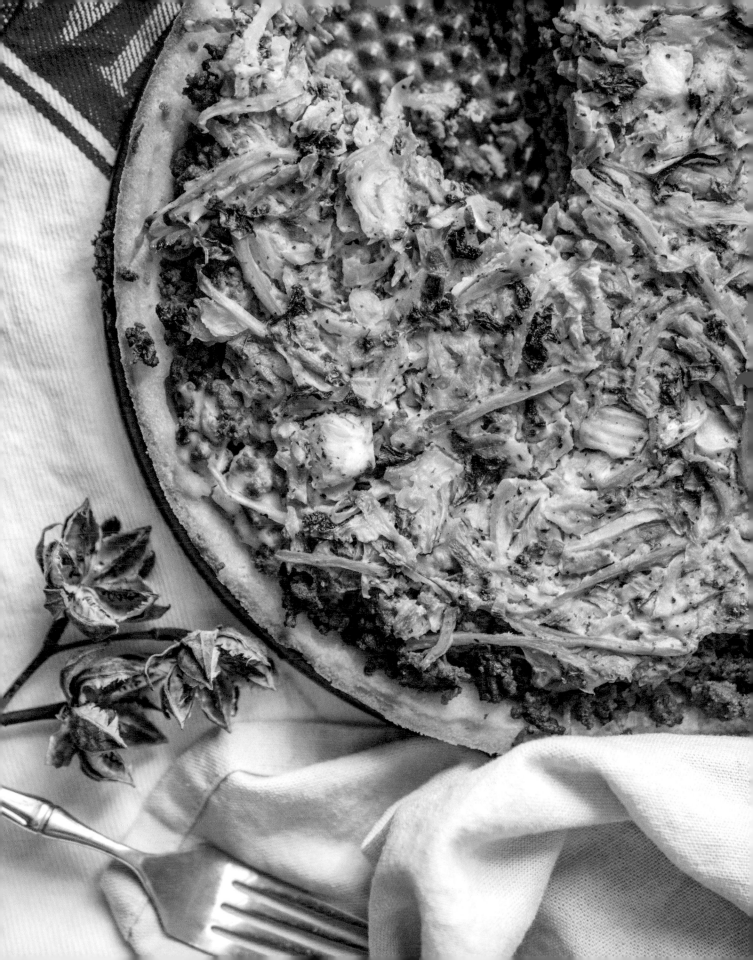

flank steak pinwheels

Don't let their fancy appearance fool you; the only tricky part of making these pinwheels is slicing the steak, and it's really not that tricky. All you need is a sharp knife, and I will walk you through it. This is a great way to make a pound of steak go a long way. I love these frugal fancy dishes—great for feeding a crowd, serving at parties, or taking to the next potluck. The combination of beef, cheese sauce, and green beans just screams comfort food! You can use any veggies you like here; I recommend choosing vegetables that can take a lot of heat without getting mushy.

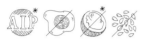

1 to 1½ pounds flank steak

¼ cup Cheesy Yellow Sauce (page 68)

½ pound fresh green beans, trimmed

½ teaspoon fine Himalayan salt

½ teaspoon garlic powder

6 to 8 slices thick-cut bacon

6 sprigs fresh oregano

1 head garlic

2 tablespoons avocado oil

SUBSTITUTIONS: To make this dish AIP-compliant, use asparagus, carrot sticks, or another AIP-friendly vegetable instead of green beans.

Makes 4 servings
PREP TIME: 20 minutes   COOK TIME: 40 minutes

○ Preheat the oven to 400°F.

○ Lay the steak flat on a cutting board. Place one hand on it and press down gently. Starting at the thickest end, cut into the meat horizontally about ¼ inch from the top and slice all the way through, going under your hand. After you have a good flap cut out, you can gently pull up on the flap as you continue to cut across the steak. You will need to keep steady pressure on the knife and make sure you don't angle it too much so the thickness remains consistent. Cut until the knife comes out the other side and you have a thin, sheetlike layer of beef.

○ If your steak is not very thick, you might be able to cut it only once. If it is very thick, cut it twice so you have three thin sheets of beef.

○ Lay the slices of beef flat on the cutting board. Cover them with a piece of plastic wrap and pound them with the smooth side of a mallet or a heavy-bottomed pot to even out the thickness and to tenderize. Do not pound so hard that you make holes in the meat.

○ Smear some sauce on one slice of steak, then add fifteen to twenty green beans. Spread them out for 2 to 3 inches along the steak, starting 1 inch from the top. Sprinkle with the salt and garlic powder. Starting at the top, roll the meat inward and over the green beans. Keep rolling until you have a burritolike tube. Holding the roll closed, wrap two or three slices of bacon tightly around it. Place the roll seam side down on a large skillet or sheet pan. Repeat with the remaining steak.

○ Top each bacon-wrapped roll with a sprig of oregano. Place the rest of the oregano between the rolls on the skillet or sheet pan.

○ Trim the top off of the head of garlic so the cloves inside are exposed. Place it on top of the oregano sprigs. Drizzle the avocado oil over everything.

○ Roast for 40 minutes, or until the bacon is cooked and slightly browned.

PER SERVING: Calories **413** · Fat **27.2g** · Total Carbohydrate **4.3g** · Dietary Fiber **4.5g** · Protein **37.5g**

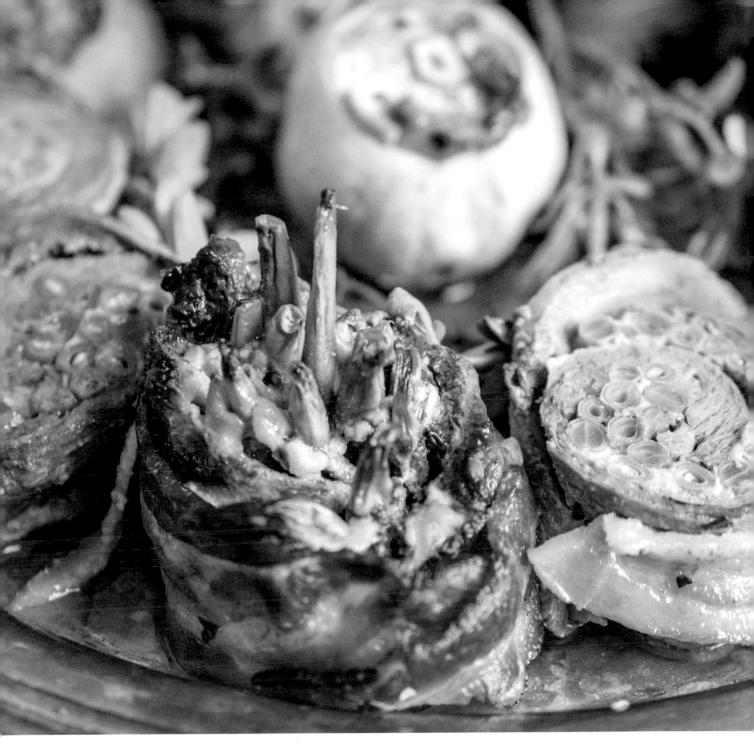

○ Let the rolls rest for 5 minutes, then use a sharp knife to cut each roll into four slices. Serve with the roasted garlic cloves and crispy oregano, with the pan sauce spooned over them.

○ Store leftovers in an airtight container in the fridge for up to 5 days. To reheat, cover with foil and bake in a preheated 350°F oven for 10 to 15 minutes.

multinational beef + rice

I started with beef bourguignon and then went a little off plan with warm spices and creamy sunflower seed butter. I added riced cauliflower at the end, and the result was a dish that transcends expectations and borders—a recipe with European roots, South Asian inspiration, and Latin American tendencies. Rich and elegant, this dish is delicious and eclectic. It's the kind of slow-cooked meal that gets better with age, so make a big batch and enjoy leftovers, because this saucy goodness tastes even better the next day.

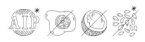

Makes 4 servings
PREP TIME: 15 minutes   COOK TIME: 15 minutes, plus 4 hours in a slow cooker

2 tablespoons avocado oil

1 large onion, diced

3 ribs celery, diced

5 cremini mushrooms, sliced

4 cloves garlic, minced

2 sprigs fresh thyme

1½ teaspoons garam masala

1 teaspoon fine Himalayan salt

1 teaspoon ginger powder

1 teaspoon ground black pepper

1 pound stew meat

2 tablespoons sunflower seed butter

1 tablespoon red wine vinegar or coconut vinegar

1 cup Roasted Beet Marinara (page 78)

2 cups riced cauliflower (see Note, page 140)

Fresh herbs or Coconut Yogurt (page 96), for garnish (optional)

○ Heat a large skillet over medium heat. When it's hot, pour in the avocado oil and add the onions and celery. Sauté, stirring often, until tender, about 5 minutes.

○ Add the mushrooms, garlic, and thyme sprigs. Sauté until the mushrooms are browned, 3 to 5 minutes. Add the garam masala, salt, ginger powder, pepper, and stew meat. Stir well and cook for 5 to 6 minutes, until the beef is lightly browned. Mix in the sunflower seed butter, making sure to coat the meat.

○ Transfer everything to a slow cooker. Mix in the vinegar and marinara. Cook on low for 3½ hours, then mix in the riced cauliflower and cook for 30 more minutes.

○ Serve garnished with fresh herbs or dollops of coconut yogurt. Store leftovers in an airtight container in the fridge for up to 5 days. To reheat, bring to a simmer on the stovetop.

TIME-SAVING TIP: You can also make this recipe in a pressure cooker. Use the sauté function for the browning and then cook on high pressure for 20 minutes. Release the pressure, stir in the riced cauliflower, and cook on low pressure for 2 minutes, then release the pressure manually. Stir well, then serve.

CHEF'S NOTE: If you don't have a slow cooker, use a Dutch oven. Brown the meat on the stovetop as instructed, then cook in a preheated 300°F oven for 4 hours.

SUBSTITUTIONS: To make this dish AIP-compliant, omit the garam masala and pepper; instead, use 1 teaspoon each of ground cinnamon and turmeric powder. In addition, replace the sunflower seed butter with coconut cream and use the AIP-compliant version of the marinara.

PER SERVING: Calories **471** · Fat **36.1g** · Total Carbohydrate **14.4g** · Dietary Fiber **5.1g** · Protein **27g**

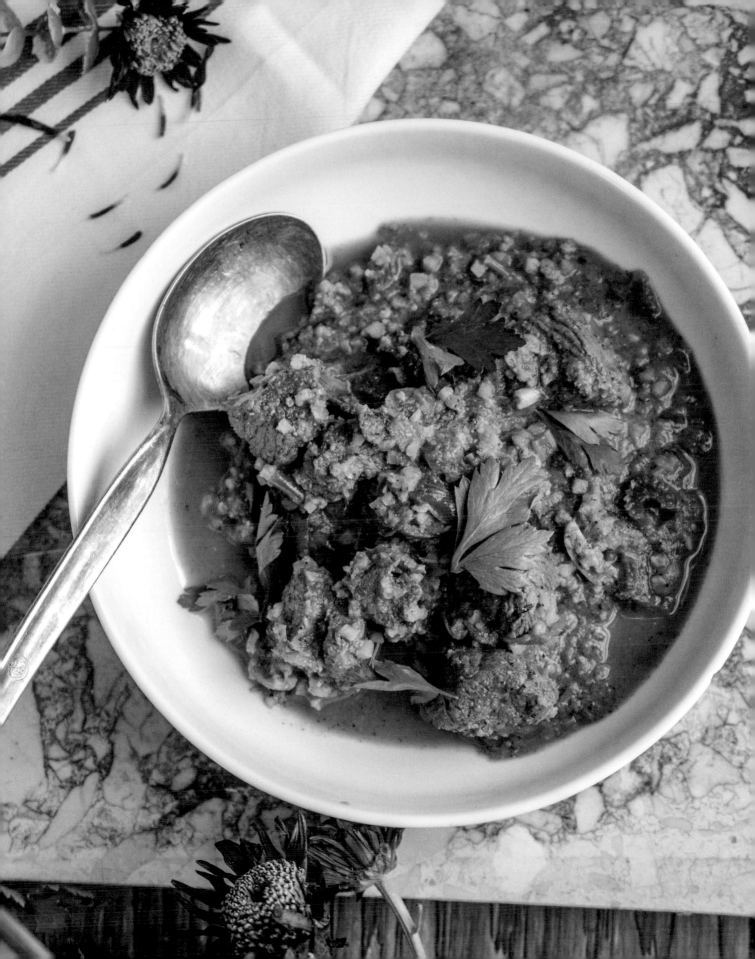

vaca frita

Vaca frita is a traditional Cuban dish whose name translates to "fried cow." I know, not that appetizing, but Spanish is a romance language, so it just makes everything sound better. In any case, this crispy shredded beef is absolutely divine. Tossed with sautéed onions and drenched in citrus, it delivers an addicting combination of flavors and textures. You can use any affordable piece of meat you can find, but chuck roast is my favorite. Slow-cooking the meat ahead of time makes this recipe practically effortless when it comes to frying up and serving the meat. Serve it over greens or in Egg Drop Soup (page 146), or add it to a bowl of ramen (page 276). For a more traditional experience, serve it with Creamy Cilantro Rice (page 342).

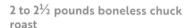

2 to 2½ pounds boneless chuck roast

2½ teaspoons fine Himalayan salt, divided

2 bay leaves

1 tablespoon white vinegar

3 tablespoons coconut oil or avocado oil

1 large onion, cut into ¼-inch slices

Juice of 2 lemons, divided

½ bunch fresh cilantro, minced (½ cup), divided

TIME-SAVING TIP: Cook the meat in a pressure cooker on high for 50 minutes instead of in a slow cooker.

Makes 4 servings
PREP TIME: 20 minutes   COOK TIME: 20 minutes, plus 8 hours in a slow cooker

○ Rub the roast with 2 teaspoons of the salt. Place in a slow cooker and add the bay leaves and vinegar. Add water until the beef is just submerged. Cook on low for 8 hours.

○ Remove the meat from the slow cooker and discard the liquid. Place the beef in a storage container, cover, and set in the refrigerator until you're ready to make and serve this dish. If you're making it right away, set the beef under a fan to cool before shredding.

○ Heat a large skillet over medium heat. When it's hot, place the oil in the skillet and add the onion slices. Cook for 10 minutes, stirring occasionally. The onions will become tender, translucent, and sweet.

○ While the onions cook, shred the meat by hand, removing any unsightly chunks of fat. Make sure to shred it into fine threads. The thinner the pieces are, the more they will crisp up!

○ Remove the onions from the skillet and set aside. Don't clean the pan. Add half of the shredded beef to the skillet over medium heat. Cook for 8 minutes, stirring once halfway through. After 8 minutes, there should be some pieces of meat stuck to the bottom of the pan; add the juice of 1 lemon and use a spatula to scrape them up.

○ Mix in half of the cilantro and half of the cooked onions. Stir to combine and immediately remove from the skillet. Repeat with the remaining shredded beef, lemon juice, cilantro, and onions.

○ Place both batches of vaca frita in a serving bowl and toss with the remaining ½ teaspoon of salt before serving.

○ Store leftovers in an airtight container in the fridge for up to 5 days. Reheat in a skillet over high heat for 5 to 10 minutes, until crispy again.

PER SERVING: Calories **639** · Fat **50g** · Total Carbohydrate **1.4g** · Dietary Fiber **1g** · Protein **44g**

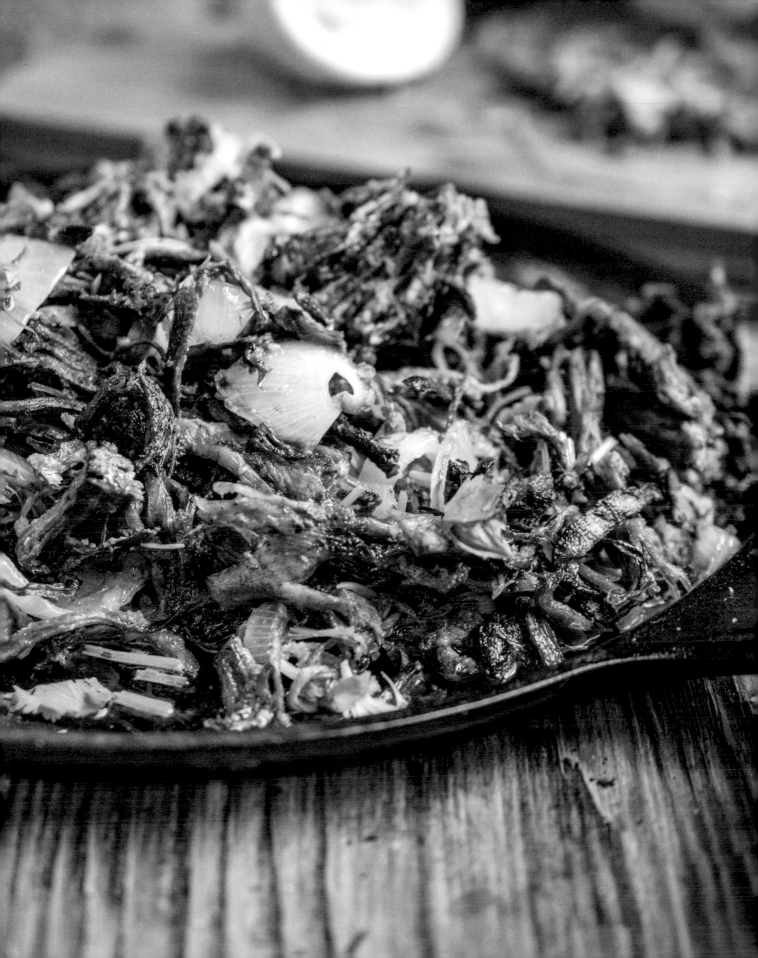

stuffed cabbage, dolmas-style

Dolmas (stuffed grape leaves) originated in various cultures around the Mediterranean and surrounding regions, from Russia to the Middle East. Ground beef seasoned with herbs and citrus is tossed with rice and rolled into small grape leaves, which are then simmered in a citrus solution for an hour. Here, I've made them in cabbage leaves for entrée-sized portions, with ingredients that you can find at any grocery store. Not quite the hearty Irish stuffed cabbage and not quite the light and tangy Mediterranean appetizer, this meal is truly a multinational creation.

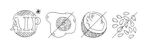

1 large head green cabbage or savoy cabbage

2 pounds ground beef (85% lean)

4 cloves garlic, minced

1 large onion, minced

2 cups riced cauliflower (see Note, page 140)

¼ cup minced fresh mint, plus more for garnish

1 tablespoon minced fresh oregano

2 teaspoons fine Himalayan salt

2 teaspoons ground black pepper

3 lemons, divided

1 cup water

2 tablespoons ghee, avocado oil, or lard

Makes 12 large dolmas (2 per serving)
PREP TIME: 30 minutes
COOK TIME: 20 minutes in a pressure cooker or 1 hour on the stovetop

◦ Turn the cabbage over so you're looking at the base. Take a paring knife and cut in an inward angle all around the core of the cabbage, then pull it out. Discard the core and set the cabbage aside.

◦ Bring a large pot of water, one big enough to fit the whole head of cabbage, to a boil. While you wait for it to boil, prepare the filling: Crumble the ground beef into a large bowl. (If you don't want to handle it, you can add it to the bowl and then use a whisk to break up the beef until it's crumbled.) Add the garlic, onions, cauliflower, mint, oregano, salt, and pepper. Juice a lemon into the mix as well, catching the seeds with your hands or a fine-mesh sieve. Then use your hands to mix the ingredients thoroughly.

◦ Once the water has begun to boil, squeeze the juice from a lemon into it. Use tongs to submerge the head of cabbage and hold it there for a minute or two, then let it go and cook for another 3 minutes. Use the tongs to carefully remove the cabbage from the water and set it in a bowl, cored side up. Carefully peel away the loose, tender cabbage leaves with the tongs. They should come off effortlessly; if they don't, put the cabbage back in the hot water for a few more minutes.

◦ Stack the cabbage leaves on a plate or cutting board. You will need room to roll the dolmas.

◦ Place a leaf in the center of your work area. Use the paring knife to trim the thickest part of the leaf, where it meets the stem, cutting out a little triangle shape. Spoon a generous amount of the meat mixture onto the leaf; the exact amount depends on the size of the cabbage, but you will get a feel for it after you've rolled one or two. With a large head of cabbage, I can fit up to a cup of filling in one dolma. Position the filling in the center toward the bottom, where you trimmed the leaf.

PER SERVING: Calories **361** · Fat **22g** · Total Carbohydrate **7.6g** · Dietary Fiber **7.2g** · Protein **32g**

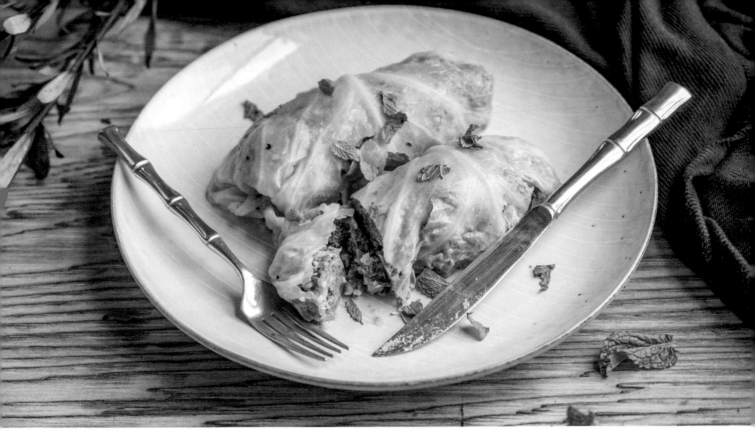

CHEF'S NOTE: These dolmas are
a meal all on their own, full of
flavor and very tender. But I'm
a sauce person, so sauce is a
welcome addition to any plate, in
my opinion. I like adding Pistou
(page 74) or Toum (page 72) to this
dish.

SUBSTITUTIONS: To make these
dolmas AIP-compliant, omit
the pepper. If you want to
make them with another kind
of protein, that's fine, but be
sure to compensate for the fat,
as poultry is much leaner—add
2 tablespoons of fat to the
ground protein mixture.

◦ Fold the leaf upward once, then fold in the sides and continue
rolling forward until you have a burrito-like roll. Make sure to apply
pressure with your hands as you roll it so it stays closed. Set aside,
seam side down, and repeat with the remaining filling and cabbage
leaves.

◦ **Pressure cooker instructions:** Arrange the dolmas in the bowl of
a pressure cooker, seam side down. Four should fit at the bottom;
continue to stack them in up to three layers. Add the cup of water
and the juice of the third lemon. Drizzle in the ghee and seal the
lid. Set the pressure to low (no higher than 3.0 psi) and the time
for 20 minutes. When the pressure cooker has finished, release the
pressure manually and carefully open the lid.

◦ **Stovetop instructions:** Place the dolmas in a large pot, layering
them on top of one another. Pour in the cup of water and the juice
of the third lemon. Drizzle in the ghee. Bring to a simmer over
medium-low heat. Cover with a tight-fitting lid and cook on low for
60 to 70 minutes. Check occasionally; if the water has evaporated,
add a second cup of water.

◦ Use a slotted spoon to remove the dolmas from the pot. The
lower ones will be delicate, so you may need to use two spoons to
remove them. Serve hot, garnished with more fresh mint.

◦ Unless you're feeding six adults, you will have leftovers. Store
them in an airtight container, in a single layer, in the refrigerator
for up to 5 days. To reheat, bake in a preheated 350°F oven for
10 to 15 minutes.

carne molida

The versatility of this ground beef dish is endless. I like to make a big batch of it weekly. We put it on salads and in tacos (duh), eat it right out of the skillet, or pile it on an avocado and call it lunch. Yeah, we're big fans of this beef in my house. It's super flavorful, cooks down to crispy perfection, and is made with just a handful of ingredients. I know this recipe will quickly become a staple in your home, too.

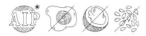

Makes 4 servings (about 3 cups)
PREP TIME: 5 minutes   COOK TIME: 20 minutes

2 tablespoons lard or avocado oil

2 pounds ground beef (85% lean)

1 tablespoon granulated garlic

2 teaspoons dried parsley

2 teaspoons fine Himalayan salt

2 teaspoons ground black pepper

2 teaspoons onion powder

1 teaspoon ground cumin

Juice of 1 lime

Chopped fresh cilantro, for garnish (optional)

◦ Melt the lard in a large pot over medium heat. Quickly add the ground beef, crumbling it in with your hands.

◦ Sprinkle all the seasonings over the ground beef and stir to combine. Use a spatula or whisk to break up the meat as you stir so that it continues to crumble and there are no large chunks.

◦ Cook, stirring occasionally, for 10 to 15 minutes. The beef will brown, then release some liquid; let that liquid boil away. Increase the heat to medium-high. Keep cooking and stirring until the beef is glossy and dark brown. Once you begin having to scrape it from the bottom of the pot, it's crispy. Turn off the heat. Squeeze in the lime juice and mix.

◦ Serve hot! A little chopped fresh cilantro for garnish goes really well, but it's not necessary.

SUBSTITUTIONS: To make this recipe AIP-compliant, omit the pepper and cumin. I recommend adding a little grated lime zest to up the tanginess. A hint of horseradish adds a welcome kick, too!

PER SERVING: Calories **326** · Fat **22.8g** · Total Carbohydrate **5.5g** · Dietary Fiber **0.7g** · Protein **24.3g**

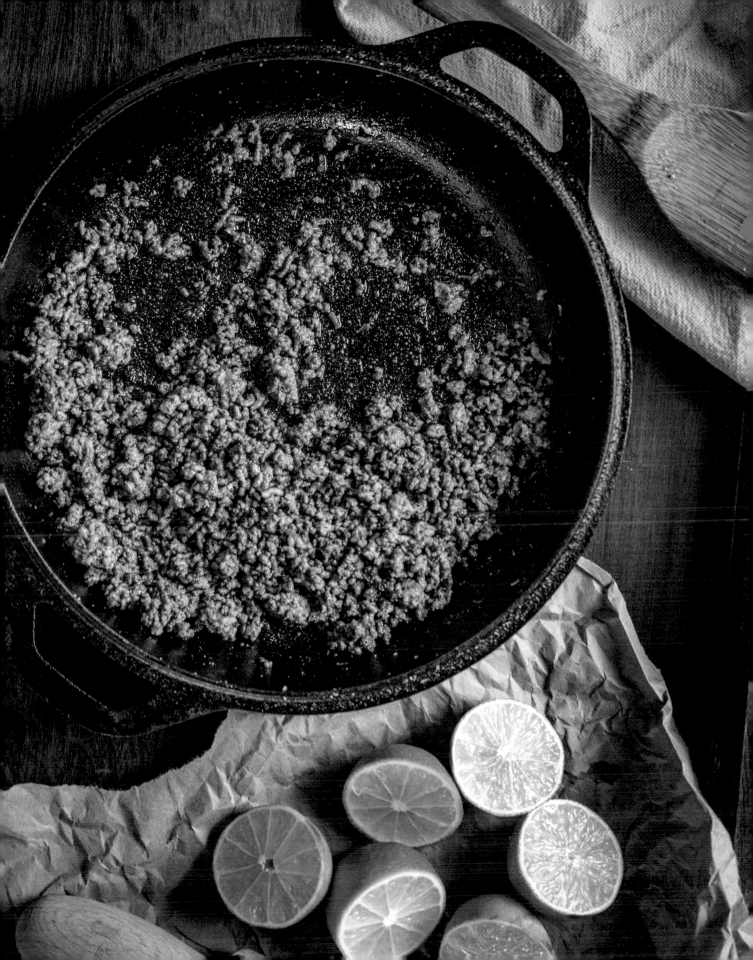

beef carnitas

When I chose to give up nightshades (primarily peppers and tomatoes) for health reasons, I thought Mexican food was forever out of my reach. Fortunately, the flavors of Mexican cuisine are complex and delicate, and with a little creativity and clean ingredients, I have been able to enjoy a few of my favorite foods—carnitas and soft, warm tortillas being two of them! Slow-cooked in its own juices with citrus, bacon, and onion, this shredded beef is bursting with flavor. I've opted for beef because pastured pork roasts are so hard to come by, but if you've got a hookup, this recipe works with pork shoulder, too! Pile it high on soft tortillas with Pickled Red Onions (page 88) and Fiesta Guacamole (page 90), and you've got yourself a legitimate taco spread.

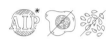

4 slices bacon, diced

1 large onion, diced

4 cloves garlic, minced

3 to 4 pounds chuck shoulder roast

1 tablespoon fine Himalayan salt

2 teaspoons dried oregano

2 teaspoons ground black pepper

2 teaspoons ground cumin

3 tablespoons coconut oil

1 cup bone broth (page 100)

Juice of 3 limes

¼ cup coconut aminos

2 bay leaves

FOR SERVING:

6 Street Taco Tortillas (page 332), warm

Fiesta Guacamole (page 90; optional)

Pickled Red Onions (page 88; optional)

CHEF'S NOTE: I'm a sucker for a loaded taco. Other fun things to add to this spread are Coconut Yogurt (page 96), which doubles as sour cream, and Hard Cheese (page 70), which will melt right over the hot carnitas. (Okay, my mouth is officially watering.)

Makes 8 servings
PREP TIME: 20 minutes   COOK TIME: 20 minutes plus 10 hours in a slow cooker

- Heat a large skillet over medium-high heat. Cook the bacon, onions, and garlic in the skillet for 5 minutes, until lightly browned, then transfer the mixture to a slow cooker. Keep the skillet hot.

- While the bacon mixture cooks, cut the roast into two equal-sized pieces and lay them flat on the cutting board. Mix the salt, oregano, pepper, and cumin in a small bowl and rub the mixture all over the roast. Scoop any seasonings left behind on the cutting board into the slow cooker.

- Melt the coconut oil in the skillet and sear the meat for 2 minutes on all sides. Once the meat is browned, place it in the slow cooker. Pour the broth into the skillet to quickly deglaze it, scraping up any seasonings and pieces of meat that are stuck to the pan. It doesn't have to simmer, just as long as you can lift the flavorful pieces off the skillet. Pour the broth into the slow cooker.

- Add the lime juice and coconut aminos to the slow cooker. Turn the beef over a few times in the bacon-onion mixture and broth.

- Place the bay leaves on top of the meat and place the lid on the slow cooker. Cook on low for 10 hours.

- Remove the meat from the slow cooker and place on a sheet pan. Use two forks to shred the beef. Pour 2 ladlefuls of liquid from the slow cooker over the beef and broil for 8 minutes, or until it reaches the desired crispiness.

- To build the perfect taco, pile carnitas in the middle of a tortilla, spoon on some guacamole, and garnish with pickled onions.

- Store leftovers in an airtight container in the fridge for up to 5 days or in the freezer for up to 30 days. To reheat, sauté in a skillet over medium heat.

PER SERVING (carnitas alone): Calories 213 · Fat 11g · Total Carbohydrate 5.6g · Dietary Fiber 0.8g · Protein 23.2g

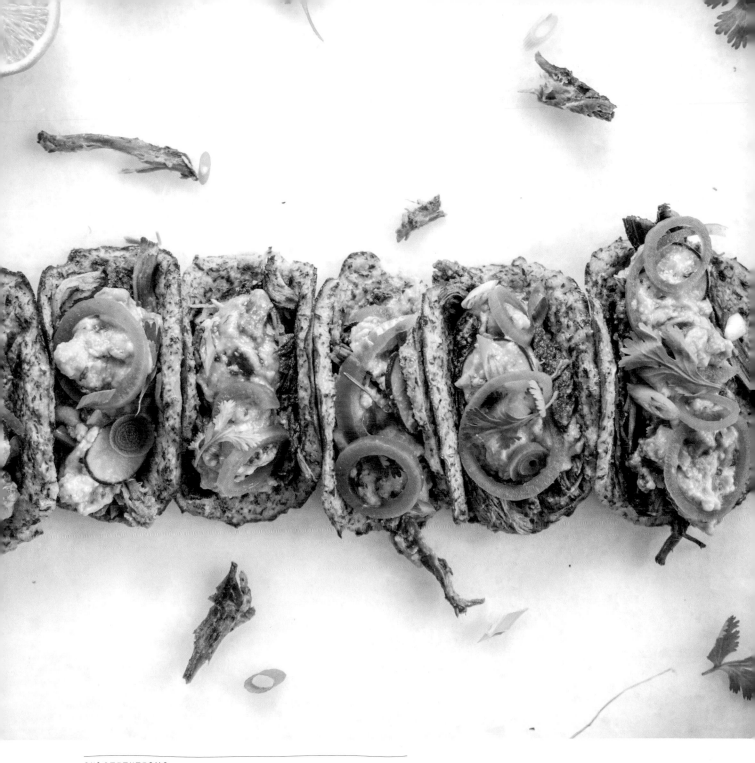

SUBSTITUTIONS: Unfortunately, I don't have an AIP-friendly tortilla option, but a thin slice of jicama works really well instead! It's not the lowest-carb option, but it's very tasty and easy to make. To make the carnitas AIP-compliant, omit the cumin and pepper and add 1 teaspoon horseradish and extra lime juice to boost the flavor. To make this dish pork-free, use turkey bacon!

spaghetti + meatballs

What's not to love about this classic family favorite? Noodles to slurp up and juicy meatballs and sauce to bring it all together. Made with zucchini noodles, which I like to call "zoodles," and Roasted Beet Marinara (page 78), this isn't your Nona's spaghetti and meatballs. It's super colorful and pleasing to the palate and the eyes. (Eating is a multisensory experience, after all!) To save time and get a superfine texture, I use my food processor to mince the vegetables and work them into the meat, creating a seasoned beef paste that has a fantastic flavor while hiding any chunks of vegetables, but you can also use a knife to mince the vegetables as finely as you can. The meatballs are pan-seared for a crispy browned exterior and finished off in the oven, freeing you up to finish the rest of the meal.

Makes 4 servings (plus extra meatballs)
PREP TIME: 20 minutes   COOK TIME: 40 minutes

FOR THE MEATBALLS:

(makes 20)

4 slices bacon

4 cloves garlic

3 ribs celery, roughly chopped

2 pounds ground beef (85% lean)

2 large eggs

2 tablespoons Italian herb blend

1 tablespoon fine Himalayan salt

2 teaspoons ground black pepper

2 cups Roasted Beet Marinara (page 78)

FOR THE NOODLES:

2 large zucchini

½ teaspoon fine Himalayan salt

FOR GARNISH:

¼ cup shelled hemp seeds (aka hemp hearts)

Chopped fresh parsley

○ Preheat the oven to 400°F.

○ Heat a large cast-iron skillet over medium heat. When it's hot, cook the bacon, flipping halfway through, until it has become crispy and rendered most of its fat, about 10 minutes.

○ In the meantime, place the garlic and celery in a food processor and pulse until minced. Add the ground beef, eggs, herb blend, salt, and pepper and pulse to combine.

○ Remove the bacon from the skillet, leaving the fat in the pan. Roughly chop the bacon, then add it to the food processor as well.

○ Process the bacon and beef mixture until a paste has formed. You might have to stop and use a spatula to move things along a few times. Once the meat mixture has an even texture and color, it's ready.

○ Using your hands, shape the meat mixture into 1-inch meatballs; you should get about twenty meatballs.

○ Set the skillet with the bacon fat over medium-high heat. Brown the meatballs in the bacon fat, six to eight at a time, for 6 minutes total, turning them every 2 minutes, then transfer the meatballs to a sheet pan. After all the meatballs are browned, bake them for 10 minutes to finish cooking them.

VARIATIONS: This dish works well with Cauliflower Alfredo (page 86), Cheesy Yellow Sauce (page 68), or Pistou (page 74). You can even make it with kelp noodles instead of zoodles. Omit the hemp seeds to make this dish AIP-compliant.

TIME-SAVING TIP: Many grocers now carry spiral-sliced vegetables. Pick up a package and save time on the zoodles! You can also prepare the zoodles ahead of time and keep them in the fridge wrapped in a kitchen towel for up to 5 days so they're ready to use when you need them.

PER SERVING (zoodles with ½ cup sauce and 3 meatballs): Calories **425** · Fat **29g** · Total Carbohydrate **9g** · Dietary Fiber **5.9g** · Protein **31.3g**

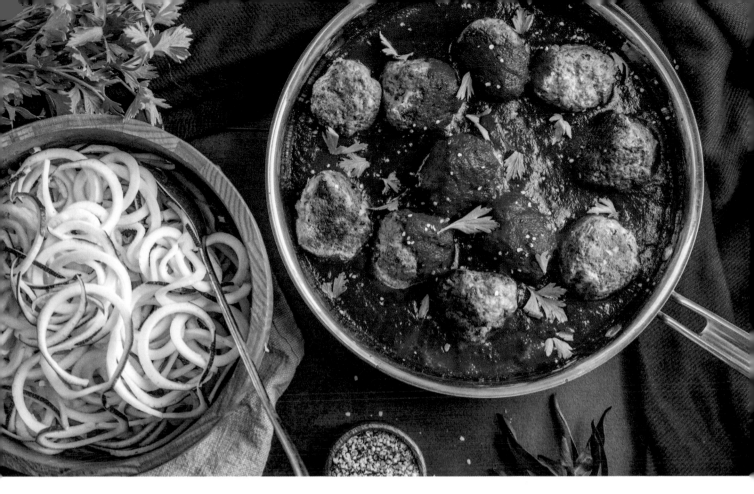

If you do not have a food processor, mince the garlic and celery and massage them into the beef with your hands to make a paste. *Warning:* Do not wear white while preparing this dish; the beautiful pink sauce will show up on light colors!

The extra meatballs will keep in an airtight container in the fridge for up to 6 days. Reheat them on the stovetop over medium heat in more marinara or in Cheesy Yellow Sauce (page 68) or Cauliflower Alfredo (page 86). Another great way to use up leftover meatballs is to slice them and pan-fry them in a little oil until they are browned and crispy. Serve the fried meatball rounds with fried eggs over Spinach Salad (page 348) or toss them with Creamy Kale Noodles (page 320) for a quick meal!

◦ While the meatballs are in the oven, prepare the rest of the ingredients.

◦ Heat the marinara in a large skillet over low heat.

◦ Using a spiral slicer, slice the zucchini into noodles. If you do not have a spiral slicer, use a vegetable peeler to make ribbons. Toss the noodles into a bowl with the salt and set a clean kitchen towel over them, tucking the towel underneath the noodles. The towel will soak up any liquid they release. Set aside at the back of the stove or in another warm area of your kitchen to take the chill off of them.

◦ In a small skillet over high heat, toast the hemp seeds for 2 to 3 minutes, moving quickly, until they begin to smell like popcorn.

◦ When the meatballs are ready, remove from the oven and add twelve meatballs to the sauce, spooning a little marinara over them. Let the other meatballs cool before storing in the fridge.

◦ Give the zucchini noodles a squeeze in the towel. Shake them out of the towel and divide among four serving plates. Spoon three meatballs and some sauce over each serving of zoodles and garnish with fresh parsley and toasted hemp seeds.

churrasco + chimichurri

My father is a butcher and my stepfather is Argentine. Needless to say, grilling meats is in my blood. Family gatherings usually include pounds of churrasco grilled up, sliced thin, and passed around on trays as we graze and talk for hours. I hope the guys don't mind, but I've changed up the cooking method a bit here. Grilling just isn't possible year-round in most regions, so I've switched things up for the perfect stovetop churrasco. Scoring the meat and quickly searing it in a blazing-hot skillet will produce a tender steak, served with al dente asparagus and loads of chimichurri!

1 pound skirt steak

1 teaspoon fine Himalayan salt

1 pound asparagus (about 15 spears)

1 tablespoon avocado oil

½ cup Chimichurri (page 80)

Makes 4 servings
PREP TIME: 10 minutes   COOK TIME: 16 minutes

○ Heat a large cast-iron skillet over medium heat until it's really hot, about 10 minutes.

○ Meanwhile, score the meat, making shallow cuts on the underside in a crisscross pattern. Skirt steak usually comes in foot-long strips; cut the strip into three or four pieces that fit in the skillet. Sprinkle the meat with the salt.

○ When the skillet is hot, fit as many strips of steak as you can in the skillet without overcrowding it—you may need to cook them in two batches. Sear the steak for 4 minutes on each side, or until well browned with charred bits. The meat will be crispy on the outside and medium on the inside. For medium-well steak, cook for another minute on each side.

○ When there's enough space in the skillet—usually when you're on the last batch of steak strips—throw the asparagus in there, too. Drizzle with the oil and cook for 4 minutes, turning once.

○ Serve with chimichurri spooned over everything. Store leftovers in an airtight container in the fridge for up to 4 days. To reheat, sear in a hot skillet for 2 minutes on each side.

CHEF'S NOTE: You're going to want to turn on the range hood and the ceiling fan and maybe open a window, too. Cooking steak on cast iron can really smoke up the joint.

PER SERVING (with 2 tablespoons chimichurri): Calories **333** · Fat **20.8g** · Total Carbohydrate **2.3g** · Dietary Fiber **2.7g** · Protein **31.8g**

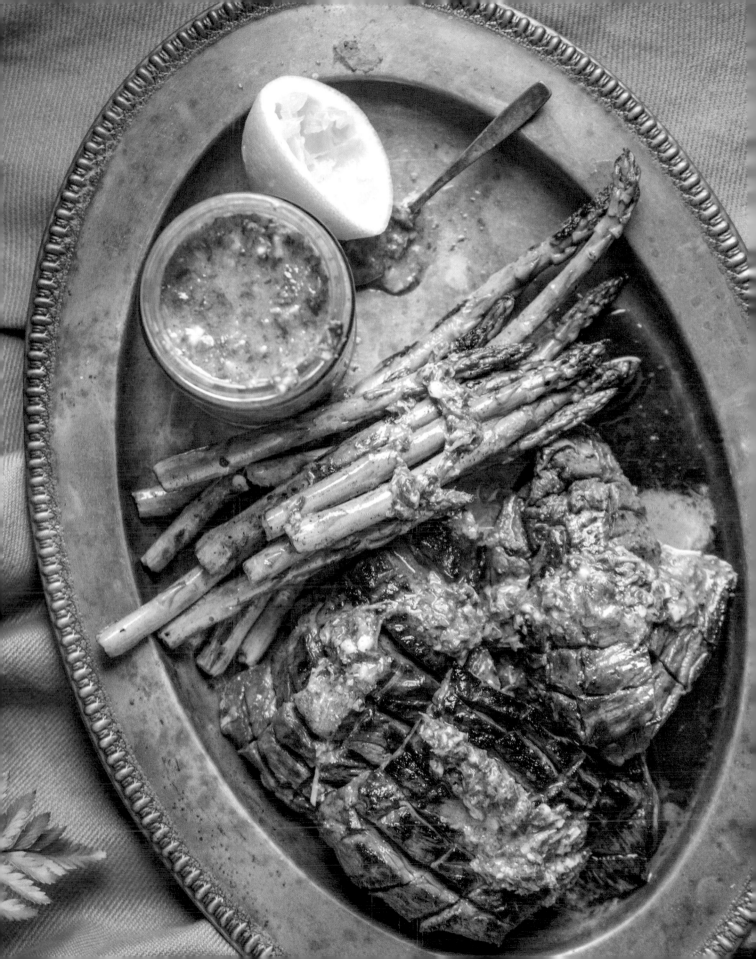

suya stir-fry

Suya is West African street food: sirloin skewers crusted with spices and crushed roasted peanuts. Yes, I know, holy cow, that sounds amazing. While in the past I've re-created these skewers with a combination of toasty seeds and warm nightshade-free spices, they were quite labor-intensive. I wanted the crunchy, nutty, warm goodness of suya without the hours of work, so I took those flavors and made a totally weeknight-worthy stir-fry. I used tri-tip steak because it tends to be more affordable, but feel free to use sirloin. The steak is tossed in a toasty seedy seasoning and sautéed with onions and green beans for a one-skillet meal that is bursting with flavor! The flax reacts wonderfully with the liquid in the recipe to create a sauce with a fantastic mouthfeel. The meat is flavorful and tender while the green beans remain crisp.

2 tablespoons raw pumpkin seeds

2 tablespoons whole flax seeds or flaxseed meal

2 tablespoons avocado oil, lard, or unsalted butter

1 medium onion, sliced

3 cloves garlic, minced

1 pound tri-tip or sirloin steak

1½ teaspoons fine Himalayan salt, divided

1 teaspoon garlic powder

1 teaspoon ginger powder

1 teaspoon ground black pepper

¼ teaspoon ground cloves

½ cup bone broth (page 100)

2 tablespoons coconut aminos

½ teaspoon liquid smoke (optional)

½ pound fresh green beans, trimmed and halved

Makes 4 servings
PREP TIME: 15 minutes   COOK TIME: 25 minutes

◦ Place the seeds in a coffee grinder, blender, or mortar and pestle and grind to a coarse crumble. Set aside.

◦ Heat a large skillet over medium heat. When it's hot, add the avocado oil, onions, and garlic. Sauté, stirring occasionally, until tender, about 8 minutes.

◦ Meanwhile, cut the beef into ½-inch pieces and place in a bowl with ¾ teaspoon of the salt, the garlic power, ginger powder, pepper, ground cloves, and ground seeds. Toss to combine and coat the beef.

◦ When the onion is tender, add the beef and all of the seedy seasoning mix to the skillet. Sauté, stirring often, until the meat is browned, about 8 minutes. As you stir, a lot of the seasoning will begin to stick to the bottom of the skillet; that's okay.

◦ Stir in the broth, coconut aminos, and liquid smoke (if using) and bring to a quick simmer. Use a spoon or spatula to gently scrape all the seasonings off of the bottom of the skillet and stir them in.

◦ Add the green beans to the skillet and sauté, stirring often, for another 4 to 5 minutes. Sprinkle in the remaining ¾ teaspoon of salt.

◦ Stir well and serve! Store leftovers in an airtight container in the fridge for up to 5 days. Reheat in a skillet over medium heat for 5 minutes or in the microwave on high for 1 to 2 minutes.

CHEF'S NOTE: If you really want to boost the nutty flavor, toast the seeds in a skillet until aromatic before grinding.

PER SERVING: Calories **410** · Fat **26.9g** · Total Carbohydrate **15.4g** · Dietary Fiber **6.1g** · Protein **28.2g**

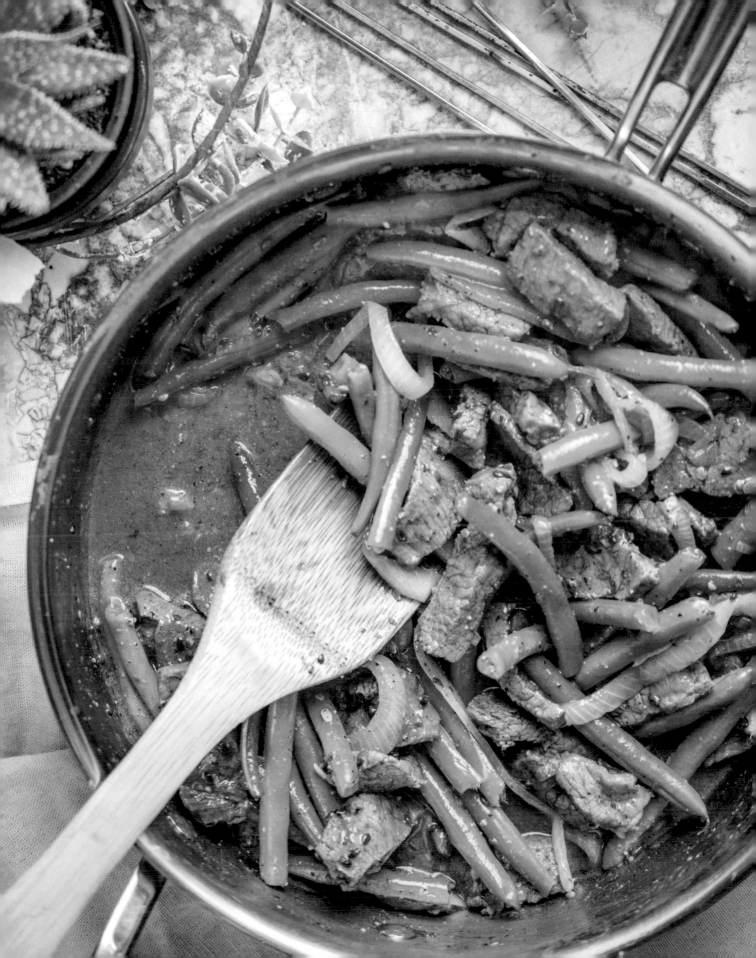

bacon-wrapped meatloaf

If you haven't baked your meatloaf like a log on a sheet pan, you're missing out. I never understood the appeal of a mushy meatloaf baked in a loaf pan, swimming it its own juices. I like my food with a proper brown on it, flavor and texture all over, and if I can make it look nice, too, then I call it a win. Not only is this recipe super easy, but it's good-looking, too! It goes great with Spiced Broccolini with Cool Cilantro Sauce (page 336) or Loaded Roasted Carrots (page 334).

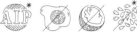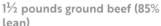

Makes 6 servings
PREP TIME: 10 minutes   COOK TIME: 50 minutes

1½ pounds ground beef (85% lean)

½ large red onion, minced

4 cloves garlic, minced

2 teaspoons dry mustard

2 teaspoons garlic powder

1½ teaspoons fine Himalayan salt

1 teaspoon ground black pepper

1 teaspoon onion powder

2 tablespoons avocado oil

2 tablespoons flaxseed meal

2 tablespoons red wine vinegar

½ pound bacon (7 or 8 slices)

○ Preheat the oven to 400°F. Line a sheet pan with parchment paper.

○ Place the ground beef, onions, garlic, dry mustard, garlic powder, salt, pepper, and onion powder in a large bowl and mix thoroughly to combine.

○ Add the avocado oil, flaxseed meal, and vinegar and mix again until thoroughly combined.

○ On one side of the sheet pan, shape the meat mixture into a loaf about 8 inches long and 3 to 4 inches tall. Lay the bacon slices in the center of the sheet pan and line them up so the sides overlap by ¼ inch. Lay the meatloaf in the center of the bacon. Bring the bacon slices up, wrapping them around the meatloaf and creating a seam at the top. Make sure to wrap tightly. Quickly flip the meatloaf over so the bacon seam is on the bottom. Fix the bacon slices if needed to make sure there are no gaps.

○ Bake the meatloaf for 50 minutes, or until the bacon is browned and crispy. Remove from the oven and let cool for 10 minutes.

○ Cut the meatloaf into slices the same width as the bacon slices. Serve right away.

○ Store leftovers in an airtight container in the fridge for up to a week. Reheat the slices in a skillet over medium heat until warm.

SUBSTITUTIONS: If you can't do flaxseed meal, you can omit it and use 1 large egg instead. To make this dish AIP-compliant, replace the dry mustard and pepper with 1 teaspoon ginger powder, and replace the flaxseed meal with 1 teaspoon coconut flour and 1 tablespoon unflavored grass-fed beef gelatin.

PER SERVING (1.5 slices): Calories **523** · Fat **39.2g** · Total Carbohydrate **4.9g** · Dietary Fiber **1.8g** · Protein **36.6g**

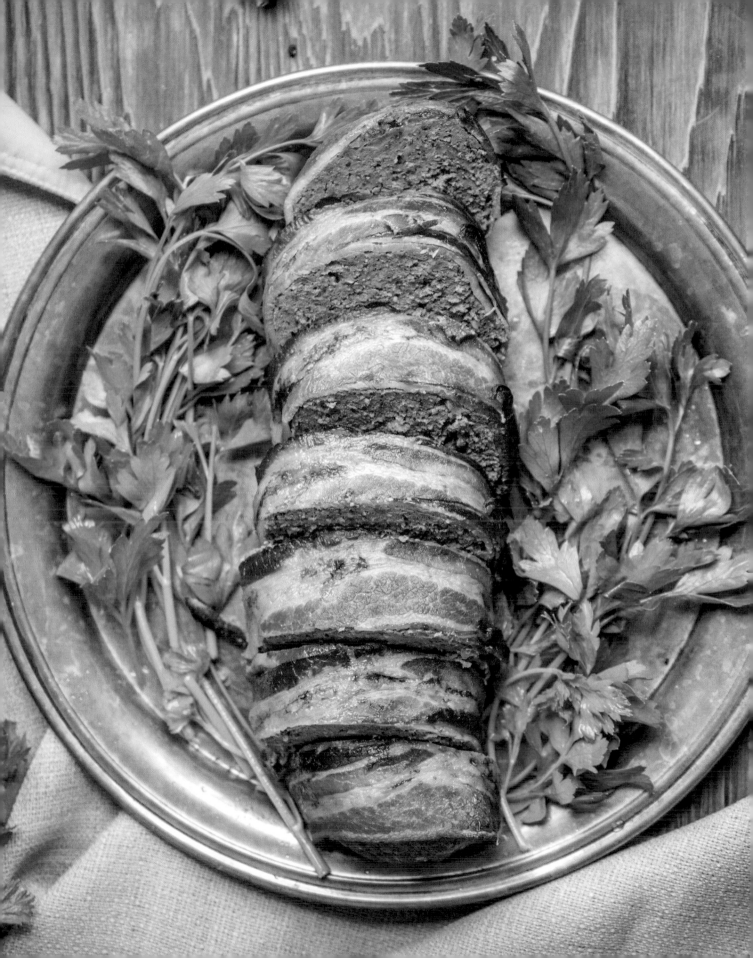

braised short ribs

The first time I made these short ribs was for an audience. I was hosting the Whole30 Recipes Instagram account, and I had spent the week kitchen-foraging and creating in-the-moment meals on Instagram Stories for the kind folks following along. What a studious crowd—several people took notes and made this dish themselves. Turns out, even some southerners gave this their seal of approval—high praise from connoisseurs of braised meats and comfort foods. I had to scramble to write notes about what I did afterward so I could remake it—you know, just to taste it, quality control and all that (wink wink). This hearty meal needs no accompaniment, but it is quite delicious over cauliflower rice or with Creamy Cauliflower Mash (page 318).

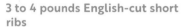

3 to 4 pounds English-cut short ribs

½ cup Greek Marinade + Dressing (page 108)

½ cup diced celery

½ cup diced red onions

4 cloves garlic, minced

3 teaspoons fine Himalayan salt, divided

2 teaspoons dried rosemary needles

2 teaspoons ground black pepper, divided

3 cups shredded cabbage or collard greens

1 cup frozen blueberries

2 cups bone broth (page 100)

¼ cup red wine vinegar

2 tablespoons nutritional yeast, for garnish (optional)

Special equipment:

Dutch oven

CHEF'S NOTE: To make this recipe in a pressure cooker, do the stovetop cooking as instructed using the sauté function of your pressure cooker. Then close the lid and cook on high for 50 minutes.

Makes 6 servings
PREP TIME: 15 minutes, plus at least 30 minutes to marinate   COOK TIME: 3½ hours

○ In a large bowl, toss the short ribs with the marinade. Cover and put in the refrigerator to marinate for at least 30 minutes or up to overnight.

○ Preheat the oven to 325°F.

○ Heat a Dutch oven over medium heat. When it's hot, use tongs to remove the short ribs from the marinade and place them in the pot, reserving the marinade. Brown the short ribs on all sides, about 3 minutes per side. You may have to do so in batches if they don't all fit at the same time. When seared, remove from the pot and set aside.

○ The pot should have accumulated fat from the short ribs on the bottom. Add the celery and onions and sauté until translucent and aromatic. Add the garlic, 1½ teaspoons of the salt, the rosemary, and 1 teaspoon of the pepper. Cook, stirring continuously, for 2 to 3 minutes, until fragrant.

○ Add the shredded cabbage and sauté until it begins to wilt. Return the short ribs to the pot and add the reserved marinade, blueberries, remaining 1½ teaspoons of salt, and remaining teaspoon of pepper. Use the tongs to mix as well as possible. Pour in the broth and vinegar, bring to a rapid boil, and cook for 10 to 15 minutes, until the liquid has reduced by half.

○ Cover the pot and place it in the oven. Cook for 3 hours. Remove from the oven and use tongs and a spoon to shred the meat and fish out the bones. Stir well and serve! Garnish with the nutritional yeast, if desired.

○ Store leftovers in an airtight container in the fridge for up to 5 days or in the freezer for up to 30 days. To reheat, bring to a simmer on the stovetop.

SUBSTITUTIONS: To make this dish AIP-compliant, omit the pepper. (Remember to omit it from the marinade as well.)

PER SERVING: Calories **704** · Fat **55g** · Total Carbohydrate **7.5g** · Dietary Fiber **1.9g** · Protein **47g**

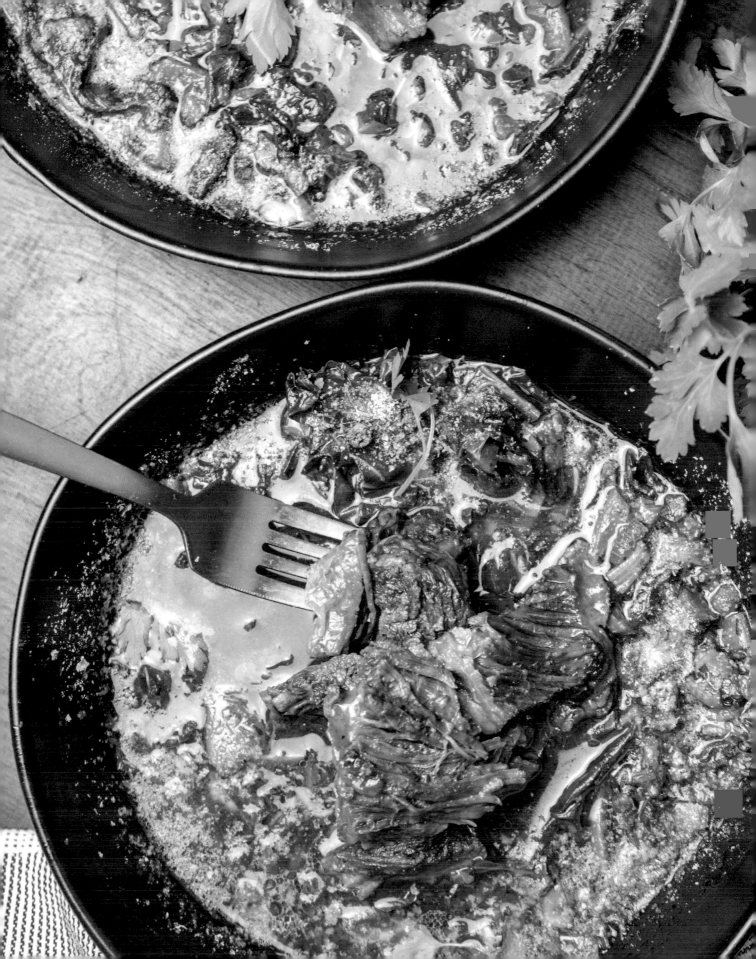

saucy seasoned liver

Offal isn't awful! I remember eating higado *(liver) when I was a kid, especially at my aunt's house. My Tia Silvy, who was never a health-food connoisseur (until recently), has always loved liver. She would prepare it* a lo Italiano, *which is how my* abuela *always made it—marinated with lemon and cooked up with lots of pepper and onions. The way she truly enjoyed eating liver made me love eating it, too. Somewhere in my twenties, I lost that love for liver, but during my healing journey I learned that what you do eat is just as important as what you don't eat— and organ meat is the gold standard for nutrient density! This recipe is for my Tia Silvy, who reminded me how delicious liver can truly be.*

1 pound pastured beef liver, cut into ½-inch cubes (see Notes)

1 sweet onion, thinly sliced

Juice of 2 limes

1 teaspoon granulated garlic

1 teaspoon ground black pepper

2 tablespoons ghee or other cooking fat (see page 53)

1 tablespoon coconut aminos

1 tablespoon Dijon mustard

1 teaspoon fine Himalayan salt

1 recipe Tender Kale Salad (page 344), for serving

Makes 4 servings
PREP TIME: 10 minutes   COOK TIME: 8 minutes

○ Heat a large skillet over medium heat.

○ While the skillet heats up, place the liver, onion slices, lime juice, granulated garlic, and pepper in a large bowl. Toss to combine and let the liver marinate for a few minutes.

○ When the skillet is hot, melt the ghee. Remove the liver from the marinade, reserving the onions and marinade, and place the liver in the skillet. Sauté, stirring occasionally, for about 5 minutes.

○ Add the onions and marinade and continue to sauté for another 3 minutes. Liver should be cooked to medium, brown on the outside and just pink in the center. Well-done liver is very tough to chew.

○ Stir in the coconut aminos and mustard. Remove from the heat, sprinkle with the salt, and serve right away with the salad.

○ I do not recommend storing liver; reheating would overcook it, making it tough and chewy.

CHEF'S NOTES: I am a huge proponent of consuming organ meat. If sautéed liver isn't your thing, try the liver pâté recipe on my blog, *The Castaway Kitchen.* What you do eat is just as important as, or more important than, what you don't. Nothing compares to organ meat when it comes to nutrient density.

Sourcing pastured organ meats is key; you want liver from grass-fed cows, not grain-fed cows. If you don't eat grains, why eat an animal that ate them? I find frozen beef livers at my local Whole Foods. You can also order pastured meats online from US Wellness Meats.

SUBSTITUTIONS: Omit the mustard and pepper to make this AIP-compliant.

PER SERVING (without salad): Calories **227** · Fat **10.6g** · Total Carbohydrate **8.4g** · Dietary Fiber **0.9g** · Protein **23.7g**

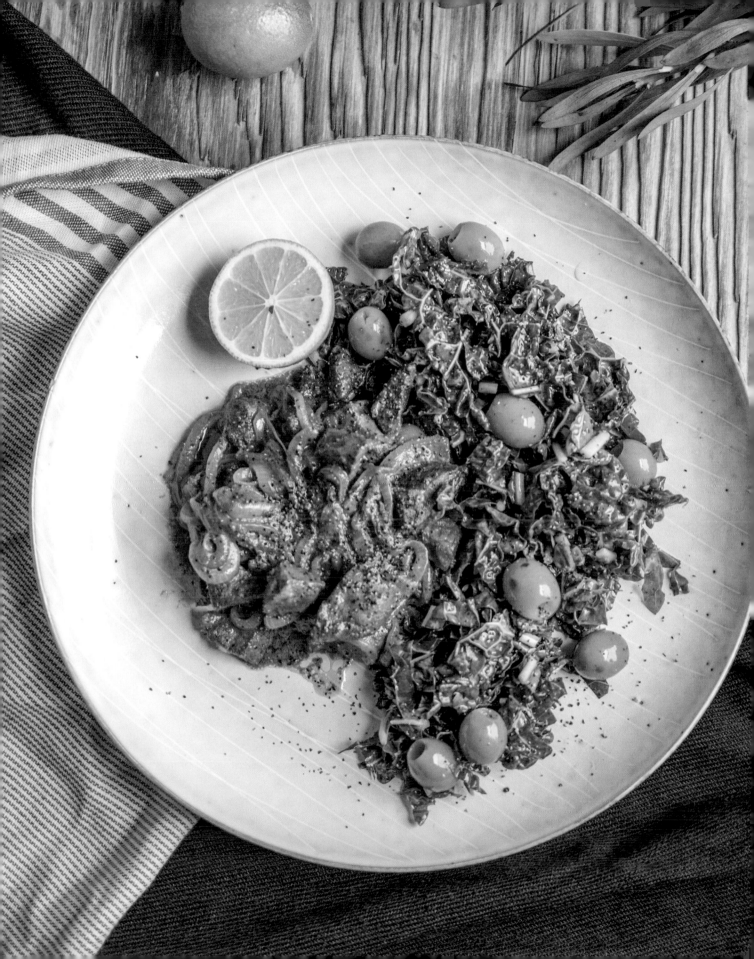

party meatballs

What is it about tiny food that is just so damn festive? Maybe it's the one-bite, toothpick-friendly thing. Making these meatballs took me back to my catering days, but I'll share a little secret: you don't have to have a party to make these! They are great for make-ahead meals and the perfect size for lunch boxes and little fingers. The most tedious thing about this recipe is shaping all the mini meatballs, but a small cookie scoop or ice cream scoop makes short work of it.

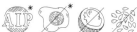
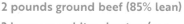

Makes 50 mini meatballs (5 per serving)
PREP TIME: 20 minutes   COOK TIME: 10 minutes

2 pounds ground beef (85% lean)

3 large egg whites, beaten (see Notes)

2 tablespoons red wine vinegar

1 tablespoon nutritional yeast

2 teaspoons dried dill weed

2 teaspoons dried parsley

2 teaspoons fine Himalayan salt

2 teaspoons garlic powder

2 teaspoons ground black pepper

2 teaspoons onion powder

1 cup coconut oil or other cooking fat (see page 53), or more if needed, for frying

Ranch Dressing (page 94) or Fiesta Guacamole (page 90), for serving (optional)

◦ Arrange the oven racks in the middle and bottom positions. Preheat the oven to 400°F. Line two sheet pans with parchment paper.

◦ Place all the ingredients except the coconut oil and dressing in a large bowl. Mix well with your hands. Shape the meat mixture into ½-inch meatballs. Use a small scoop or teaspoon to measure, then roll them between your hands to shape them. Place on the prepared sheet pans and bake for 10 minutes.

◦ While the meatballs bake, heat a large pot over medium-high heat. Pour in the coconut oil—it should be 1 inch deep—and heat until the oil sizzles around the end of a wooden spoon handle when it's inserted in the oil. Add about fifteen meatballs at a time to the pot and cook for 3 to 5 minutes, using a slotted spoon to move and turn the meatballs as they cook. Then use the spoon to remove them from the oil and set on a paper towel–lined plate to drain. Repeat until all of the meatballs are browned and crispy.

◦ Serve the meatballs with toothpicks and ranch dressing, guacamole, or another sauce for dipping, if desired.

◦ Store leftovers in an airtight container in the fridge for up to 5 days. To reheat, bake in a preheated 350°F oven for 10 minutes.

SUBSTITUTIONS: To make these meatballs egg-free, use 2 tablespoons flaxseed meal instead of the egg whites. To make them AIP-compliant, replace the pepper and egg whites with 1 teaspoon coconut flour and 1 tablespoon unflavored grass-fed beef gelatin.

CHEF'S NOTES: If you are preparing these meatballs ahead of time, you can bake them and store them par-cooked in the fridge for up to 3 days, then fry them per the recipe instructions to heat and serve.

After you separate out the egg whites, use the yolks to make Homemade Mayo (page 82) or Hollandaise (page 196).

PER SERVING: Calories **305** · Fat **24.5g** · Total Carbohydrate **0.8g** · Dietary Fiber **0.6g** · Protein **20.2g**

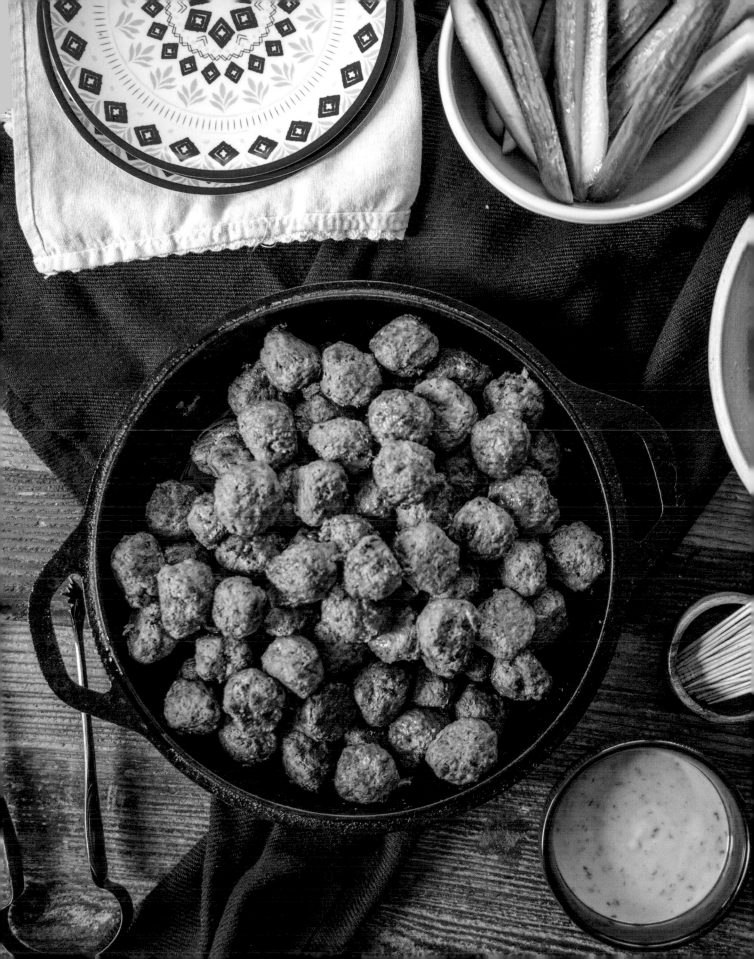

gyro skillet sausages

I'm all about recipe mash-ups, borrowing flavors from various cultures and mixing them up to create one tasty meal. These crispy gyro-inspired sausages are great over salads or in tacos. Dip them in Tzatziki (page 98) or pour it on top; these two were made for each other.

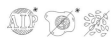

1 pound ground beef (85% lean)

1 pound ground lamb

1 tablespoon dried oregano

2 teaspoons fine Himalayan salt

2 teaspoons ground black pepper

1 teaspoon ground cumin

1 small onion, roughly chopped

½ cup chopped fresh parsley or cilantro

2 large eggs

2 tablespoons coconut flour

1 tablespoon cooking fat (see page 53), or more if needed

Makes 12 sausages (2 per serving)
PREP TIME: 20 minutes   COOK TIME: 45 minutes

○ In a large bowl, mix together the ground beef and lamb using your hands. Add the oregano, salt, pepper, and cumin and mix thoroughly. Set aside.

○ Place the onions, parsley, and eggs in a food processor or blender. Pulse until the parsley and onion are finely minced and almost pureed. Add this to the meat mixture along with the coconut flour. Mix thoroughly.

○ Heat a large cast-iron skillet over medium heat. While it heats, shape the sausages: Take about ¼ cup of the meat mixture and roll it into a cylindrical shape no more than 2 inches in diameter and 3 inches long. Repeat with the rest of the meat mixture.

○ When the sausages are ready and the skillet is hot, heat the cooking fat in the skillet. Add four sausages, or as many as will fit without crowding the pan, and cook for 15 minutes, using tongs to gently turn the sausages every 3 to 5 minutes so they brown on all sides. When they have a nice dark crust on all sides, transfer them to a paper towel–lined plate.

○ Repeat with the next two batches of sausages, adding more cooking fat as needed between batches. There might be quite a bit of splatter, so use a splatter screen if you have one to avoid a mess.

○ Store leftovers in an airtight container in the fridge for up to 4 days. To reheat, bake in a preheated 350°F oven for 5 minutes.

VARIATIONS: If you're not a lamb lover, use 2 pounds ground beef or a mixture of ground beef and pork instead.

SUBSTITUTIONS: To make these sausages AIP-compliant, omit the cumin, pepper, and eggs and add 1 tablespoon lemon juice or vinegar and 1 tablespoon unflavored grass-fed beef gelatin to the meat mixture.

CHEF'S NOTE: You can mince the onion and parsley by hand and whisk them with the eggs rather than pureeing them in a blender. I prefer the puree mainly because I have a picky eater at home who will sit there and pick out all the pieces of onion. But also, the smoother the onion-parsley-egg mixture, the more structural integrity the sausages will have.

PER SERVING: Calories **312** · Fat **18.4g** · Total Carbohydrate **2.2g** · Dietary Fiber **2.3g** · Protein **32.7g**

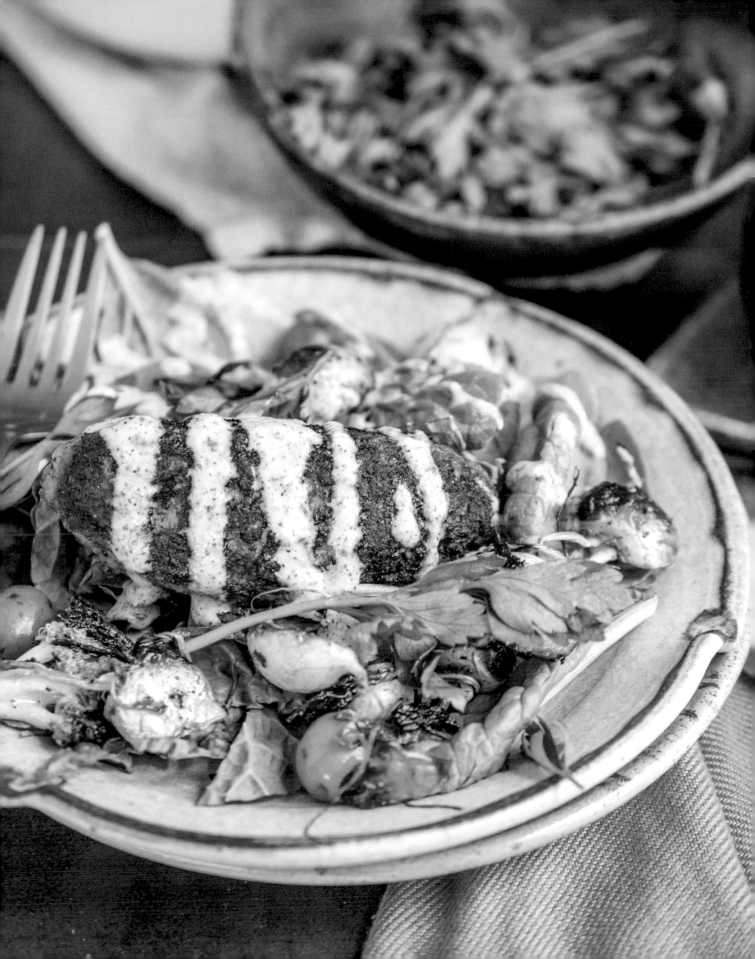

protein fried rice

This one-pan meal is inspired by my friend ChihYu, who blogs over at I Heart Umami. The mixture of beef and pork cooked with sesame oil and fresh aromatics is her signature flavor. The crispy morsels of meat outnumber the grains of cauliflower rice, and the dish is studded with tender green vegetables for a dinner that everyone will love. I like to top it with sliced avocado and sesame seeds. If you have a picky eater like I do, there is time to separate a portion of plain browned meat before adding the veggies, and not an onion in sight. Parents everywhere, you're welcome.

Makes 6 servings
PREP TIME: 10 minutes   COOK TIME: 25 minutes

1 pound ground beef (85% lean)

1 pound ground pork

3 tablespoons sesame oil, divided

3 tablespoons coconut aminos, divided

1 tablespoon coconut oil or lard

3 ribs celery, diced

3 cloves garlic, minced

2 green onions, sliced

1 tablespoon peeled and minced fresh ginger

½ cup chopped asparagus spears

1 tablespoon fish sauce

1 teaspoon fine Himalayan salt

1 teaspoon ground black pepper

1 teaspoon onion powder

1½ cups riced cauliflower (see Note, page 140)

Sesame seeds, for garnish (optional)

◦ In a large bowl, mix together the ground beef and pork using your hands. Pour in 1 tablespoon of the sesame oil and 1 tablespoon of the coconut aminos. Gently mix and set aside.

◦ Heat a large skillet over medium heat. When it's hot, melt the coconut oil in the skillet. Add the celery, garlic, green onions, and ginger. Sauté, stirring often, for 5 minutes, then remove the mixture from the skillet and set aside. Don't wash the skillet.

◦ Add the meat mixture to the skillet, using your fingers to crumble it. Cook, using a whisk to break it up and stir it frequently, until browned and crumbled, 3 to 5 minutes. Continue to cook, stirring occasionally, until any fluid the meat released has evaporated, about another 10 minutes. It will smell divine, and there will be dark brown bits among the meat.

◦ Add the cooked aromatics to the skillet, along with the asparagus, the remaining 2 tablespoons of sesame oil, the remaining 2 tablespoons of coconut aminos, the fish sauce, salt, pepper, and onion powder. Immediately mix in the riced cauliflower, stir, and cook for another 5 minutes, until the rice is thoroughly combined and heated. Garnish with sesame seeds, if desired.

◦ Serve hot! Store leftovers in an airtight container in the fridge for up to 5 days. To reheat, sauté in a skillet over medium heat.

CHEF'S NOTE: For a super-boosted flavor and a creamy consistency, pour some Ginger Sauce (page 102) over this fried rice. There is something about creamy rice that is just so satisfying.

VARIATIONS: You can use all beef or all pork if you like. You can even use ground chicken or turkey. If using a leaner meat, mix 1 tablespoon cooking fat into it.

SUBSTITUTIONS: To make this dish AIP-compliant, omit the sesame oil and pepper and use 3 tablespoons garlic-infused avocado oil or bacon fat for flavor. If you're avoiding coconut, use lard and replace the coconut aminos with aged balsamic vinegar or a balsamic vinegar reduction.

PER SERVING: Calories **463** · Fat **35.3g** · Total Carbohydrate **6.6g** · Dietary Fiber **3g** · Protein **30.2g**

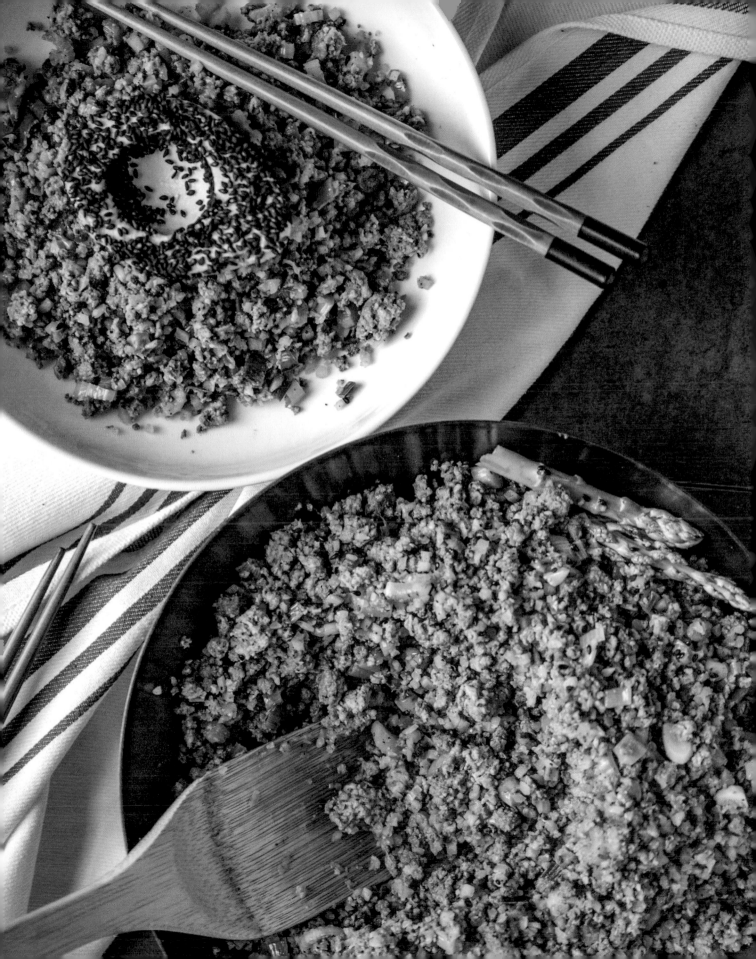

pan-seared rib-eye with arugula

When I graduated from college, my parents graciously sent me to Europe to travel a bit. It was really an elaborate ploy to get me to chaperone my little sister's middle-school trip—not what I had in mind. I did, however, get to spend some days with a friend who was doing a study-abroad program in Florence. Her boyfriend was local, and his family invited us to Easter luncheon. It was like something out of a movie: A rustic restaurant on a mountainside looking out over chianti vineyards. Courses and courses of food coming to the table. Heavy wooden boards overflowing with meats, olives, and cheeses. Of all the rich foods to grace my palate that day, my favorite was the steak—thin slices of rare meat, perfectly cooked and served simply with a pile of arugula on top. I have re-created that dish for you here. A big bone-in rib-eye is perfect for feeding a family. Cook one massive steak, top it with arugula, and feed a crowd.

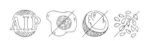

1 (1½- to 2-pound) bone-in rib-eye steak

2 tablespoons ghee or lard, divided

2 teaspoons fine Himalayan salt

5 cloves garlic, peeled

3 sprigs fresh oregano, thyme, or sage

2 cups fresh arugula

Makes 4 servings
PREP TIME: 5 minutes   COOK TIME: 15 minutes

○ Set the rib-eye out to come to room temperature about 30 minutes before you begin cooking.

○ Place a large cast-iron skillet in the oven and preheat the oven to 425°F.

○ While the oven heats, brush the steak with 1 tablespoon of the ghee and sprinkle it with the salt.

○ When the oven has come to temperature, remove the skillet and set it on the stovetop over medium heat. Place the steak in the skillet and sear for 2 minutes. Flip the steak with tongs and top it with the garlic and herbs. Sear for 2 minutes on the other side, then place the skillet with the steak in the oven for 8 to 10 minutes, depending on the thickness of the steak and the desired doneness.

○ Remove the skillet from the oven and return it to the stovetop over medium heat. Move the herbs and garlic to the side of the pan and dollop the remaining tablespoon of ghee over them.

○ Carefully tilt the skillet so the fat pools with the garlic and herbs. Using a small spoon, repeatedly pour this pooled fat over the steak as it cooks for 2 minutes.

○ Remove the steak from the skillet and set it on a cutting board to rest for 5 minutes. When ready to serve, run a sharp knife along the inside of the bone to separate the meat, then slice the steak against the grain in very thin slices.

○ Divide the steak slices among four plates. Add ½ cup arugula to each plate and spoon the pan sauce all over the arugula. Enjoy!

○ It's a shame to eat meat this good as leftovers—it's just not the same. But if you have extra, cut it up into small pieces and store in an airtight container in the fridge for up to 4 days. Reheat in a hot skillet. Rib-eye is fatty, so it will be nice and crispy; toss it with eggs or greens for a beef hash.

PER SERVING: Calories **586** · Fat **47g** · Total Carbohydrate **2g** · Dietary Fiber **0g** · Protein **38g**

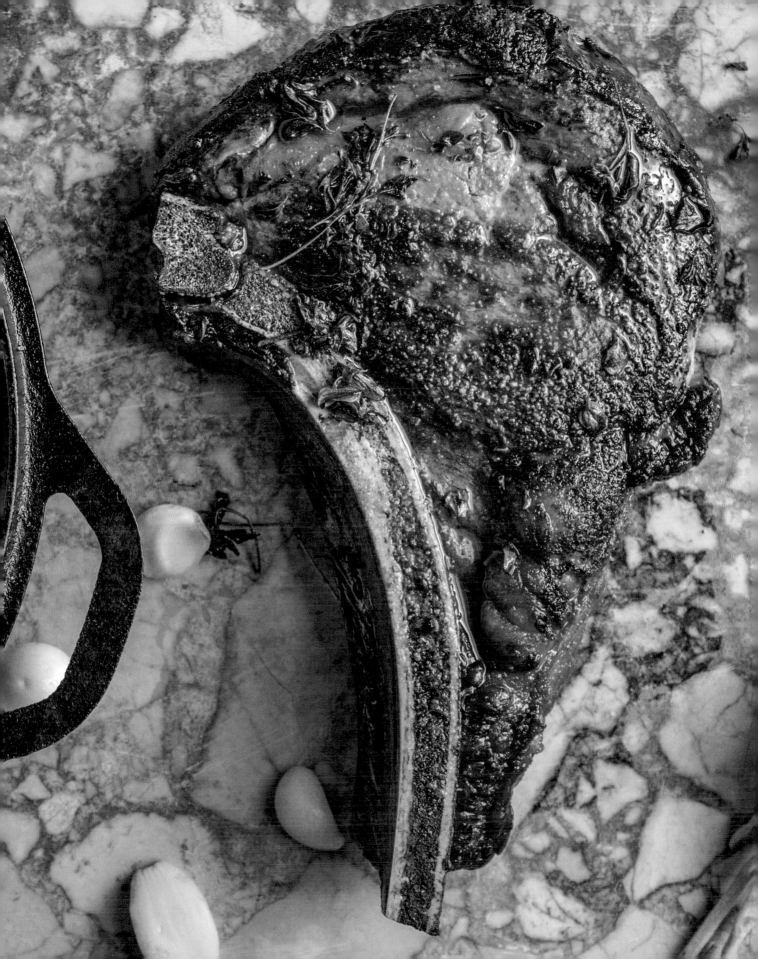

lazy moco

Loco moco is a dish I came to know when I moved to Hawaii. It's traditionally made with rice, a hamburger patty, a fried egg, and gravy. However, if I ordered it at a restaurant, my order would go something like this: "May I please have the loco moco, extra beef patty, no rice, over greens, hold the gravy (because it's not gluten-free)? Thanks!" Eventually, I thought to myself, girl, you can make this at home with cauliflower rice and Paleo gravy, and so I did. It was a lot of work, a meal with four separate hands-on components. So I changed it up and added a little sheet pan action to the dish, and you know what? It's easy and super quick. It's even a little lazy.

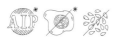

4 cups riced cauliflower (see Note, page 140)

2 tablespoons bacon fat, lard, or ghee, divided

2 teaspoons fine Himalayan salt, divided

1 pound ground beef (85% lean)

FOR THE GRAVY:

3 tablespoons ghee or lard

2 tablespoons coconut flour

1 cup bone broth (page 100)

1 tablespoon coconut vinegar

3 sprigs fresh thyme or rosemary

½ teaspoon fine Himalayan salt

½ teaspoon ground black pepper

4 large eggs

CHEF'S NOTE: The flavor and thickness of this gravy is delicious, but it's not as smooth as traditional gravy. The coconut flour gives it a slight grainy mouthfeel because coconut flour does not dissolve like cornstarch or tapioca starch. I think having a healthy, low-carb gravy that tastes amazing is a fair trade-off!

SUBSTITUTIONS: To make this dish AIP-compliant, use lard, omit the pepper, and skip the fried eggs.

Makes 4 servings
PREP TIME: 10 minutes   COOK TIME: 15 minutes

∘ Preheat the oven to 425°F.

∘ Spread the cauliflower on a sheet pan so that it takes up about three-quarters of it. Drizzle 1 tablespoon of the bacon fat over the cauliflower and sprinkle with 1 teaspoon of the salt.

∘ Form the beef into four patties about ¼ inch thick and make an indentation in the center of each patty. Coat the patties with the remaining tablespoon of fat and sprinkle with the remaining teaspoon of salt. Line them up next to the riced cauliflower in the empty space on the sheet pan. Place in the oven and roast for 15 minutes.

∘ Meanwhile, make the gravy: Melt the ghee in a small saucepan over medium-high heat. Whisk in the coconut flour and keep whisking until the flour is browned and smells toasty, almost like popcorn. This will take only a few minutes. Then pour in the broth and vinegar and stir until the mixture is smooth and fluid. Add the thyme sprigs, salt, and pepper and bring to a boil. Reduce the gravy for 5 to 8 minutes, whisking occasionally, until it becomes thick. When it's ready, it will coat a back of a spoon. Remove the gravy from the heat and discard the thyme sprigs.

∘ When the patties have about 5 minutes left to cook, heat a large skillet over medium heat. When it's hot, lightly grease the skillet, then crack in the eggs. Cook, undisturbed, until the whites are cooked through. Remove from the heat. Use the edge of the spatula to separate the eggs.

∘ Assemble four plates, each with a cup of riced cauliflower topped with a burger patty, a generous amount of gravy over the patty, and a fried egg. Enjoy!

∘ Store leftovers in an airtight container in the fridge for up to 5 days. To reheat, place in a skillet over medium heat, and fry the egg to order.

PER SERVING: Calories **541** · Fat **45.2g** · Total Carbohydrate **8.5g** · Dietary Fiber **5.1g** · Protein **30.9g**

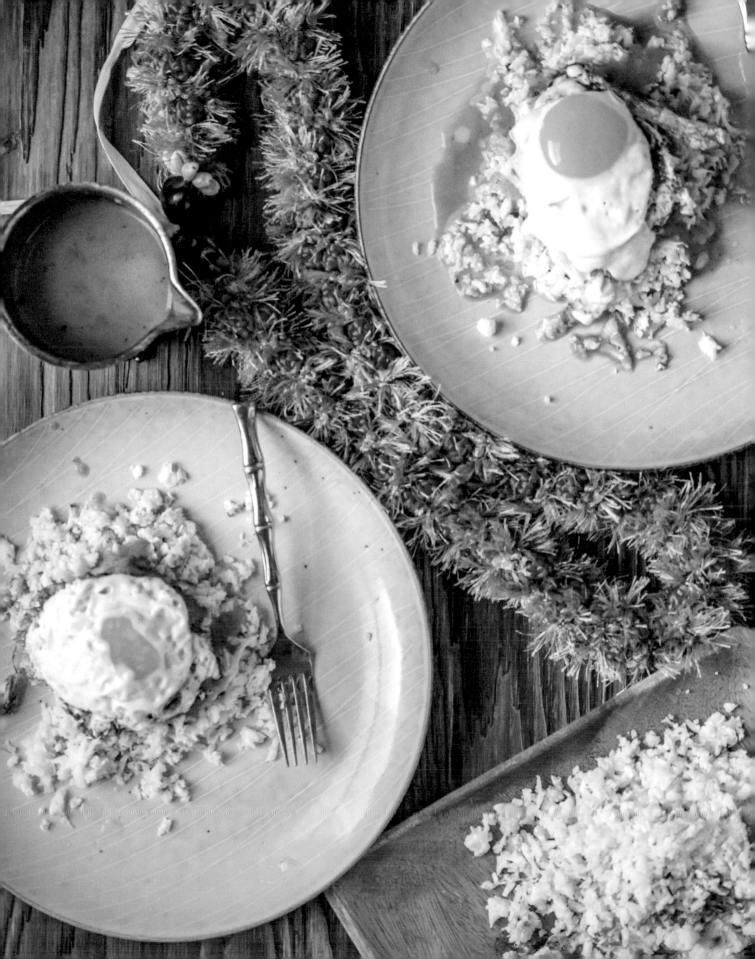

slow cooker shawarma

All the bold, delicious flavors of shawarma, made easy, tender, and juicy. This slow cooker rendition is absolutely divine, aromatic and bursting with flavor, with minimal hands-on time! I love to serve it with cauliflower rice, or you can get jazzy with Creamy Cilantro Rice (page 342) or pile it on crispy rounds of Crispy Thin Flatbread (page 134). Pickled Red Onions (page 88) are quite delicious as a garnish.

1 tablespoon fine Himalayan salt

1 tablespoon ground black pepper

1 tablespoon ground cumin

1 teaspoon ground cardamom

½ teaspoon ground nutmeg

3 pounds boneless chuck short rib or shoulder

¼ cup coconut vinegar or red wine vinegar

3 tablespoons avocado oil

5 cloves garlic, peeled

1 large onion, quartered

1 lemon, quartered

1 navel orange, quartered

Makes 5 or 6 servings
PREP TIME: 10 minutes, plus overnight to marinate
COOK TIME: 8 hours in a slow cooker

○ In a small bowl, mix together the salt, pepper, cumin, cardamom, and nutmeg. Rub the spice mixture all over the meat.

○ Place the meat in a large bowl and drizzle the vinegar and oil all over it. Add the garlic, onion, and citrus. Toss to combine, squeezing some juice out of the fruit. Cover and set in the refrigerator to marinate overnight.

○ When you're ready to cook, put everything in the slow cooker, meat on the bottom, citrus and onion quarters on top. Cook on low for 8 hours.

○ Discard the large pieces of citrus. Use two forks to shred the beef. If you like crispy beef, you can spread it on a sheet pan and broil it for 5 minutes to get delicious crispy tips. Divide the shredded beef among five or six plates, spoon the delicious slow cooker sauce over the meat, and serve.

○ Store leftovers in an airtight container in the fridge for up to 5 days or in the freezer for up to 30 days. To thaw and reheat, place in a preheated 400°F oven for 10 to 20 minutes.

PER SERVING (5 servings): Calories **496** · Fat **28.1g** · Total Carbohydrate **7.9g** · Dietary Fiber **1.6g** · Protein **53.9g**

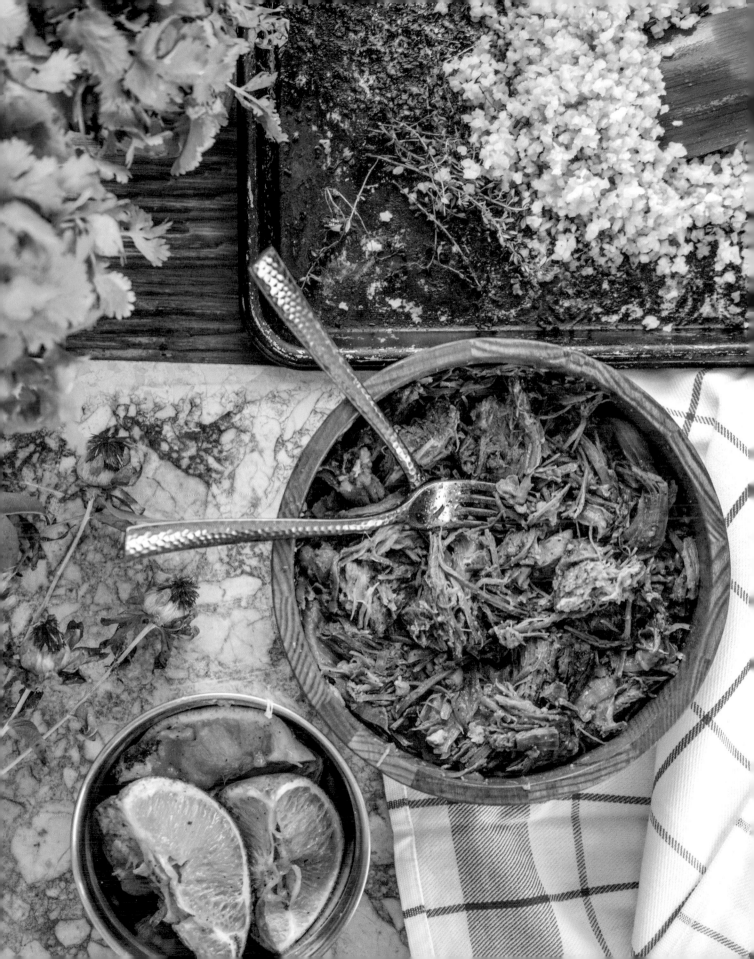

sticky pistou meatballs

Another meatball recipe made in a whole other way, because there is more than one way to make a delicious meatball and variety is the spice of life. The best thing about these sticky meatballs is how easily and quickly they come together. The second-best thing is how flexible this recipe is. You can make it as written with Pistou (page 74) for a salty herb flavor, or use Ginger Sauce (page 102) for teriyaki-inspired meatballs, or use Chimichurri (page 80) or Greek Marinade + Dressing (page 108). The stickiness that makes these slightly addictive comes from using gelatin in the mix—a great replacement for breadcrumbs or eggs in ground beef recipes!

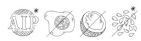

1⅓ pounds ground beef (85% lean)

¼ cup Pistou (page 74)

2 tablespoons unflavored grass-fed beef gelatin

1 teaspoon ground cumin

½ teaspoon fine Himalayan salt

Makes 12 meatballs (2 per serving)
PREP TIME: 10 minutes   COOK TIME: 25 minutes

∘ Preheat the oven to 425°F. Line a sheet pan with parchment paper.

∘ Crumble the ground beef into a large bowl. Add the remaining ingredients and mix with your hands until well combined.

∘ Shape the meat mixture into twelve 2-inch meatballs and place them on the prepared sheet pan. Bake for 15 minutes, use tongs to gently turn the meatballs over, and then bake for another 10 minutes. Remove from the oven and serve hot.

∘ Store leftover meatballs in an airtight container in the refrigerator for up to 5 days. To reheat, microwave on high for 1 minute or sauté over medium heat for 8 minutes.

CHEF'S NOTE: The oven temperature and cooking time are perfect for throwing in a sheet pan of broccoli florets, seasoned as instructed in the Chicken + Broccoli Bowls recipe (page 230), and cooking your side dish simultaneously. It's great for dinner in a pinch!

SUBSTITUTIONS: To make this recipe AIP-compliant, follow the AIP modifications for the pistou on page 74 and omit the cumin.

PER SERVING: Calories **470** · Fat **34.5g** · Total Carbohydrate **0.1g** · Dietary Fiber **0.6g** · Protein **38g**

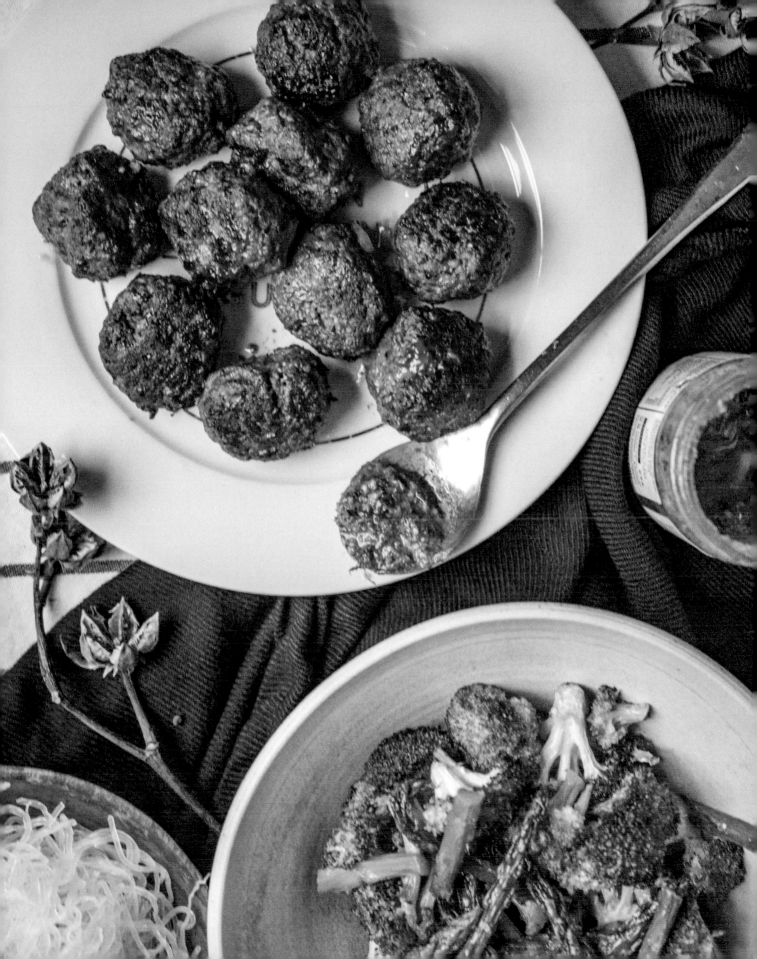

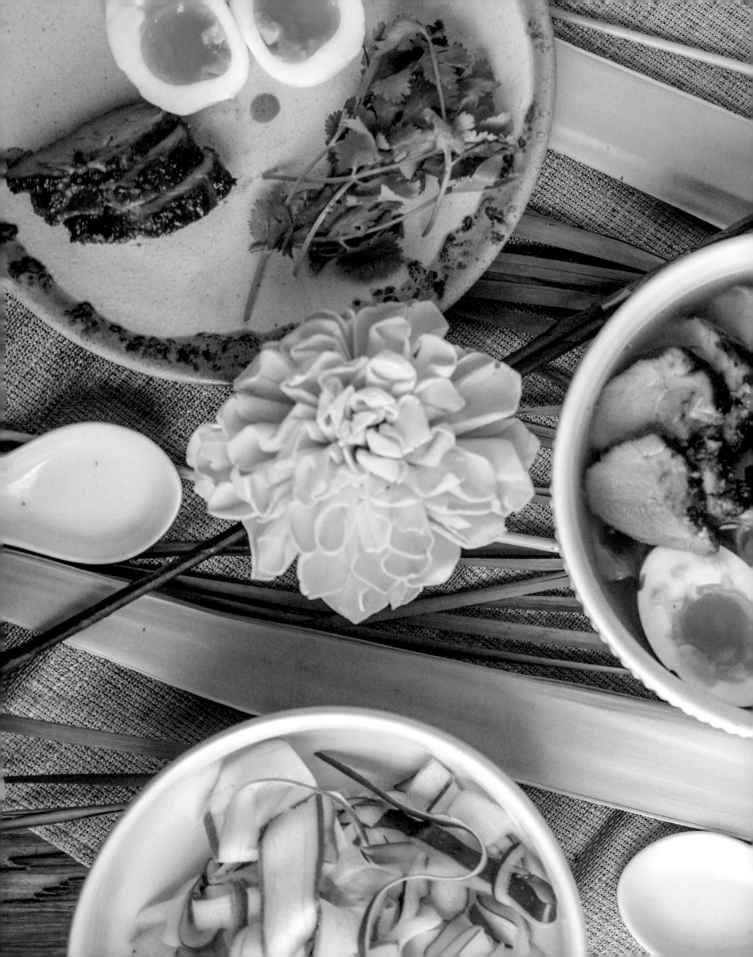

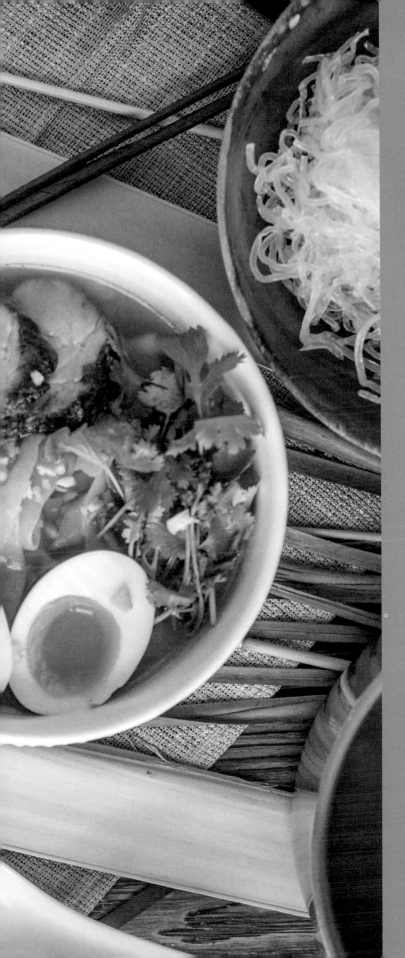

PORK

I'm Cuban, and we eat a lot of pork. However, besides my love of pork rinds, I don't really prepare too many traditional Cuban pork dishes. That's not to say I haven't picked up some skills through my restaurant and blogging work. This chapter highlights my favorite ways to cook pork to be fun, tender, flavorful, and doable on any budget or time frame.

pork char siu + ramen

Char siu is a Cantonese barbecue method known for its bright red sauce. This glazed, sticky, sweet pork is tender and bursting with flavor. Traditional recipes use a combination of soy, tomato, chili-based pastes, and sugar to create this flavor. Here, I have MacGyvered together an equally delicious sauce with coconut aminos, fish sauce, blackberries, and a little magic. After an overnight marinade and a quick stint in the oven, you have sticky, finger-licking-good pork. It's the ideal protein to go over a bowl of ramen made of your noodle of choice, some flavorful bone broth, a jammy egg, and a whole lot of ginger. Forget takeout; one bite of this sweet pork and you'll be hooked.

Makes 6 servings
PREP TIME: 30 minutes, plus at least 3 hours to marinate
COOK TIME: 30 minutes

FOR THE CHAR SIU:

1½ to 2 pounds pork tenderloin

1 teaspoon fine Himalayan salt

½ cup blackberries

4 tablespoons coconut aminos, divided

3 tablespoons lard, bacon fat, or ghee

2 tablespoons coconut vinegar

1 tablespoon Dijon mustard

1 tablespoon fish sauce

2 teaspoons ginger powder

1 teaspoon Chinese five-spice powder

1 teaspoon garlic powder

2 teaspoons granulated erythritol or other low-carb sweetener (see page 38)

FOR THE RAMEN:

6 cups bone broth (page 100)

4 cloves garlic, minced

1 (1-inch) piece fresh ginger, peeled and minced

2 tablespoons sesame oil (optional)

1 teaspoon coconut aminos

1 teaspoon fish sauce

1 teaspoon fine Himalayan salt

6 cups shirataki noodles

6 large eggs (optional)

½ ounce fresh cilantro or basil, trimmed, for garnish

○ Place the pork tenderloin in a freezer bag or airtight container. Sprinkle with the salt.

○ Heat a small saucepan over medium heat. Combine the blackberries, 2 tablespoons of the coconut aminos, lard, vinegar, mustard, fish sauce, ginger powder, Chinese five-spice powder, and garlic powder in the saucepan. Bring to a simmer and cook, stirring occasionally, for 8 to 10 minutes. When the blackberries have turned red, mash them.

○ Pour the sauce through a fine-mesh sieve into a small bowl, using a spoon to mash the berries and scraping the sieve to get as much out as possible. Let the sauce cool to room temperature.

○ Add the sauce to the pork and rub it all over, then seal the bag or container. Place in the fridge to marinate for at least 3 hours or up to overnight.

○ Set the pork out to come to room temperature 30 minutes before cooking. Preheat the oven to 350°F. Line a sheet pan with parchment paper and place a baking rack on it.

○ Remove the pork loin from the marinade and place it on the rack, reserving the marinade. Mix the marinade with the remaining 2 tablespoons of coconut aminos and the erythritol.

○ Place the pork on the middle rack of the oven and roast for 15 minutes, then spoon half of the marinade over it. Roast for another 7 to 10 minutes, until the internal temperature is 145°F. Spoon the remaining half of the marinade all over it. Broil for 2 minutes.

○ Remove the pork from the oven and let it rest for 5 minutes, then cut it into ¼-inch-thick slices.

PER SERVING: Calories **499** · Fat **21.7g** · Total Carbohydrate **7g** · Dietary Fiber **1g** · Protein **51.5g**

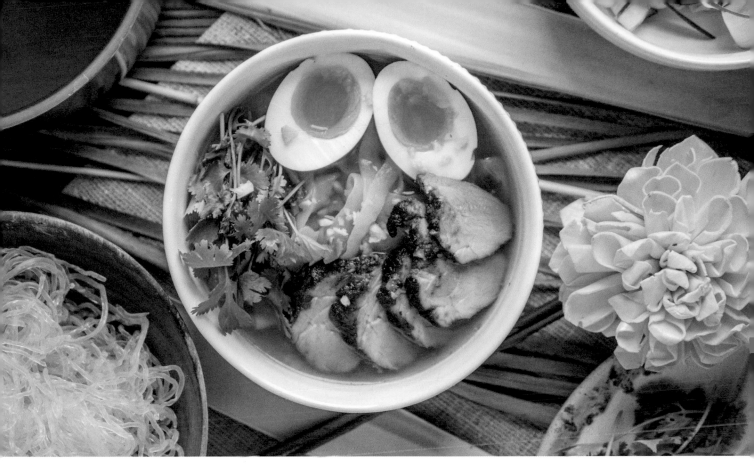

CHEF'S NOTE: Ramen is a completely satisfying meal. You can keep it simple with just broth, noodles, and pork or dress it up even more with bacon, sesame seeds, extra veggies—whatever your heart desires. Plus, this pork is amazing with just about any dish; try it over cauliflower rice or even in a salad.

VARIATIONS: Use kelp noodles! To prepare the kelp noodles, rinse them in cool water, then add them to the simmering broth to soften. You can also use fresh zucchini noodles.

TIME-SAVING TIP: Make the char siu ahead of time, as well as the hard-boiled eggs. If you have a dozen hard-boiled eggs in the fridge, they are ready for anything from Baked Scotch Eggs (page 178) to Fried Hard-Boiled Eggs (page 116) to this ramen!

○ While the pork roasts, prepare the ramen: In a large pot, mix the broth with the garlic, ginger, sesame oil (if using), coconut aminos, fish sauce, and salt. Bring to a simmer and cook for 8 minutes, then reduce the heat and keep warm until the pork is done.

○ Rinse the shirataki noodles in a fine-mesh sieve, drain, and set aside.

○ If including hard-boiled eggs, bring a large pot of water to a rapid boil. One at a time, add the eggs to the water. Boil for 7 minutes, then quickly drain all the water from the pot and cover the eggs with ice and cold water. Let them sit for 2 minutes. Peel the eggs under the cold water or under a fine stream of running water. Make sure to remove that fine film under the shell; this will ensure the egg whites won't break off.

○ Assemble the ramen bowls: Place 1 cup of noodles in each of six bowls, then add 1 cup of hot broth to each bowl. Add a hard-boiled egg (if using), a few sprigs of cilantro, and three or four slices of char siu pork. Serve hot and dig in!

○ The best way to store this is to pack each component of the meal in a separate airtight container. The pork will keep in the fridge for 3 to 4 days, the broth a week, and the eggs 5 days. Prepare the noodles to order.

berry bliss slow cooker pork

The easy version: dump a cup of Raspberry Vinaigrette (page 104) and four seared pork chops in a slow cooker and cook on low for six hours. The full version: grab all the ingredients you need to make the raspberry vinaigrette—though note that some of the amounts are different— and add everything to your slow cooker with some seared pork and bone broth. This is a truly simple meal with complex flavor that serves up beautifully!

Makes 4 servings
PREP TIME: 10 minutes   COOK TIME: 6 minutes, plus 6 hours in a slow cooker

4 thick-cut boneless pork chops (about 4 ounces each)

1 teaspoon fine Himalayan salt

½ teaspoon ground black pepper

2 tablespoons avocado oil

2 cups raspberries or blackberries

½ cup bone broth (page 100)

½ cup chopped red onions

¼ cup chopped fresh parsley

¼ cup red wine vinegar

1 teaspoon peeled and minced fresh ginger

Pinch of ground nutmeg

Dash of ground cinnamon

10 drops liquid stevia (optional)

○ Heat a large skillet over medium heat, or heat an electric pressure cooker on sauté mode. Sprinkle the pork chops with the salt and pepper. When the skillet or pressure cooker is hot, pour in the oil and sear the chops for 3 minutes on each side.

○ Place the seared pork chops in the slow cooker so they are all lying flat. Add the remaining ingredients. Cover and cook on low for 6 hours.

○ Remove the lid from the slow cooker and use tongs to carefully remove the pork chops. Serve with the tender berries and sauce spooned on top of the chops. It's quite lovely.

○ Store leftovers in an airtight container in the fridge for up to 4 days. Reheat in a covered skillet over medium heat for 5 to 10 minutes.

CHEF'S NOTE: The pork chops will be almost fall-apart tender. If you use a cup of raspberry vinaigrette rather than the individual ingredients, I recommend shredding the pork before serving.

SUBSTITUTIONS: To make this dish AIP-compliant, omit the pepper and stevia and add 1 tablespoon coconut aminos.

VARIATIONS: You can use any kind of berry in this recipe— whatever you have on hand or is in season will work.

PER SERVING: Calories **303** · Fat **19.2g** · Total Carbohydrate **3.2g** · Dietary Fiber **4.5g** · Protein **29.5g**

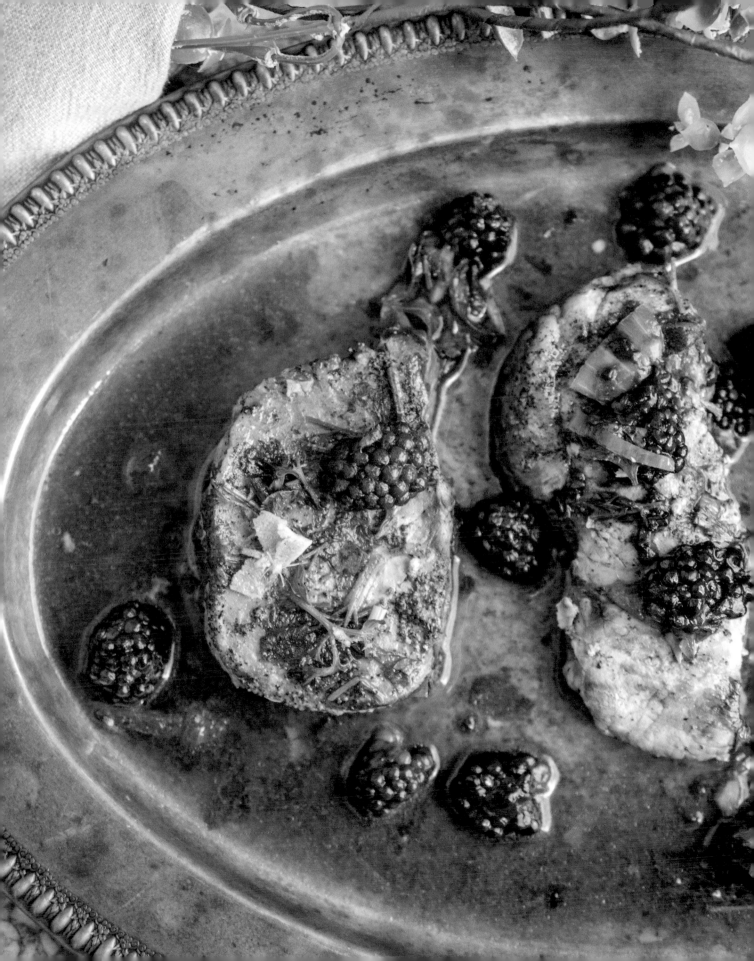

pork sausage

When you begin to clean up your plate, sausage is one of those foods that can go from a staple of your diet to completely gone. So many store-bought sausages are packed with weird ingredients, sweeteners, gluten, and so on. Luckily, ground pork is pretty cheap, and making your own sausage is not hard at all. Make a batch of these juicy spiced patties to have around for quick meals. They're divine with leftover roasted veggies, with Fried Hard-Boiled Eggs (page 116), or over Spinach Salad (page 348).

Makes 10 patties (1 per serving)
PREP TIME: 10 minutes   COOK TIME: 15 minutes

2 pounds ground pork

2 ribs celery, minced

4 cloves garlic, minced

2 teaspoons Dijon mustard

2 teaspoons fine Himalayan salt

1 teaspoon dried thyme leaves

1 teaspoon ground black pepper

¼ teaspoon ginger powder

¼ teaspoon ground cinnamon

Pinch of ground nutmeg

○ Place all of the ingredients in a large bowl and mix thoroughly with your hands.

○ Heat a large cast-iron skillet over medium heat. While it heats, shape the pork mixture into patties, about ¼ cup per patty.

○ When the skillet is hot, place four or five patties in the pan, without crowding the pan. Cook the patties for 6 minutes per side, or until the internal temperature reaches 165°F. Repeat with the remaining patties.

○ This sausage stores well side by side in an airtight container in the refrigerator for up to 5 days or in the freezer for up to 30 days. To reheat, place in a preheated 350°F oven for 8 to 10 minutes.

SUBSTITUTIONS: If you don't eat pork, you can make this sausage with ground turkey instead; be sure to use dark meat for juicy sausage. To make this sausage AIP-compliant, omit the mustard, pepper, and nutmeg.

PER SERVING: Calories **157** · Fat **12g** · Total Carbohydrate **2g** · Dietary Fiber **0.3g** · Protein **9g**

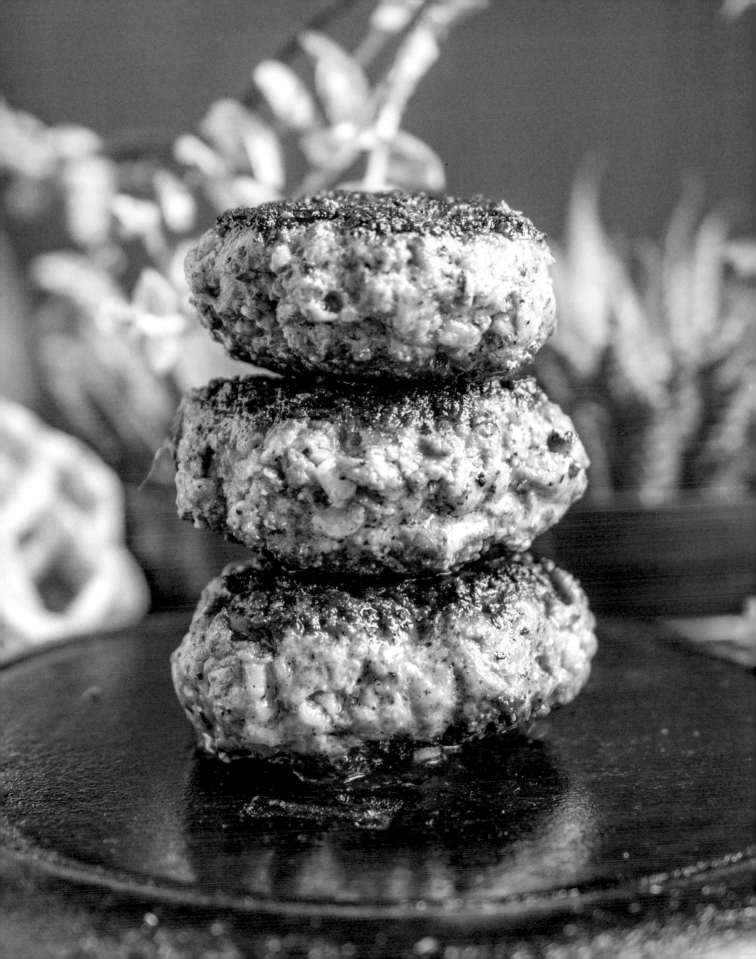

crispy kalua pork + korean vegetable salad

When we moved to Hawaii, I fell in love with kalua pork, a juicy, smoky pork that traditionally is wrapped in banana leaves and slow-cooked over hot lava rocks. This recipe is much simpler, and since I don't think you'll find hot lava rocks at the store, you can use a slow cooker instead. I add liquid smoke, onion, banana peel, and salt to re-create the simple smoky flavors, then crisp up the pork in a cast-iron skillet because everything tastes better crispy—fact. At our favorite neighborhood restaurant, Uahi Island Grill, I always order the kalua pork crisped up and served with a double side of Korean slaw. This recipe is inspired by that dish.

Makes 6 servings
PREP TIME: 20 minutes   COOK TIME: 10 minutes, plus 10 hours in a slow cooker

FOR THE KALUA PORK:

3 pounds bone-in pork shoulder

1 tablespoon fine Himalayan salt

2 tablespoons liquid smoke

1 sweet onion, quartered

1 cup water

1 banana peel (optional)

FOR THE VEGETABLE SALAD:

4 cups water

4 cups chopped watercress, ong choy, or broccoli florets

1 tablespoon minced garlic

1 teaspoon peeled and minced fresh ginger

1 tablespoon coconut aminos

1 tablespoon coconut vinegar

1 tablespoon sesame oil

1 teaspoon fine Himalayan salt

1 teaspoon ground black pepper

SUBSTITUTIONS: To make this dish AIP-compliant, omit the pepper and sesame oil from the salad. Check the labels and make sure the liquid smoke contains just water and smoke concentrate.

◦ Pat the pork shoulder dry and stand it up on a flat surface with the layer of fat facing up. Score the fat with a very sharp knife, gently cutting slits into it in a diagonal pattern.

◦ Sprinkle the salt all over the pork shoulder, then rub in the liquid smoke until the pork is well covered.

◦ Place the onion quarters in the slow cooker. Add the water and banana peel (if using). Place the pork shoulder fat side up on top of the onions. Cook on low for 9 to 10 hours.

◦ When it's done, transfer the pork to a large bowl. Remove the bone and use two forks to shred the meat. Spoon 2 to 3 tablespoons of the liquid from the slow cooker onto the shredded pork.

◦ Crisp up the shredded pork: Heat a large cast-iron skillet over medium heat. When it's hot, add the shredded pork in one even layer. Let it cook undisturbed for 5 minutes. Stir well, flatten again, and cook undisturbed for another 5 minutes. Then use a spatula to scrape it up from the bottom of the skillet and stir.

◦ While the pork is crisping, blanch the vegetables for the salad: Bring the water to a simmer in a large pot over medium heat. Add the watercress, garlic, and ginger, cover, and cook for 3 minutes. Prepare a large bowl of ice water. Remove the vegetables from the steaming water and quickly place in the ice bath for 2 to 3 minutes. Drain and pat dry.

◦ Place the coconut aminos, vinegar, sesame oil, salt, and pepper in a small bowl. Add the blanched vegetables and gently toss to combine. Serve the crispy pork with this delicious cold salad.

◦ Kalua pork keeps well. Store the pork in an airtight container in the fridge for up to 5 days. Store the salad in a separate airtight container in the fridge for no more than 2 days.

PER SERVING: Calories **536** · Fat **36.3g** · Total Carbohydrate **6g** · Dietary Fiber **2g** · Protein **43.8g**

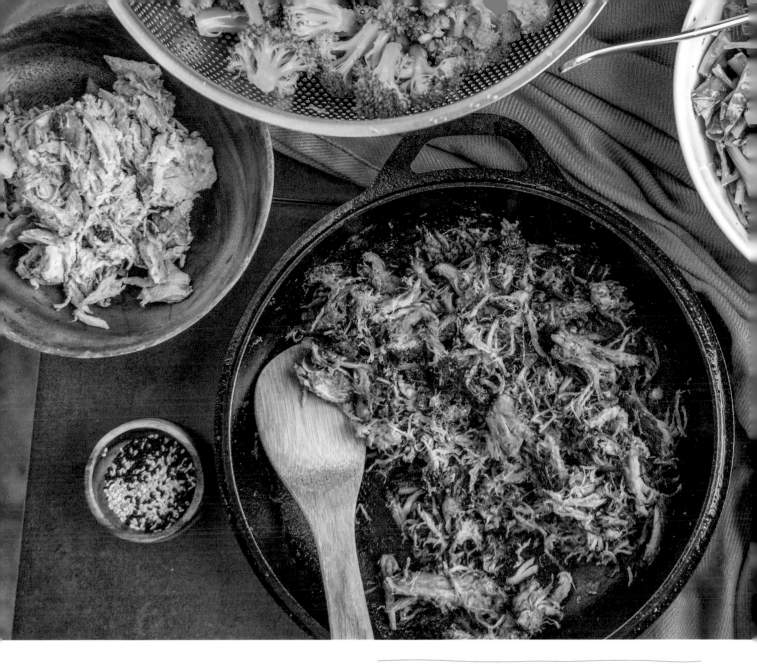

TIME-SAVING TIP: You can slow-cook the pork ahead of time and store it in an airtight container in the fridge for up to 5 days or in the freezer for up to a month. Thaw in the refrigerator and follow the crisping instructions with the cold pork. The salad can be made ahead of time and stored in an airtight container in the refrigerator, with the dressing on the side, for a day or two.

CHEF'S NOTES: At Uahi Island Grill, the Korean slaw also contains shaved carrots and bean sprouts. I jazzed up the sauce but simplified the salad to keep things easy, but feel free to add these if you like. This chilled vegetable dish is delightful with any meal; I also recommend enjoying it with Scallion Pork Patties (page 286). If you prefer soft, juicy pork to crispy pork, enjoy the kalua pork straight from the slow cooker!

cauliflower carbonara

Using premade cauliflower rice lets you make this Italian meal in less than twenty minutes! I'm not going to tell you how to live your life, but if you're cooking for date night, make this creamy and decadent dish.

Makes 2 servings
PREP TIME: 5 minutes   COOK TIME: 20 minutes

2 tablespoons unsalted butter, ghee, or avocado oil

8 ounces boneless ham steak, diced

6 cloves garlic, minced

1 tablespoon capers (optional)

4 cups riced cauliflower (see Note, page 140)

1 teaspoon fine Himalayan salt

½ teaspoon ground black pepper

½ cup bone broth (page 100)

½ cup coconut cream (see Note, page 144)

2 tablespoons nutritional yeast (optional)

4 large egg yolks, divided

2 tablespoons minced fresh parsley, for garnish

○ Heat a large skillet over medium heat. Melt the butter in the skillet, then add the ham, garlic, and capers (if using). Sauté, stirring often, until the ham is lightly browned and sweet and the garlic is aromatic, about 6 minutes.

○ Add the cauliflower, salt, and pepper. Mix well and sauté for 5 minutes. If the cauliflower is still frozen, stir often and cook until the rice has thawed and any liquid it releases has evaporated, 5 to 8 minutes.

○ Add the broth, coconut cream, and nutritional yeast (if using). Increase the heat to medium-high and simmer for 8 to 10 minutes, until the liquid is reduced by half.

○ Turn off the heat. One at a time, mix in two of the egg yolks until completely incorporated. The carbonara should smell savory and have a golden color and creamy texture.

○ Divide the carbonara between two shallow bowls. Smooth out the surface and make a shallow divot in the center of each bowl. Gently place a fresh egg yolk in each divot and sprinkle minced parsley all around it.

○ Stir the egg yolks into the hot carbonara and dig in! If you're making this dish to enjoy later, add all of the yolks while the carbonara is on the stove and mix until fully combined. This way, the yolks will cook gently, reducing the risk of foodborne illness.

○ Store leftovers in an airtight container in the fridge for up to 3 days. Reheat in a small skillet over medium-low heat.

VARIATION: Use noodles in place of the cauliflower for a noodle carbonara! Any kind of noodle will work—see page 54 for more information.

CHEF'S NOTE: Consuming raw or undercooked foods always carries the risk of foodborne illness. The risk of salmonella in fresh egg yolks is slim, but it's there. I suggest you mix in the egg yolks while the dish is very hot, which cooks them gently.

SUBSTITUTIONS: If you can't find quality ham or just don't like it, bacon works really well with this recipe. Use 8 slices of bacon and omit the butter. Chop the bacon and cook over medium heat until crispy, then add the garlic and capers and continue with the recipe as written. If you want to omit the coconut cream, use an additional ½ cup bone broth (1 cup total) instead.

PER SERVING: Calories **580** · Fat **38.6g** · Total Carbohydrate **19.7g** · Dietary Fiber **7.2g** · Protein **39.5g**

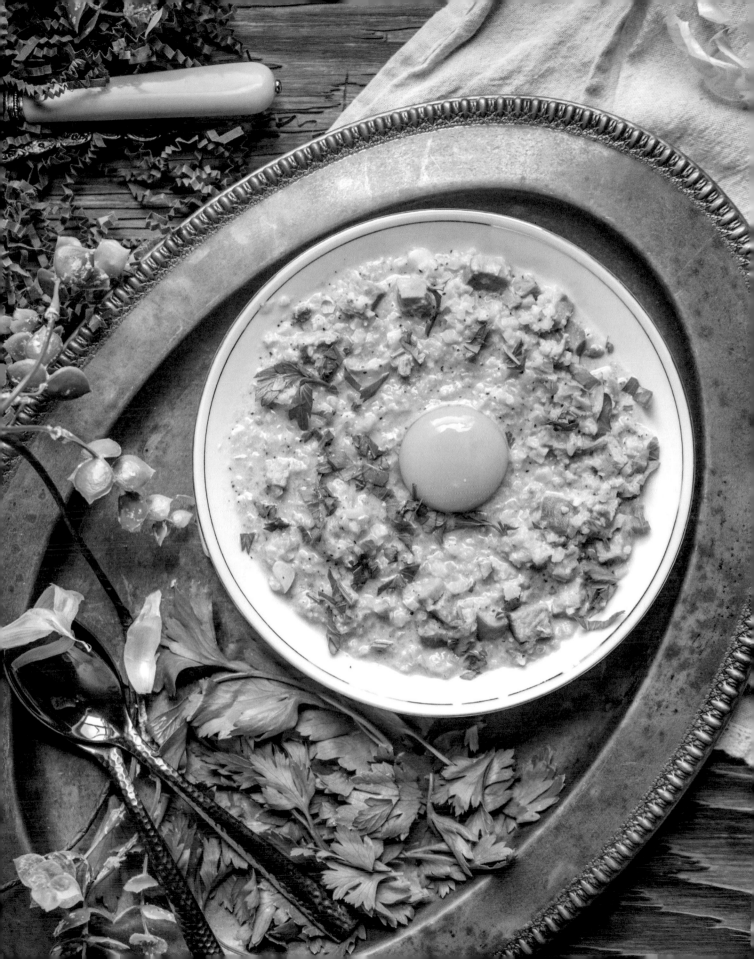

scallion pork patties with ginger sauce

If you don't know, now you do: I have more than ten burger recipes on my blog, from beef to turkey to pork. I love making fun, flavorful burger variations. They are always a hit with the family, they store and reheat really well, and it's a cinch to make a big batch of them. These juicy Asian-inspired burgers are packed with your favorite takeout flavors and served with my favorite Ginger Sauce (page 102). These are sure to become a staple in your home.

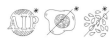

Makes 8 patties (1 per serving)
PREP TIME: 10 minutes   COOK TIME: 20 minutes

2 pounds ground pork

2 cloves garlic, minced

2 green onions, minced, plus more for garnish

2 ribs celery, minced

1 tablespoon coconut aminos

1 tablespoon sesame oil

1 teaspoon fine Himalayan salt

1 teaspoon ground black pepper

3 large eggs

1 tablespoon coconut flour

1 tablespoon unflavored grass-fed beef gelatin

1 tablespoon cooking fat (see page 53), plus more if needed

Sesame seeds, for garnish

½ cup Ginger Sauce (page 102), for serving

◦ In a large bowl, crumble the ground pork. Add the garlic, green onions, celery, coconut aminos, sesame oil, salt, and pepper and mix thoroughly with your hands.

◦ Add the eggs and mix with your hands until well combined. Add the coconut flour and gelatin and mix until the meat mixture feels like a sticky dough.

◦ Heat a large cast-iron skillet over medium heat.

◦ While the pan heats, shape the pork mixture into eight large patties. Place the cooking fat in the hot skillet. Add three or four patties at a time and sear for 5 minutes per side, or until the centers feel firm, like the palm of your hand, and both sides are browned. Repeat with the remaining pork patties, adding more cooking fat to the skillet as needed between batches.

◦ Garnish the patties with sesame seeds and more green onion slices and serve with the sauce on the side.

◦ Store leftover patties in an airtight container, stacked or standing up in rows. Reheat in a preheated 350°F oven for 5 to 10 minutes.

SUBSTITUTIONS: To make these patties AIP-compliant, omit the sesame oil, pepper, eggs, and sesame seeds. Add 1 teaspoon ginger powder and an additional 1 teaspoon coconut flour to the pork mixture instead.

PER SERVING (with 1 tablespoon sauce): Calories **262** · Fat **12g** · Total Carbohydrate **3.6g** · Dietary Fiber **0.9g** · Protein **33.4g**

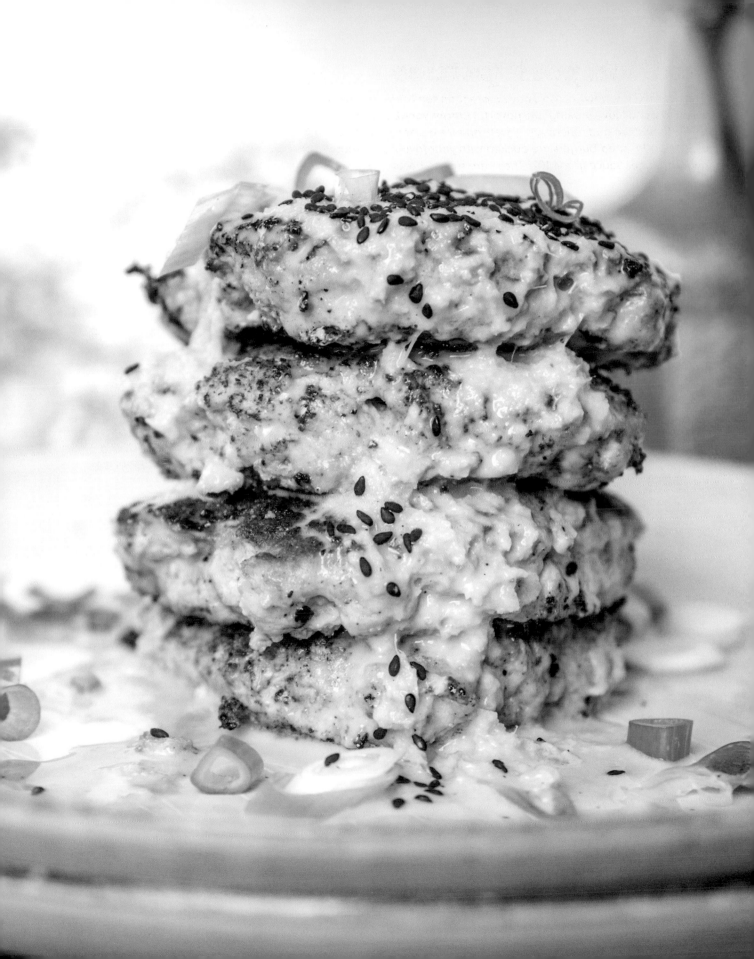

cabbage + sausage casserole

This is an old English dish. It's not fancy. It's not particularly pretty, either. But it's easy to throw together, it's filling, and most of all, it's cheap. With four ingredients, you can feed up to six mouths, making it a staple for a family on a budget. I feel a certain kinship with these old recipes from hard times. So much ingenuity comes from hardship. As you make this dish, think of mothers in the Great Depression or my grandmother, scrounging what she could to feed her family in communist Cuba. Sharing this meal pays homage to all the parents who do their best to nourish their families, even when circumstances seem dire.

4 cups water

1 large head savoy or napa cabbage

1 recipe Pork Sausage (page 280), uncooked

2 tablespoons butter, ghee, or avocado oil

½ teaspoon fine Himalayan salt (optional; omit if using salted butter)

Leaves from 2 sprigs fresh thyme (optional)

Makes 6 to 8 servings
PREP TIME: 30 minutes   COOK TIME: 3 hours

○ Bring the water to a simmer in a large oven-safe sauté pan (no more than 12 inches across) with a tight-fitting lid.

○ While the water heats, fill a large bowl with ice water, then core the cabbage and gently pull apart the leaves without tearing them.

○ Put half of the cabbage leaves in the simmering water, cover, and blanch for 1 minute. Use tongs to quickly remove the leaves and transfer them to the bowl of ice water. Repeat with the remaining leaves.

○ Remove the cabbage leaves from the ice water and pat them dry. I like to lay them on clean kitchen towels. This allows me to choose my leaves carefully for the casserole. Save six to eight of the biggest leaves for the top layer.

○ Preheat the oven to 300°F.

○ Pour the water out of the pan, dry the pan, and lightly grease it. Place a thin layer of cabbage leaves on the bottom.

○ Spread one-third of the sausage over the cabbage leaves in a thin, even layer, making sure to spread it all the way to the sides of the pan. Add another layer of cabbage leaves, dot the leaves with some butter, sprinkle with a pinch of salt (if using), and add another layer of sausage. Repeat again: one more layer of cabbage leaves and one more layer of sausage.

○ Top the final sausage layer with the cabbage leaves that you set aside for the top, making the thickest layer of cabbage yet. Dot the leaves with butter and cover the pan with the lid.

○ Place the pan in the oven and bake the casserole for 2½ hours. Uncover and bake for another 30 minutes. Remove from the oven and sprinkle with the thyme leaves (if using). Use a large spoon to serve this soft casserole.

VARIATIONS: To change up this casserole, add Pickled Red Onions (page 88) or crispy bacon between the layers, add pumpkin or hemp seeds to the top layer for crunch, or serve it with Cheesy Yellow Sauce (page 68)!

SUBSTITUTIONS: To make this casserole AIP-compliant, prepare the AIP-compliant version of the pork sausage and use avocado oil.

PER SERVING (6 servings): Calories **452** · Fat **36.3g** · Total Carbohydrate **2.4g** · Dietary Fiber **5.6g** · Protein **26.6g**

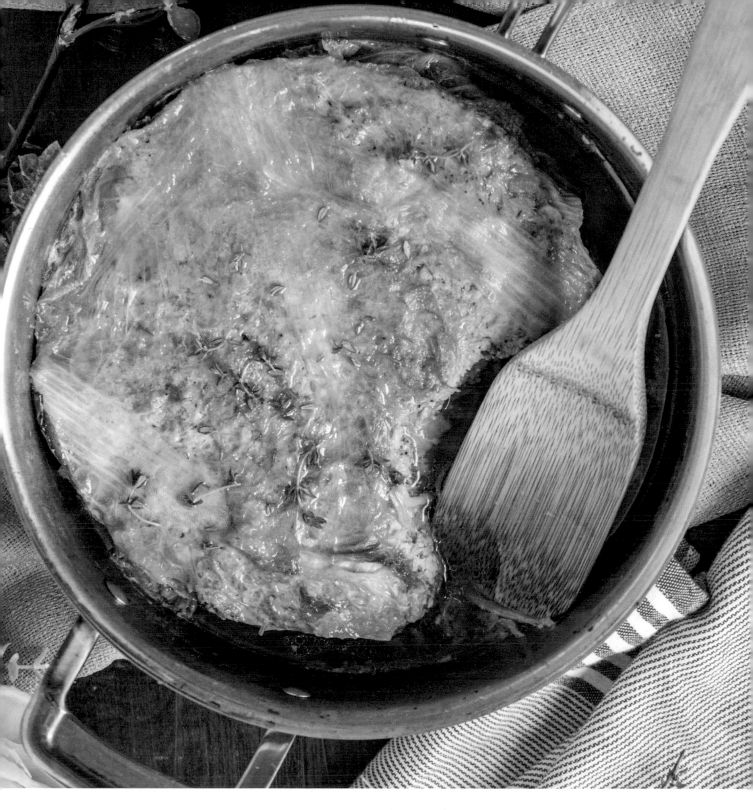

○ Serve with toasted slices of Nut-Free Keto Bread (page 324) or Everything Flaxseed Meal Crackers (page 326) for a warm, hearty meal any time of the year.

○ Store in an airtight container in the fridge for up to 5 days. Reheat in a preheated 350°F oven, uncovered, for 10 to 20 minutes.

braised pork chops with creamy green beans

This recipe was born one night when I was making dinner in a rush, flustered and with a ton of work waiting for me. Yet, as we sat down to eat, the whole family relaxed into this meal. There was silence as we all got lost in the comforting flavors on our plates. For a moment there was peace, and I realized that I had to write down exactly what I had done. Since then I have made and shared a few variations of this recipe; after all, pork chops are a classic. This combination, however, with creamy green beans and red onions, has never left my kitchen—until now.

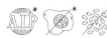

Makes 4 servings
PREP TIME: 10 minutes   COOK TIME: 40 minutes

FOR THE CREAMY GREEN BEANS:

1 medium head cauliflower, roughly chopped

1½ cups bone broth (page 100)

¼ cup Garlic Confit (page 76), or 4 cloves garlic, peeled

2 tablespoons cooking fat (see page 53)

2 cups fresh green beans, trimmed

1 red onion, sliced

2 teaspoons fine Himalayan salt, divided

2 large egg yolks

FOR THE PORK CHOPS:

2 teaspoons fine Himalayan salt

1 teaspoon garlic powder

1 teaspoon ground black pepper

1 teaspoon onion powder

5 sprigs fresh thyme

4 boneless thick-cut pork chops

2 tablespoons avocado oil

¼ cup bone broth (page 100)

2 tablespoons coconut aminos

2 tablespoons red wine vinegar

TIME-SAVING TIP: Make the cauliflower puree ahead of time, or substitute Cauliflower Alfredo (page 86) if you have some already made.

○ Make the creamy green beans: Place the cauliflower, broth, and garlic confit in a medium-sized pot and bring to a simmer over medium heat. Cover and cook until the cauliflower is fork-tender, about 20 minutes.

○ Meanwhile, heat a large skillet over medium heat. When it's hot, heat the cooking fat in the skillet. Add the green beans, red onion slices, and 1 teaspoon of the salt. Sauté, stirring occasionally, for 10 minutes, until the beans begin to brown and the onions are tender and translucent. Reduce the heat to medium-low.

○ By now the cauliflower should be done. Transfer it and all of the broth to a blender, add the remaining teaspoon of salt, and blend until smooth. While the blender is running, open the lid vent and drop in the egg yolks one at a time.

○ Once well combined, pour the cauliflower cream over the green beans and onions in the skillet. Stir, cover, and remove from the heat, but keep the pan on the stove or in the oven so it stays warm.

○ Prepare the pork chops: Heat a large skillet over medium heat. While the skillet heats, combine the salt, garlic powder, pepper, onion powder, and thyme sprigs in a small bowl. Rub the seasoning mixture all over the pork chops, making sure they are evenly coated.

○ Melt the oil in the hot skillet. Add the chops, spacing them so they do not touch. Cook undisturbed for 5 minutes, then flip the chops over and cook for 3 minutes on the other side.

○ Add the broth, coconut aminos, and vinegar to the skillet with the pork chops. Cover and cook for 3 minutes. Use your finger to gently press on the center of a chop; when it's done, it should feel like the palm of your hand, firm but with a little give, and the internal temperature should be 165°F. Remove from the heat.

○ Let the pork chops rest for a few minutes, then pour the pan sauce over the chops. Serve with the creamy green beans.

○ Store leftovers in an airtight container in the fridge for up to 5 days. Reheat in a large skillet, covered, over medium-low heat for 8 to 10 minutes.

PER SERVING: Calories **563** · Fat **27.9g** · Total Carbohydrate **18.1g** · Dietary Fiber **6.3g** · Protein **59.1g**

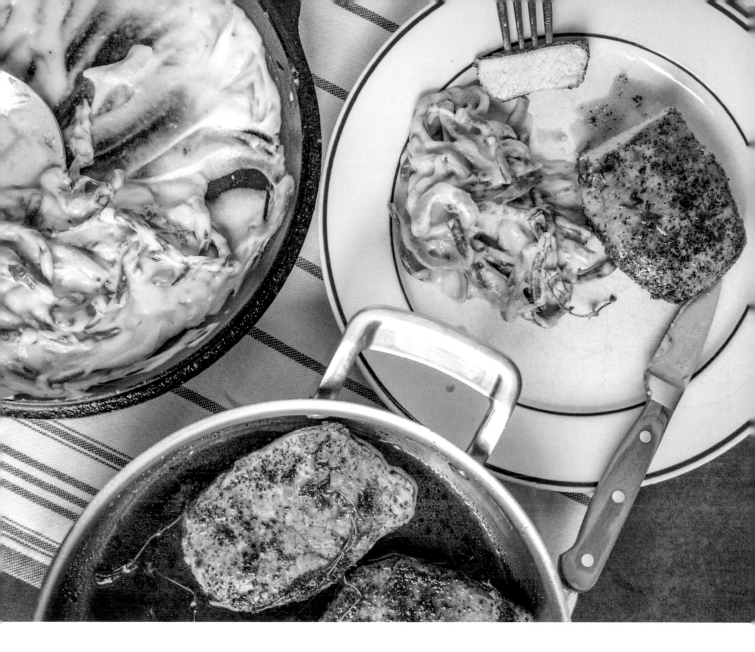

CHEF'S NOTE: If you want to make this dish simpler, or if you just don't like green beans, double the cauliflower, bone broth, and garlic and serve the chops over the puree. It's equally delicious!

SUBSTITUTIONS: Feel free to tweak the seasonings on the pork chops and use whatever herb you have on hand. For an AIP-compliant version, omit the egg yolks and pepper, add 1 tablespoon lard to the cauliflower puree, and serve the chops over a smooth cauliflower puree (see the Note for instructions).

spiced pork tenderloin with rustic mushroom sauce

When I want to chef it up for my toddler on a weeknight, this is my go-to meal. It looks fancy and tastes restaurant-worthy, but it takes just twenty minutes to make. I love cutting pork tenderloin into medallions; it's a great way to get super-juicy pork without worrying about roasting it too long or drying it out. Bonus: the medallions cook super fast! A quick sear followed by a quick pan sauce and boom, dinner is ready. This pork goes well with Creamy Kale Noodles (page 320), Everything Flaxseed Meal Crackers (page 326), and Tender Kale Salad (page 344).

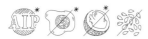

1 teaspoon fine Himalayan salt

1 teaspoon garam masala

1 teaspoon ground black pepper

1 teaspoon ground cumin

1 teaspoon onion powder

1 teaspoon granulated erythritol or other low-carb sweetener (see page 38)

1 pound pork tenderloin, cut into 2-inch-thick medallions

2 tablespoons cooking fat (see page 53)

FOR THE SAUCE:

2 cups halved cremini mushrooms

1 sprig fresh thyme, or 1 teaspoon dried thyme leaves

1 cup full-fat coconut milk

1 large egg yolk

⅛ teaspoon fine Himalayan salt

Makes 4 servings
PREP TIME: 10 minutes   **COOK TIME:** 10 minutes

○ Heat a large skillet over medium heat.

○ In a large bowl, combine the salt, garam masala, pepper, cumin, onion powder, and erythritol. Add the pork medallions and toss until evenly coated. Gently flatten the medallions so they cook evenly.

○ When the skillet is hot, add the cooking fat and swirl it around. Arrange the medallions in the skillet so they do not touch. Sear for 3 minutes on each side, then use tongs to turn the medallions and give the sides a quick sear. Lay the medallions flat again, cover the skillet, and cook for another 2 to 3 minutes. When the centers feel firm, like the palm of your hand, or when the internal temperature of the pork reaches 145°F, remove the medallions from the skillet and set aside to rest while you make the sauce. Do not wash the pan.

○ Make the sauce: Add the mushrooms and thyme to the hot skillet and sauté, stirring often, for 3 to 5 minutes, until the mushrooms are tender and browned. Add the coconut milk and bring to a simmer. Whisk in the egg yolk and salt. Whisk continually until the sauce thickens, which will happen rapidly.

○ Remove the skillet from the heat. Pour the sauce over the medallions or serve it on the side.

○ Store leftovers in an airtight container in the fridge for up to 5 days.

SUBSTITUTIONS: If you want to omit the coconut milk and egg from the sauce, use cauliflower puree: Simmer 1 cup cauliflower florets with ¼ cup bone broth until tender, then blend with 1 tablespoon cooking fat until smooth. Add this puree to the mushrooms in place of the coconut milk.

To make this AIP-compliant, follow the above instructions for a cauliflower puree. In addition, omit the garam masala, pepper, and cumin, and replace them with 1 teaspoon ground ginger, ½ teaspoon ground cinnamon, and a pinch of cloves.

PER SERVING: Calories **384** · Fat **26.4g** · Total Carbohydrate **5.3g** · Dietary Fiber **1.8g** · Protein **33g**

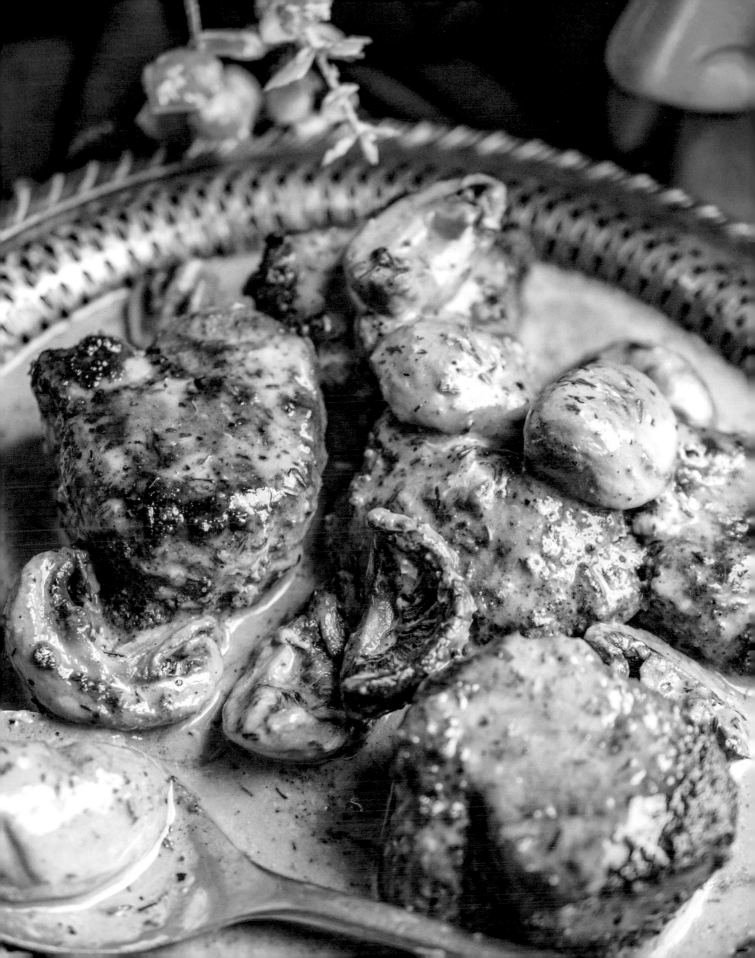

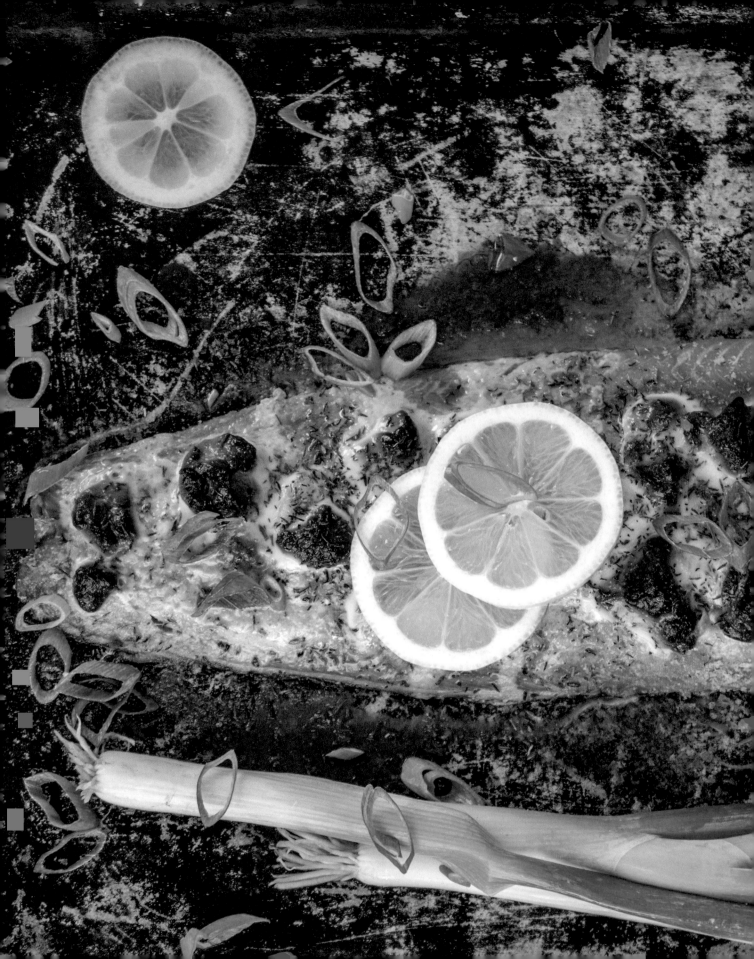

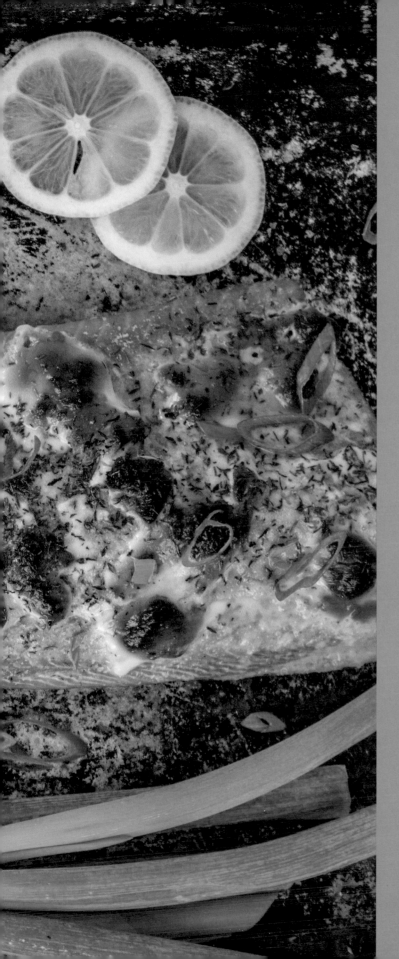

SEAFOOD + FISH

Perhaps it was growing up in South Florida and all the fishing trips to the Keys, but seafood has always been a part of my diet! It surprised me to discover, as an adult, how many people avoid cooking seafood, mostly because they don't know how to prepare it. These dishes are simple and solid, and I promise that even if you've never cooked fish or seafood before, you'll soon feel like a pro!

shrimp + grits

This recipe has it all: loud flavor, tons of texture, subtle complexities—and it plates really nicely, too. But the best part? It's easy to make. This is the dish to make when you want to impress folks at a dinner party without working up too much of a sweat in the kitchen. The grits are made of cauliflower (our champion) with a buttery toasted coconut base that adds a welcome richness, and the shrimp are spicy and crispy, with beautiful color. Finish it off with a handful of greens, and voilà!

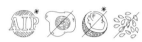

Makes 4 servings
PREP TIME: 20 minutes   **COOK TIME:** 20 minutes

FOR THE GRITS:

3 tablespoons coconut butter

2 tablespoons ghee, unsalted butter, or lard

3 cloves garlic, minced

1 (1-inch) piece lemon peel

5 cups riced cauliflower (see Note, page 140)

1 cup bone broth (page 100)

1 teaspoon fine Himalayan salt

FOR THE SHRIMP:

1 teaspoon fine Himalayan salt

1 teaspoon ground black pepper

1 teaspoon ground cumin

1 teaspoon minced fresh rosemary

½ teaspoon ginger powder

1 pound fresh shrimp, peeled and deveined (preferably tail-on)

5 slices bacon, diced

Juice of 1 lemon

2 tablespoons coconut aminos

Fresh arugula or parsley, for garnish

○ Make the grits: Heat a large skillet over medium heat. When it's hot, add the coconut butter, ghee, garlic, and lemon peel. Let the fats melt and come to a simmer. Cook, stirring occasionally, for 2 to 3 minutes, until the coconut butter begins to brown. It will be light brown and smell like toasted coconut.

○ Add the cauliflower and stir to combine. If the cauliflower is frozen, cook, stirring often, until it's thawed. Then add the broth and salt. Bring to a simmer and cook undisturbed until the liquid is reduced by half, about 10 minutes.

○ Meanwhile, prepare the shrimp: Heat a second large skillet over high heat. While it heats, combine the salt, pepper, cumin, rosemary, and ginger powder in a large bowl. Add the shrimp and toss to coat the shrimp thoroughly.

○ When the skillet is hot, place the bacon in the skillet and cook, stirring often, for 8 minutes, or until well browned and almost crispy. Add the shrimp and sauté, stirring often, for 2 to 3 minutes, until the shrimp have curled and turned pink. Add the lemon juice and coconut aminos and stir quickly to deglaze the skillet and coat the shrimp in the sauce. They should be browned and caramelized, with sticky chunks and lots of crispy bacon.

○ Remove the skillet from the heat. Give the cauliflower grits a stir; they should be creamy, without too much pooling liquid. Spoon the grits into four shallow bowls and fish out the lemon peel. Add four or five shrimp to each bowl, making sure to get some chunks of bacon in there, too. Garnish with arugula or parsley.

○ Store leftovers in an airtight container in the fridge for up to 3 days. To reheat, sauté in a hot skillet for 3 to 4 minutes.

CHEF'S NOTE: To take this dish to the next level, use fish stock instead of bone broth. Follow the recipe for bone broth on page 100, but use a few fish heads in place of the animal bones.

SUBSTITUTIONS: To make this dish AIP-compliant, omit the pepper and cumin. If you're avoiding coconut, you can omit the coconut butter from the grits; in its place, I recommend stirring in 2 or 3 egg yolks at the end to make the grits rich and creamy. In addition, replace the coconut aminos with aged balsamic vinegar or a balsamic vinegar reduction.

PER SERVING: Calories **363** · Fat **20.6g** · Total Carbohydrate **13.3g** · Dietary Fiber **5.5g** · Protein **26g**

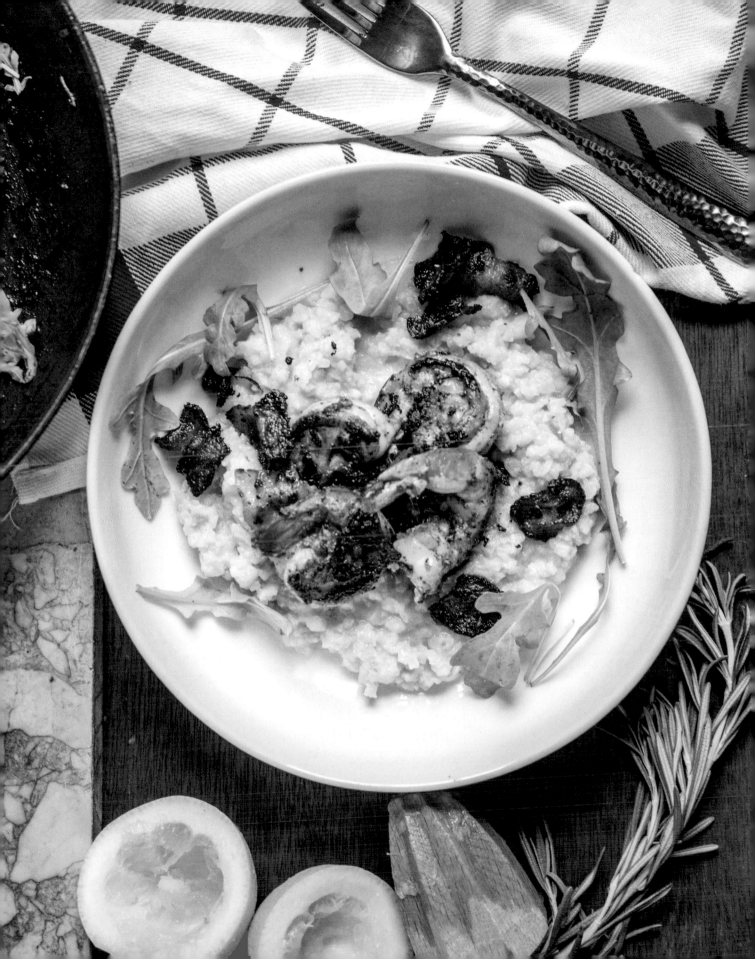

calamari two ways

Fried calamari was always my go-to when eating out. I just loved those crispy, chewy rings. But as I now know, commercially fried foods are the worst, carrying a combination of inflammatory canola oil and gluten-filled breading. I thought this dish was out of my reach forever. But when the recipe for Chicken Katsu (page 220) turned out just perfect, I knew that the coconut breading would work for calamari, too. Oh, happy day! I like to bread half of the calamari and leave the other half mostly naked, just lightly dusted in coconut flour. It lightens up the dish a bit, but it's still absolutely tasty! Pair these crispy rings with Ginger Sauce (page 102) and Roasted Beet Marinara (page 78) and serve Creamy Cilantro Rice (page 342) or Spinach Salad (page 348) on the side for an unforgettable seafood meal!

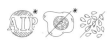

1 cup coconut oil, or more if needed, for frying

½ cup coconut flour

1 teaspoon fine Himalayan salt

1 teaspoon ground black pepper

3 large eggs

1 tablespoon red wine vinegar

1 cup unsweetened shredded coconut

1 pound cleaned calamari tubes, sliced into ½-inch rings

FOR SERVING:

2 limes, cut into wedges

½ cup Ginger Sauce (page 102)

½ cup Roasted Beet Marinara (page 78)

SUBSTITUTIONS: To make these AIP-compliant, skip the eggs and shredded coconut and omit the pepper. Add 1 teaspoon ginger powder and 1 teaspoon turmeric powder to the coconut flour mix. Toss the calamari rings in this mix and follow the instructions for frying. Garnish with toasted coconut flakes!

Makes 4 servings
PREP TIME: 20 minutes   COOK TIME: 20 minutes

○ Set a cooling rack on a sheet pan or line a plate with paper towels.

○ Heat an 8-inch heavy-bottomed pot or skillet over medium heat. Add the coconut oil—it should be 1 inch deep—and heat until the oil sizzles around the end of a wooden spoon handle when it's inserted in the oil.

○ While the oil heats, bread the calamari: In a large bowl, combine the coconut flour, salt, and pepper. In another bowl, whisk the eggs with the vinegar. Place the shredded coconut in a third bowl.

○ Add the calamari to the bowl with the flour mixture and toss to coat. Remove half of the calamari and place in a colander; shake to remove the excess flour.

○ Working with three or four rings at a time, dredge the calamari from the colander in the egg mixture and then in the shredded coconut, then place in the skillet with the hot oil. Fry until golden all over, turning once, about 4 minutes total. Use tongs to remove the crispy rings from the oil and place on the cooling rack or paper towel–lined plate.

○ Repeat until the breaded calamari are all done. The eggs and shredded coconut should be about done, too! Then remove the rest of the calamari from the coconut flour and shake to remove the excess flour.

○ Fry all the coconut flour–coated rings together for 5 to 6 minutes, turning and stirring occasionally, until they're golden around the edges and all the rings are rounded. Remove from the oil and set to drain next to the twice-breaded batch.

○ Serve right away with lime wedges and/or dipping sauces.

PER SERVING (without sauce): Calories **422** · Fat **18.9g** · Total Carbohydrate **12g** · Dietary Fiber **18g** · Protein **36g**

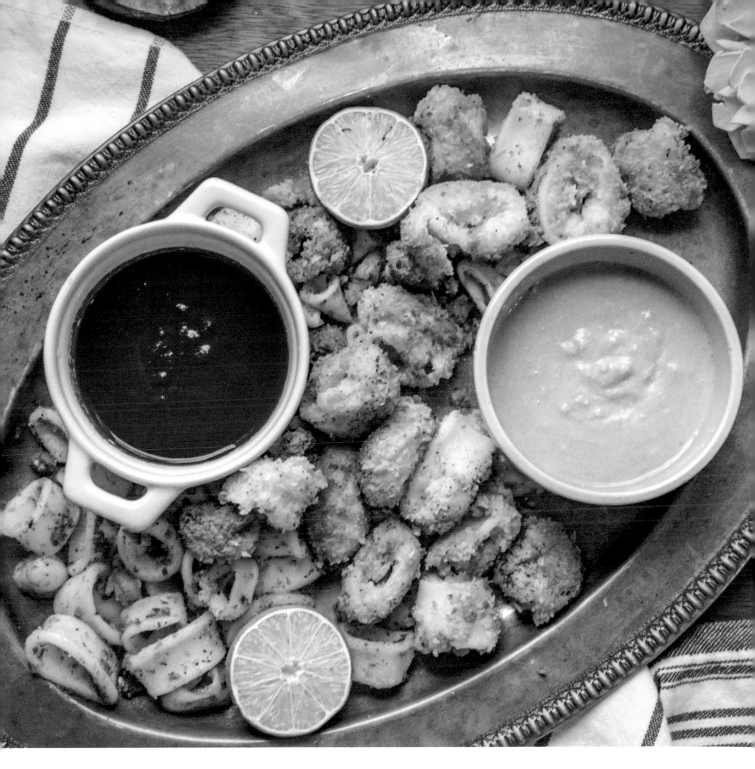

CHEF'S NOTE: You can play around with the seasonings here. Add your favorite herbs and spices to the coconut flour mixture to change things up!

◦ If you're making this recipe ahead of time, place the calamari on a cooling rack over a sheet pan and store in the oven for up to an hour. Gently heat at 300°F for 8 to 10 minutes right before serving.

pan-seared cod

Sometimes simple is just better. This is definitely the case when it comes to delicious, flaky white fish. The magic here is in the golden, crispy, buttery crust that forms on the fish during cooking. Add just a few aromatics and you have a restaurant-worthy fish dish in minutes. I love pairing this with leftover roasted vegetables or Half-Sour Pickled Salad (page 340) for a light meal. Serve it with Spiced Broccolini with Cool Cilantro Sauce (page 336) for a date-night meal that is sure to impress.

4 (6-ounce) boneless, skinless cod fillets

1 teaspoon fine Himalayan salt

3 tablespoons ghee or bacon fat

2 sprigs fresh parsley

1 green onion, sliced

1 tablespoon Garlic Confit (page 76)

Lime or lemon halves, for garnish (optional)

CHEF'S NOTE: This cooking method will work with any firm white fish. Halibut, mahi mahi, and sea bass are my favorites.

Makes 4 servings
PREP TIME: 10 minutes   COOK TIME: 10 minutes

◦ Pat the fish fillets dry and rub the salt all over them.

◦ Heat a large cast-iron skillet over medium heat until it's very hot, rotating the pan halfway every few minutes. Drip water on it to check the temperature; when the droplets dance, it's ready.

◦ Melt the ghee in the skillet. Add the fish fillets, being careful not to crowd the pan—cook two fillets at a time if you have to. Sear the fish for 4 to 6 minutes. When the edges of the fish begin to look opaque white and you can see that it is golden underneath, use a thin spatula to flip the fish.

◦ Place the parsley, green onion slices, and garlic confit around the fish. Cook for 3 to 4 minutes, until the fish is tender and flakes easily with a fork.

◦ Transfer the fish to a serving platter. Spoon the ghee mixture over the fish. Garnish with lime halves, if desired. Let it rest for 3 to 5 minutes before serving.

◦ I'm not a fan of leftover fish. Cook as many fillets as you have people to feed to avoid having leftovers. If they can't be avoided, store leftovers in an airtight container in the fridge for up to 3 days.

PER SERVING. Calories **223** · Fat **11.3g** · Total Carbohydrate **2.5g** · Dietary Fiber **0.1g** · Protein **27.5g**

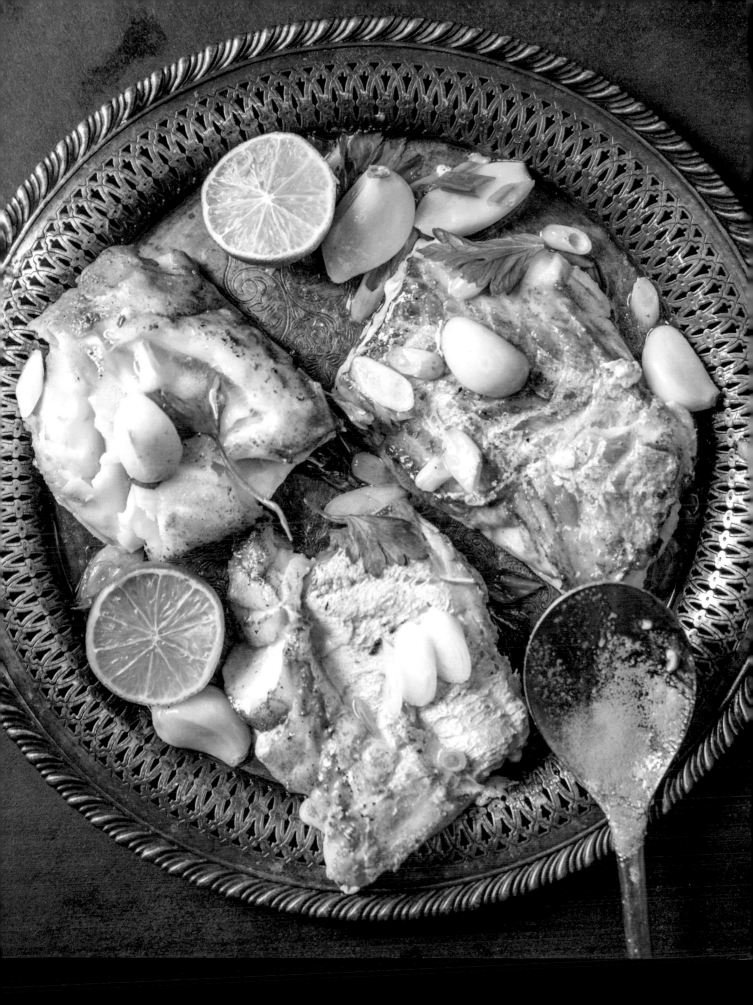

seared golden scallops *with wilted bacon spinach*

Jumbo scallops are a rare treat in my house. They're definitely on the pricey side, but they're also absolutely divine, and if you get the opportunity to cook some, this recipe will not disappoint. The scallops are seared yet saucy, with a combination of flavors that really brings out their natural sweetness. Essentially a one-skillet recipe with two parts, this simple yet beautiful dish will have you cooking scallops like a pro!

FOR THE SPINACH:

4 slices bacon, diced

1 small onion, diced

1 sprig fresh rosemary

¼ teaspoon ground nutmeg

½ pound baby spinach

2 tablespoons bone broth (page 100)

1 tablespoon nutritional yeast

2 teaspoons granulated garlic

¼ teaspoon fine Himalayan salt

FOR THE SCALLOPS:

1 tablespoon lard

8 jumbo scallops

1 teaspoon fine Himalayan salt

½ teaspoon turmeric powder

2 tablespoons coconut aminos

2 tablespoons bone broth (page 100)

CHEF'S NOTE: You can use kale, collard greens, or Swiss chard instead of spinach. The bacon is optional but highly recommended. This dish cooks quickly and needs to be served posthaste, as scallops continue to cook after they are removed from the heat. These delicate morsels are buttery and sweet but become chewy if overcooked.

SUBSTITUTIONS: To make this dish AIP-compliant, omit the nutmeg. Use a pinch of ground cloves instead.

Makes 2 servings
PREP TIME: 10 minutes   COOK TIME: 30 minutes

◦ Cook the spinach: Place the bacon in a large skillet over medium heat. Let it cook undisturbed until it begins to sizzle, about 3 minutes. Add the onions, rosemary, and nutmeg. Cook, stirring occasionally, for about 15 minutes, until the bacon is crispy and the onions are translucent. Remove the rosemary sprig. Transfer half of the bacon-and-onion mixture to a dish and set aside to use later as a garnish.

◦ Add the spinach to the skillet a fistful at a time, letting each fistful wilt before adding more. Mix in the broth, nutritional yeast, granulated garlic, and salt. Bring to a simmer and cook, stirring continuously, for 2 minutes.

◦ Transfer the spinach mixture to a large bowl, cover, and set aside, but keep it close to the stove so it stays warm.

◦ Cook the scallops: Wipe the skillet with a paper towel and set it back on the burner over medium heat. Let it heat for a minute or two, then add the lard. While the lard heats, lay the scallops on a cutting board and pat them dry with a paper towel or clean kitchen towel. Rub the salt and turmeric all over the scallops.

◦ Once the lard is hot—it should be a little bubbly but not smoking—add the scallops to the skillet, making sure not to crowd them. Let them sear undisturbed for 2 minutes, then use a very thin spatula to carefully scrape them up and flip them over, revealing a beautiful golden crust. Sear undisturbed for another 2 minutes, then add the coconut aminos to the skillet. Swirl the pan to get the coconut aminos all over the scallops, then use the spatula to remove the scallops from the skillet and set them on two serving plates.

◦ Add the broth to the skillet and bring it to a quick simmer. Use a spatula to deglaze the pan, lifting up any flavor left behind and any aminos that have caramelized on the bottom. Pour this pan sauce over the scallops.

◦ Serve right away with the spinach on the side. Garnish with the reserved bacon and onions. Enjoy!

PER SERVING: Calories **279** · Fat **11.8g** · Total Carbohydrate **13.2g** · Dietary Fiber **5.8g** · Protein **28.3g**

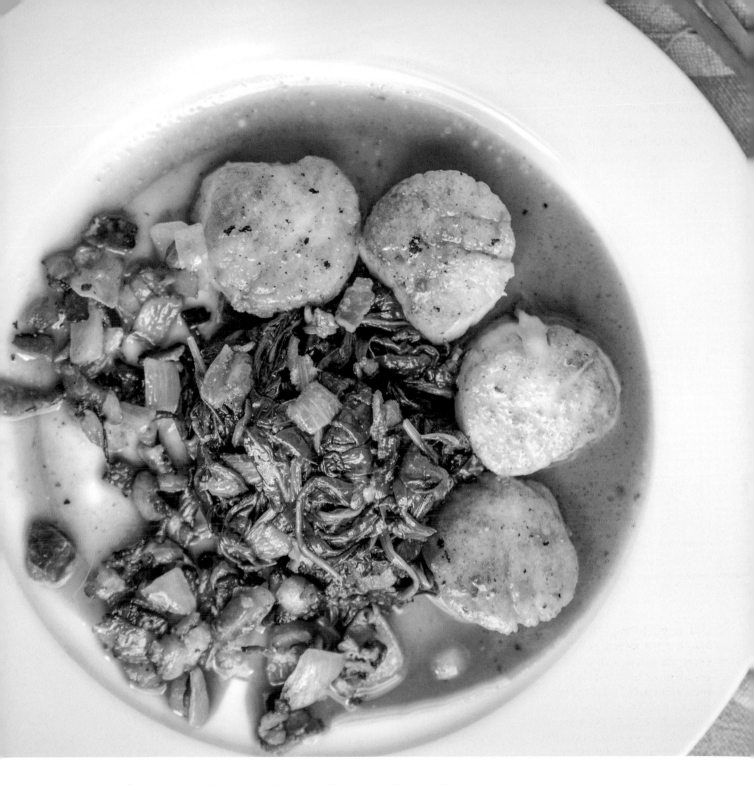

° I don't recommend eating leftover scallops, as reheating them can make them rubbery. Store leftover spinach and bacon in the fridge for up to 3 days.

camarones enchilados

This saucy and spicy shrimp dish is a Cuban classic and reminds me of my Tia Yoyi. It is traditionally made with a few kinds of peppers and a hit of saffron, but I sauté Pickled Red Onions (page 88) and Garlic Confit (page 76) and quickly simmer them in Roasted Beet Marinara (page 78) to make short work of the sofrito, the basis of the delicious, savory flavor (see the Note on page 152). Camarones enchilados are perfect over cauliflower rice, which soaks up all of the saucy goodness. This dish even got a thumbs-up from my beet-hating husband, and that's saying something.

Makes 4 servings
PREP TIME: 10 minutes, plus 20 minutes to marinate   **COOK TIME:** 10 minutes

2 cups riced cauliflower (see Note, page 140)

2 tablespoons water

1 pound jumbo shrimp, peeled and deveined

Juice of 1 lemon

1 tablespoon red wine vinegar

1 teaspoon fine Himalayan salt

1 teaspoon ground cumin

½ teaspoon ginger powder

½ teaspoon ground black pepper

1 tablespoon lard or avocado oil

⅓ cup Garlic Confit (page 76), roughly chopped

⅓ cup Pickled Red Onions (page 88)

½ cup Roasted Beet Marinara (page 78)

1 tablespoon coconut aminos

½ medium Hass avocado, sliced, for garnish

○ Heat a medium-sized saucepan over medium-low heat. Place the cauliflower and water in the saucepan, stir, and cover. Cook while you prepare the shrimp.

○ Place the shrimp, lemon juice, vinegar, salt, cumin, ginger powder, and pepper in a large bowl. Toss to combine, cover, and allow to marinate for 20 minutes.

○ Melt the lard in a large skillet over medium heat, then add the garlic confit and pickled onions. Cook, stirring continuously, for 2 to 3 minutes.

○ Remove the shrimp from the marinade, reserving the marinade. Add the shrimp to the skillet and sauté until they begin to turn pink, about 6 minutes.

○ Add the marinara, coconut aminos, and reserved marinade. Simmer, stirring occasionally, for 2 to 3 minutes, until the shrimp are fully cooked; they'll be coiled and brightly colored.

○ Divide the cooked cauliflower rice among four plates. Spoon the shrimp over the cauliflower rice. Garnish with avocado slices.

○ Store leftovers in an airtight container in the fridge for up to 3 days. To reheat, sauté over medium heat for 5 to 6 minutes.

SUBSTITUTIONS: To make this dish AIP-compliant, omit the cumin and pepper. Double the ginger and add 1 teaspoon dried oregano or your preferred herb for flavor.

CHEF'S NOTE: If you don't have garlic confit or pickled red onions on hand, you can use 4 cloves garlic, minced, and 1 red onion, sliced. Sauté in the lard for 8 minutes, or until tender, then continue with the recipe as written.

PER SERVING (with avocado): Calories **367** · Fat **22.1g** · Total Carbohydrate **12.6g** · Dietary Fiber **3.8g** · Protein **28.8g**

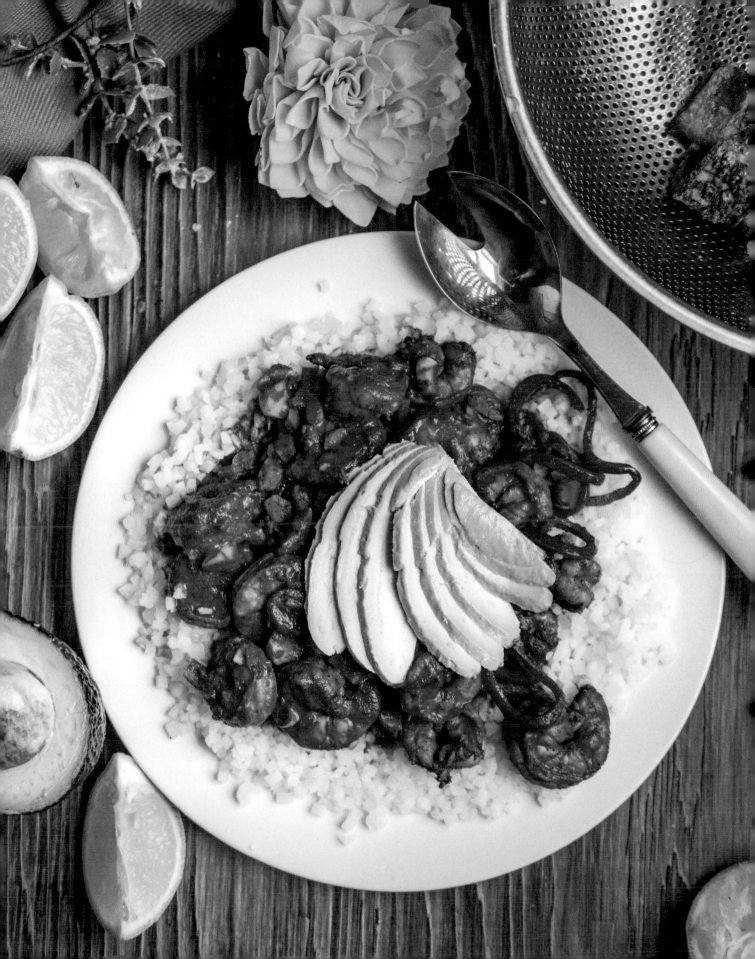

salmon zoodle casserole

I never had tuna noodle casserole until I met my husband. We had been dating for several months when he asked me to make him his childhood favorite. At first, I was perplexed by the concept of combining pasta, canned tuna, and cheese. It just didn't seem right to me—growing up with immigrant parents, I missed out on a lot of these American classics. Eventually I made him some version of a tuna noodle casserole, and years later I made a tuna zoodle (zucchini noodle) casserole for my blog. It continues to be one of the most beloved recipes there. This recipe draws from that one, but I've use Cauliflower Alfredo (page 86) and eggs to make a kind of béchamel and swapped tuna for its classier cousin, wild-caught salmon. I've also used a combination of zoodles and kelp noodles. I find the kelp noodles add body and texture to the tender casserole. However, you can use all zoodles, all kelp noodles, or even shirataki noodles! The result is a beautiful, nourishing casserole that packs tons of veggies and a little nostalgia.

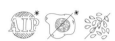

2 medium zucchini

¼ teaspoon fine Himalayan salt

FOR THE BÉCHAMEL:

1 recipe Cauliflower Alfredo (page 86)

3 large eggs

1 tablespoon Dijon mustard

1 tablespoon red wine vinegar

1 teaspoon dried dill weed

½ teaspoon fine Himalayan salt

½ teaspoon ground nutmeg

¼ teaspoon celery salt

1 (12-ounce) package kelp noodles

1 red onion, thinly sliced

3 (6-ounce) cans wild-caught or smoked salmon, boneless and skinless

4 slices bacon, cut into 1-inch pieces

Makes 9 servings
PREP TIME: 15 minutes   COOK TIME: 45 minutes

○ Preheat the oven to 375°F.

○ Using a spiral slicer, slice the zucchini into noodles; if you do not have a spiral slicer, use a vegetable peeler to make ribbons. Spread them out on a clean kitchen towel and sprinkle with the salt, then let them sit for 10 minutes.

○ Meanwhile, make the béchamel: Place all of the sauce ingredients in a blender. Blend on high until thick and smooth, about 30 seconds. Set aside.

○ Assemble the casserole: Drain and rinse the kelp noodles and spread them out in a 9 by 13-inch casserole dish. Add the onion slices. Next, wrap the zoodles up in the towel and squeeze out the excess liquid over the kitchen sink. Add the zoodles to the casserole dish with the kelp noodles and onions and toss to combine.

○ Drain the canned salmon and flake it over the noodle mixture. Pour the béchamel over the salmon and use a spatula to spread it out evenly and make sure it gets to the bottom noodles. Sprinkle the bacon pieces evenly over the casserole.

○ Bake the casserole for 40 minutes, then turn on the broiler, move the casserole dish to just under it, and broil for 2 minutes to toast the top. Remove from the oven and cut into nine rectangles. Serve warm.

○ To store leftovers, cover the casserole dish with plastic wrap or aluminum foil and refrigerate for up to 4 days. To reheat, uncover and bake in a preheated 325°F oven for 15 minutes.

PER SERVING: Calories **218** · Fat **13g** · Total Carbohydrate **9g** · Dietary Fiber **3.5g** · Protein **17g**

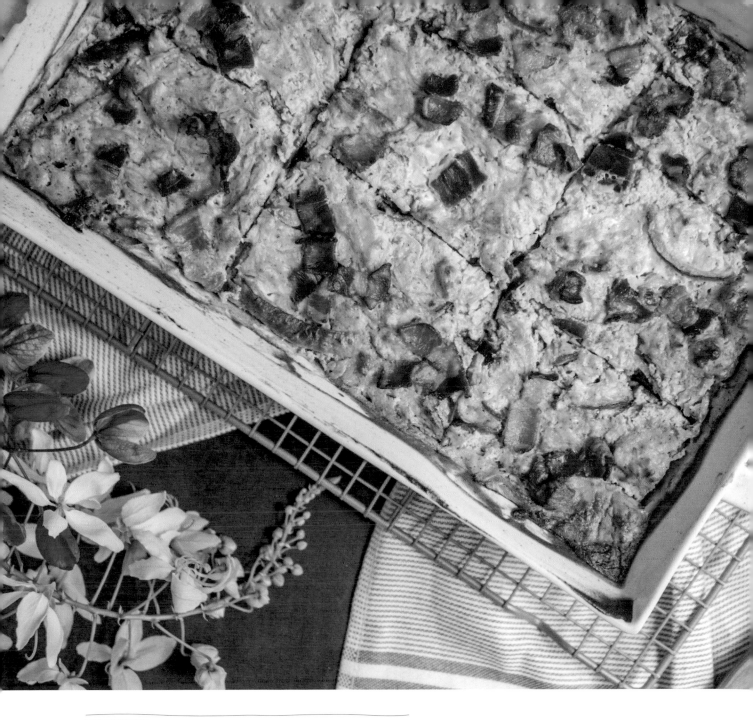

VARIATIONS: If you're really jonesing for some old-school flavor, go ahead and use tuna in this recipe. The béchamel bakes up creamy in the center and crisp on top. It will totally hit the spot. If you're not into fish, leftover pulled chicken or pork would work, too.

SUBSTITUTIONS: To make this dish AIP-compliant, omit the nutmeg and skip the eggs and mustard in the béchamel. You can use 1 tablespoon arrowroot starch if you wish to thicken it. If you can do egg yolks, which are usually less reactive than the whites, use 3 yolks.

deconstructed dragon roll

This is my favorite sushi roll, keto-fied and made into an easy-to-assemble bowl. The sticky cauliflower rice mimics sushi rice really well and is absolutely roll-worthy. If you're up for the extra work or really missing sushi rolls, go crazy and roll them up! For the rest of us (especially those who aren't super smooth in the nori-rolling department), this bowl will hit the spot. If you have access to quality seafood, like fresh ahi tuna or salmon, I highly recommend you go raw with this dish. A favorite from the blog, this Paleo sushi has been blowing minds for two years.

Makes 2 servings, with extra rice
PREP TIME: 10 minutes   COOK TIME: 20 minutes

FOR THE SUSHI RICE:

3 tablespoons coconut oil or sesame oil

4 cups riced cauliflower (see Note, page 140)

2 tablespoons apple cider vinegar or coconut vinegar

1 teaspoon fine Himalayan salt

2 heaping tablespoons unflavored grass-fed beef gelatin

⅔ cup full-fat coconut milk

FOR THE SHRIMP:

1 tablespoon coconut oil

8 large shrimp, peeled and deveined

1 teaspoon ginger powder

½ teaspoon fine Himalayan salt

2 teaspoons coconut aminos

FOR THE SUSHI BOWLS:

2 sheets nori, cut into 2-inch strips

1 medium Hass avocado, peeled, pitted, and sliced

8 spears asparagus, trimmed, or 2 small cucumbers, cut into spears

2 teaspoons sesame seeds, for garnish

Pinch of fine Himalayan salt, for garnish

2 tablespoons coconut aminos, for garnish

- Make the sushi rice: Heat a large skillet over medium heat. When it's hot, pour in the 3 tablespoons of oil, then add the cauliflower. Sauté, stirring often, for about 5 minutes, until the cauliflower is hot. If the cauliflower is frozen, sauté until any liquid has evaporated.

- Mix in the vinegar and salt. Sprinkle in the gelatin and stir well. Add the coconut milk and bring to a boil, stirring continuously. Continue to cook, stirring occasionally, for 8 to 10 minutes, until the liquid has evaporated. When you can see the bottom of the pan when you make a hole in the rice with a spoon, it's ready.

- Transfer the rice to a plate, spread it out flat, cover, and place in the fridge for at least 20 minutes to cool and get sticky while you cook the shrimp.

- Make the shrimp: Put the skillet back over medium heat and pour in the tablespoon of coconut oil. Add the shrimp, ginger powder, and salt. Stir to combine, then arrange the shrimp so they lie flat in the skillet. Cook for 2 minutes, or until the shrimp are crispy and browned, then flip them over, add the coconut aminos, and cook for 2 minutes on the other side. When they are coiled and pink and have golden crispy edges, remove them from the skillet. Set aside.

- Assemble the sushi bowls: Use a large ice cream scoop or 1-cup measuring cup to shape a single serving of sticky rice and set it on one side of a large shallow bowl. Add half of the nori strips and place half of the shrimp over them. Add half of the avocado slices and asparagus or cucumber spears next. Sprinkle everything with half of the sesame seeds and a small pinch of salt, and drizzle with 1 tablespoon of the coconut aminos. Repeat with the remaining ingredients to make a second sushi bowl.

- Store leftovers in an airtight container in the fridge for up to 3 days.

PER SERVING: Calories **496** · Fat **42.8g** · Total Carbohydrate **16.2g** · Dietary Fiber **14.1g** · Protein **25.5g**

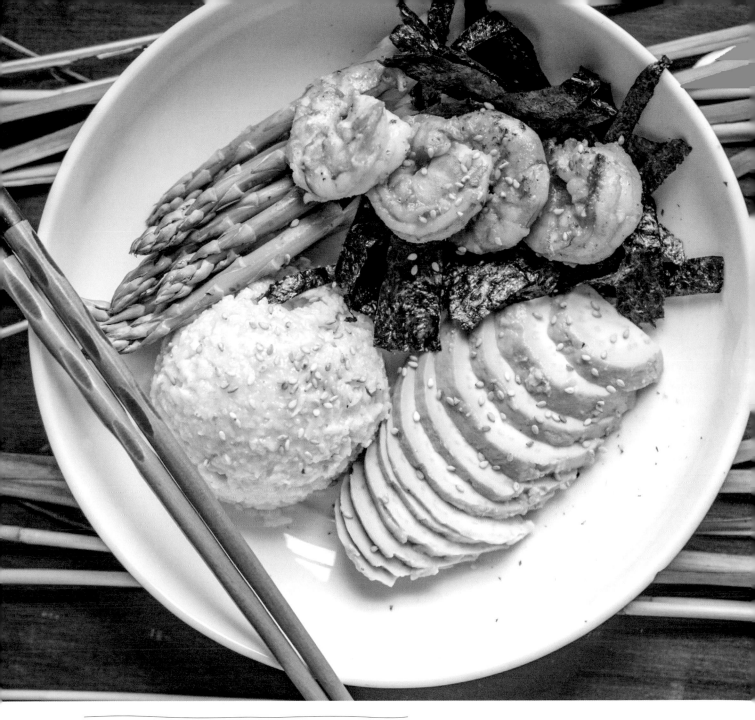

VARIATIONS: To make this a poke bowl, skip the shrimp and use raw sushi-grade ahi tuna. Mix it with 2 tablespoons sesame oil and 2 tablespoons coconut aminos. Add sliced green onions and you're good to go. I have a detailed recipe on my blog at thecastawaykitchen.com/2016/06/soy-free-ahi-poke.

SUBSTITUTIONS: To make this dish AIP-compliant, use coconut oil, not sesame oil, and omit the sesame seeds. To make it coconut-free, use bone broth (page 100) or another nondairy milk to cook the rice, omit the coconut aminos, and use avocado oil instead of coconut oil.

shrimp linguine

This was the first dish I made with kelp noodles. It was love at first bite. It's the dish I make for my family and friends when I want to show them how delicious this keto diet can be. As they slurp the last of the sauce off their plate, the meal always ends with, "Tell me more." This dish is simple enough that even a novice home cook can execute it with confidence, but the flavors are reminiscent of fine dining; it's delicate and aromatic, with lots of flavor. This recipe makes two bowls. You can serve it in a large bowl to share—maybe you'll find yourself in a Lady and the Tramp scenario.

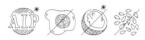

1 (12-ounce) package kelp noodles

2 tablespoons unsalted butter, ghee, or lard

5 cloves garlic, smashed with the side of a knife and then minced

8 jumbo shrimp, peeled and deveined

1 teaspoon dried thyme leaves

1 teaspoon fine Himalayan salt

1 teaspoon ground black pepper

1 cup Cauliflower Alfredo (page 86)

Makes 2 servings
PREP TIME: 10 minutes   COOK TIME: 10 minutes

○ Heat a large cast-iron skillet over medium heat. Submerge the kelp noodles in a bowl of warm water and set aside.

○ Place the butter in the hot skillet and heat until it begins to bubble, about 2 minutes. It will turn golden brown and smell slightly toasted when it's ready. Add the garlic to the butter. With a kitchen towel wrapped around the skillet's handle, tilt the skillet with one hand so the garlic and butter pool at one end. Use a spoon to keep pouring the butter over the garlic for 1 to 2 minutes, until it turns golden brown.

○ Add the shrimp to the skillet, then sprinkle in the thyme, salt, and pepper. Use a spatula to keep moving the shrimp and garlic around for 4 to 5 minutes. Once the shrimp have turned pink and most of them have just coiled, drain the kelp noodles and add them to the skillet. Use tongs to toss and combine the noodles with the shrimp. Add the Alfredo and continue to cook, stirring occasionally, for 2 to 3 minutes, until the noodles have softened. They will look and behave just like spaghetti when ready.

○ Serve immediately in large bowls with forks and spoons so you can twirl the noodles and get all the saucy goodness. Store leftovers in an airtight container in the fridge for up to 3 days. To reheat, simmer in a hot skillet for 5 to 6 minutes.

CHEF'S NOTE: I love to garnish this dish with some Garlic Confit (page 76) or Everything Bacon (page 84). For extra color and nutrition, you can also add a cup of greens at the end to wilt as the noodles soften.

SUBSTITUTIONS: To make this dish AIP-compliant, omit the pepper, use lard or coconut oil instead of butter, and use the AIP-compliant version of the Alfredo.

VARIATIONS: Use 4 cups zoodles (from 2 medium zucchini) if you're not into kelp noodles.

PER SERVING: Calories **413** · Fat **37.3g** · Total Carbohydrate **13.6g** · Dietary Fiber **5.3g** · Protein **19g**

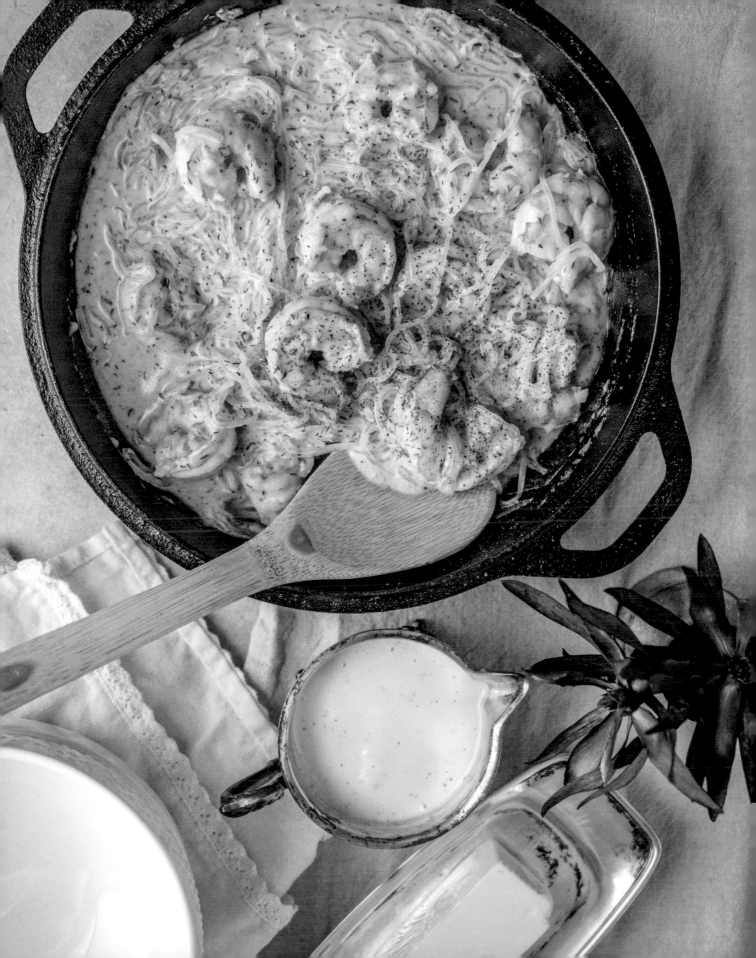

toasted coconut salmon

Choosing the right salmon is paramount for maximum flavor and high omega-3 content. Always buy wild-caught salmon. Purchasing fish in its peak season is a good way to get it for an affordable price. King salmon is available in early summer; in late summer, you'll find sockeye and then coho salmon. Look for fillets that are uniform in thickness; this will ensure even cooking. Bright and tight flesh without gaps is a good sign of freshness. This recipe cooks up in no time and really showcases the delicious taste of the salmon. Topped with coconut butter, this meal is a powerhouse of flavor and good fats and a showstopping dinner, perfect for entertaining or Sunday supper. This beautiful main dish goes well with Creamy Cauliflower Mash (page 318) or Curried Vegetable Salad (page 338).

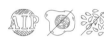

1 (1½-pound) salmon fillet

1 teaspoon fine Himalayan salt

1 tablespoon nutritional yeast

¼ cup coconut butter

1 teaspoon grated lemon zest

1 teaspoon dried thyme leaves

1 green onion, sliced, for garnish

CHEF'S NOTE: I'm obsessed with this recipe. A parent is allowed to have a favorite, right?

Makes 4 to 6 servings
PREP TIME: 10 minutes   COOK TIME: 8 minutes

○ Preheat the oven to 400°F.

○ Lay the salmon skin side down on a sheet pan. Run your fingers along the length of the fish to check for pin bones. They will be difficult to see but easy to feel. If they are present, use kitchen tweezers or pliers to pull them out.

○ Sprinkle the fillet evenly with the salt. Let it sit at room temperature while the oven preheats.

○ When the oven is ready to go, sprinkle the nutritional yeast evenly over the fillet, then spread the coconut butter over it, leaving clumps of it here and there. Sprinkle the lemon zest and then the thyme over the fillet, as evenly as possible.

○ Roast the salmon on the middle rack of the oven for 5 minutes, then set the oven to broil. Broil for 2 to 3 minutes, until the clumps of coconut butter are browned and the fish is cooked through. If you're making king salmon, which tends to be much larger, it may need to cook longer. A good indicator that the salmon is ready is that the meat flakes easily. Test this at 1-minute intervals until the thickest part of the fish easily flakes when pierced with a fork.

○ Remove the salmon from the oven. Let it rest for a few minutes, then garnish the fillet with the green onion slices. Slice the fillet into as many portions as you need and lift the pieces off of the skin with a spatula to serve.

○ Store leftovers in an airtight container in the fridge for up to 4 days. To reheat, flake and sauté the salmon in a skillet over medium heat for 4 minutes.

PER SERVING (6 servings): Calories **238** · Fat **13.9g** · Total Carbohydrate **2.9g** · Dietary Fiber **2.2g** · Protein **22.5g**

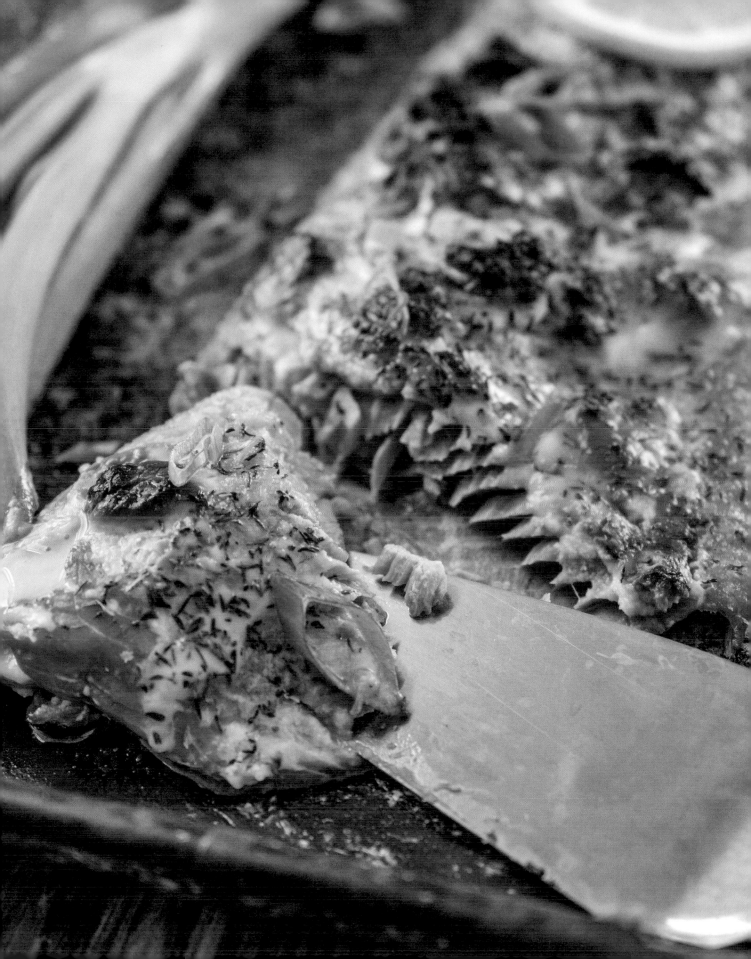

little lobster mac skillet

This isn't really a faux mac and cheese, but it's inspired by it! The word langostino is Spanish for "little lobster," and these prawns make a delicious and affordable lobster substitute. This one-skillet recipe coats sautéed broccoli florets and juicy little langostino tails in a thick, savory sauce. Baked up with crispy bacon and sweet pickled onions on top, this meal is the kind of delicious you could eat every day—as in, it serves four, but my husband and I usually polish it off in one sitting.

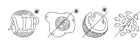

FOR THE SAUCE:

1½ tablespoons cooking fat (see page 53)

½ red onion, diced

2 medium carrots, diced

5 cloves garlic, minced

1 cup bone broth (page 100)

2 tablespoons nutritional yeast

1 tablespoon red wine vinegar

1 large egg

1½ tablespoons cooking fat (see page 53)

1 pound broccoli, cut into florets (about 3 cups)

2 tablespoons coconut butter, divided

1 pound precooked langostino tails (see Note)

1 teaspoon Dijon mustard

1 teaspoon fine Himalayan salt

1 teaspoon ground black pepper

¼ teaspoon ground nutmeg

3 slices bacon, chopped

¼ cup Pickled Red Onions (page 88)

Makes 4 servings
PREP TIME: 10 minutes   COOK TIME: 20 minutes

○ Preheat the oven to 400°F.

○ Make the sauce: Heat a large oven-safe skillet over medium heat. When it's hot, place the cooking fat in it, then add the onions, carrots, and garlic. Sauté until the onions are translucent, about 5 minutes. Add the broth, cover, and simmer for 5 minutes, or until the carrots are very tender. You should be able to mash them with a spoon.

○ Carefully transfer everything from the skillet to a blender or food processor. Add the nutritional yeast and vinegar and blend until smooth. Then, with the blender running on low, add the egg and blend until completely smooth. Set aside.

○ Put the skillet back on the stove over medium heat and add the 1½ tablespoons of fat. Add the broccoli florets and 1 tablespoon of the coconut butter, stir until well combined, and sauté for 2 minutes. Add the langostino tails, mustard, salt, pepper, and nutmeg. Sauté, stirring frequently, for 2 minutes.

○ Mix in the sauce. Top with the remaining tablespoon of coconut butter, the bacon, and the pickled onions. Set the skillet on the middle rack of the oven and bake for 8 to 10 minutes, until the bacon is crispy. Serve right away!

○ If there are leftovers (doubtful), store them in an airtight container in the fridge for up to 5 days. To reheat, sauté over high heat for 5 minutes.

CHEF'S NOTE: Costco sells a 2-pound bag of wild-caught langostino tails, fully cooked and frozen. They're delicious and affordable. If you can't find langostino tails, use precooked jumbo shrimp or pasteurized jumbo lump crabmeat. We're flexible; we've got range.

SUBSTITUTIONS: To make this dish AIP-compliant, omit the mustard and pepper and add 1 teaspoon Italian herb blend. In the sauce, omit the egg and substitute 2 tablespoons coconut cream and 1 tablespoon unflavored grass-fed beef gelatin. For a coconut-free option, use butter or ghee instead of coconut butter.

PER SERVING: Calories **348** · Fat **22.7g** · Total Carbohydrate **6.7g** · Dietary Fiber **1.6g** · Protein **27.4g**

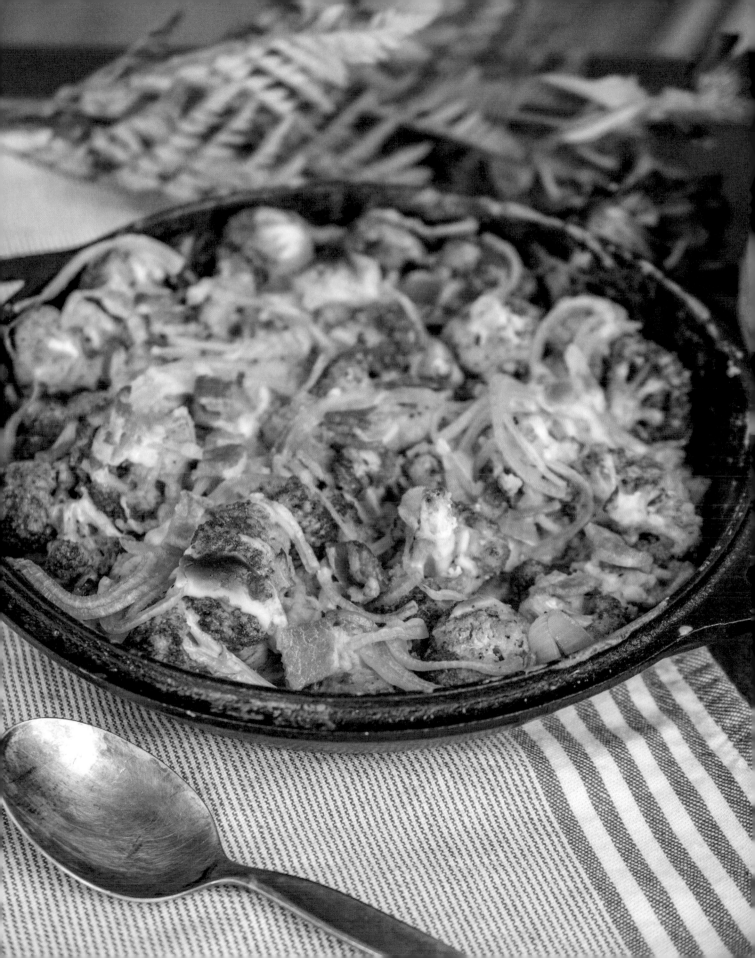

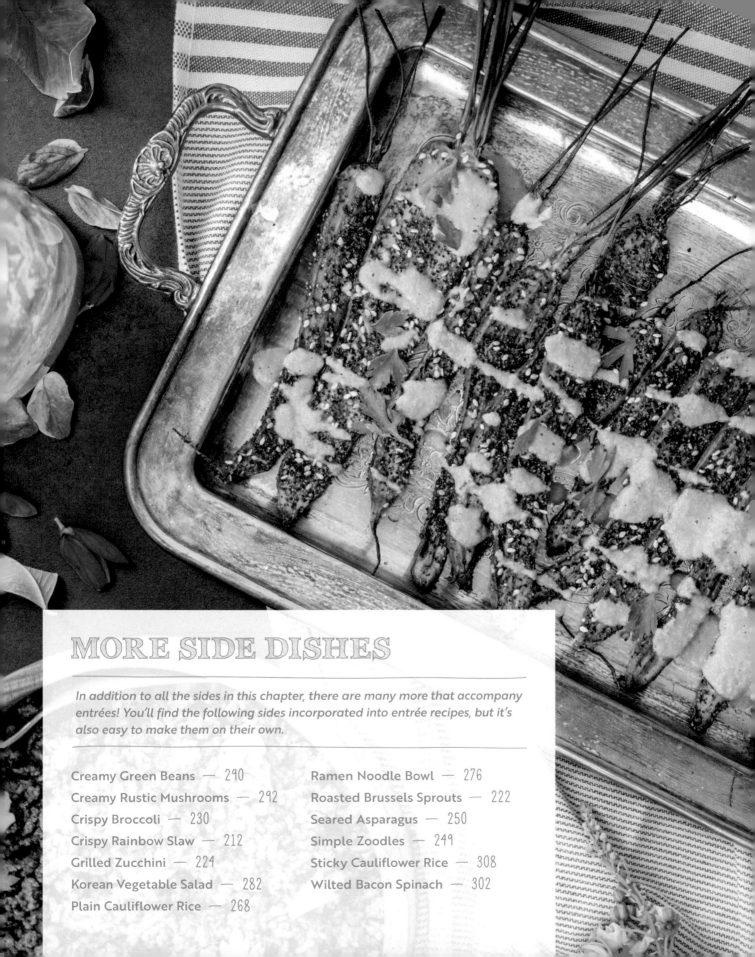

MORE SIDE DISHES

In addition to all the sides in this chapter, there are many more that accompany entrées! You'll find the following sides incorporated into entrée recipes, but it's also easy to make them on their own.

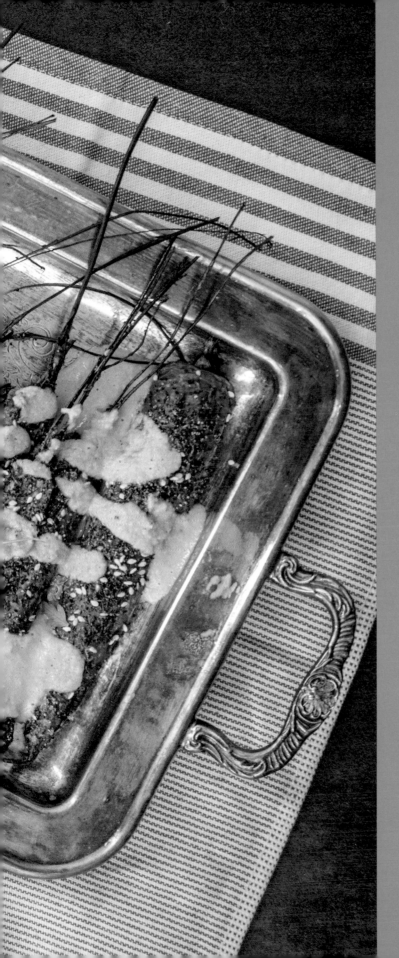

SIDES + BEVERAGES

Accompaniments and libations to complete your meals. From nutrient-dense to crave-crushing and refreshing, these pairing options will add just the right touch to your meal.

creamy cauliflower mash

The trick to thick, real-deal, potato-like cauliflower mash is to skip the steaming. You want to mimic the starchiness of potatoes, so roasting your cauliflower is the way to go. Garlic, rosemary, and bacon fat, the dream team, make this cauliflower mash steakhouse-worthy!

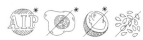

1 medium head cauliflower, cut into 1-inch pieces

5 cloves garlic

Needles from 2 sprigs fresh rosemary

2 tablespoons bacon fat, melted

1 teaspoon fine Himalayan salt

1 teaspoon ground black pepper

¼ cup coconut cream (see Note, page 144)

2 large egg yolks

Makes 4 servings
PREP TIME: 15 minutes   COOK TIME: 30 minutes

◦ Preheat the oven to 400°F.

◦ On a sheet pan, toss the cauliflower pieces with the garlic, rosemary, and bacon fat. Spread them evenly over the pan and roast for 30 minutes, until the cauliflower is toasted and the garlic is golden brown.

◦ Transfer the cauliflower, garlic, and rosemary to a food processor. Add the salt and pepper and pulse until the mixture is broken down. Add the coconut cream and egg yolks, then blend until smooth. You might need to stop and scrape down the sides once or twice. The mash will be thick and rich.

◦ Serve hot. Store leftovers in the fridge in an airtight container for up to 5 days.

SUBSTITUTIONS: To make this mash AIP-compliant, omit the pepper and replace the egg yolks with 2 tablespoons avocado oil. To make it coconut-free, omit the coconut cream and add ¼ cup Homemade Mayo (page 82).

PER SERVING: Calories **171** · Fat **13g** · Total Carbohydrate **10g** · Dietary Fiber **4g** · Protein **5g**

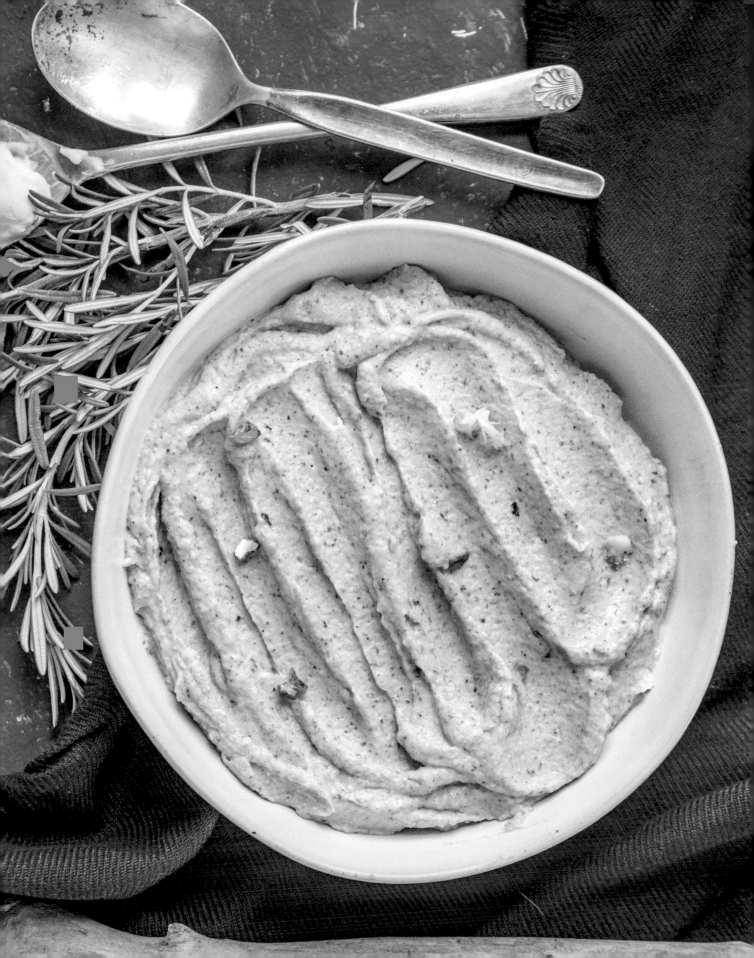

creamy kale noodles

Pasta aglio e olio used to be one of my favorite meals. Al dente spaghetti is lightly sautéed with lots of kale, even more garlic, and a generous glug of olive oil—the simplicity is perfection. It wasn't until I discovered kelp noodles that I was able to re-create my favorite pasta dishes with an authentic mouthfeel. Even better, kelp noodles are very affordable and extremely easy to prepare! You can find them at any health-food store, or better yet, you can buy them by the box online. Great eaten cold and crunchy or hot and saucy, these mineral-rich noodles just became your best friends. Here, I've prepared them simply, aglio e olio with lots of kale, then added some Cheesy Yellow Sauce (page 68) to drive home the authentic pasta flavor. Buon appetito!

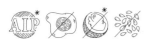

2 (12-ounce) packages kelp noodles

2 tablespoons lemon juice

6 ounces dinosaur kale

2 tablespoons unsalted butter, ghee, or lard

6 cloves garlic, minced

2 tablespoons extra-virgin olive oil

1 teaspoon fine Himalayan salt

1 cup Cheesy Yellow Sauce (page 68)

Cracked black pepper, for garnish

Makes 4 servings
PREP TIME: 10 minutes   COOK TIME: 15 minutes

○ Open the packets of kelp noodles into a large bowl. Submerge the noodles in warm water. Add the lemon juice and let soak for 10 minutes.

○ Meanwhile, wash and dry the kale and trim the stems. I like to fold the leaf in half at the vein and slice the stem at an angle. Stack the leaves and cut them into ¼-inch-wide strips. Set aside.

○ Heat a large skillet over medium-high heat. When it's hot, add the butter, garlic, and kale. Sauté, stirring often, for 5 minutes, or until the kale is wilted and browned at the edges. Gather the sautéed kale on one side of the skillet.

○ Drain the kelp noodles and add them to the skillet, away from the kale. Then transfer the kale to the bowl that held the kelp noodles. Set aside.

○ Add the olive oil and salt to the kelp noodles. Sauté for 3 to 4 minutes, until they begin soften. Stir in the cheese sauce and heat until warm. Transfer the sauced noodles to the bowl with the kale and toss to combine.

○ Garnish with a little cracked pepper and dig in! Store leftovers in an airtight container in the fridge for up to 5 days. To reheat, sauté over high heat for 3 minutes.

VARIATIONS: You can use zoodles (zucchini noodles) instead of kelp noodles: use 4 cups fresh zoodles and follow the recipe as written.

If you don't have Cheesy Yellow Sauce on hand, you can use any sauce you like: Pistou (page 74), Cauliflower Alfredo (page 86), Roasted Beet Marinara (page 78), or even just extra butter and some nutritional yeast. This recipe is a great template for preparing kelp noodles—make it your own!

CHEF'S NOTE: This dish makes the perfect accompaniment to leftover proteins for a quick weeknight dinner that is ready in 30 minutes. I love it with Sticky Pistou Meatballs (page 272).

SUBSTITUTIONS: To make this dish AIP-compliant, use bacon fat or coconut oil instead of butter and skip the cracked black pepper at the end.

PER SERVING: Calories **201** · Fat **13.6g** · Total Carbohydrate **13.9g** · Dietary Fiber **6.6g** · Protein **7.2g**

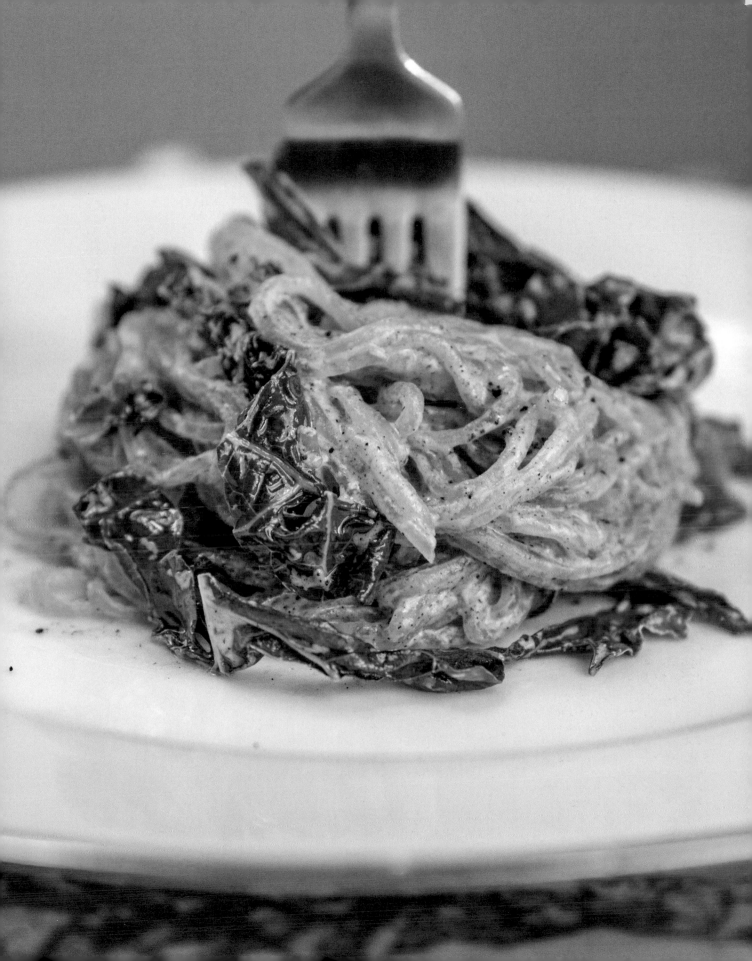

crispy bacon green beans

Turns out my kid will eat vegetables only if they are crispy. He's four, but he might be on to something. That's how this recipe was born. I knew he wouldn't eat the green beans steamed, no matter how much butter I put on them, so I fried them up in a cast-iron skillet that was hanging out with leftover bacon fat from that morning. We could not believe how delicious these crispy, bacon fat–fried green beans were. I thought I would never make them another way… until I threw them in the oven. I can't stress how easy this recipe is, yet how absolutely tasty the result. This dish is a staple in my home.

1 pound fresh green beans

5 cloves garlic, peeled

½ teaspoon fine Himalayan salt

5 slices bacon, cut into ½-inch pieces

Makes 4 servings
PREP TIME: 5 minutes   COOK TIME: 30 minutes

○ Preheat the oven to 400°F.

○ Trim the green beans. To be efficient, I like to hold a bunch in my hand and use kitchen shears to snip off the ends. Spread them out on a sheet pan so none are overlapping. Add the garlic cloves to the pan and sprinkle everything with the salt. Distribute the bacon pieces evenly over the green beans.

○ Roast for 15 minutes. Open the oven, use a kitchen towel to hold the sheet pan firmly in one hand, and give it a shake so the green beans and bacon move around a bit. Close the oven and roast the beans for another 15 minutes, or until they are slightly shriveled with crispy ends.

○ Store leftovers in an airtight container in the fridge for up to 4 days. To reheat, sauté over high heat for 5 minutes.

CHEF'S NOTE: Caution: These beans are addicting! They make the perfect side dish to any meal, but I especially love them with Toasted Coconut Salmon (page 312), Shrimp Linguine (page 310), or Party Meatballs (page 260). Or make them a meal all on their own: top a pile of these with a fried egg and call it a day!

PER SERVING: Calories **169** · Fat **10g** · Total Carbohydrate **9.7g** · Dietary Fiber **3.9g** · Protein **11.1g**

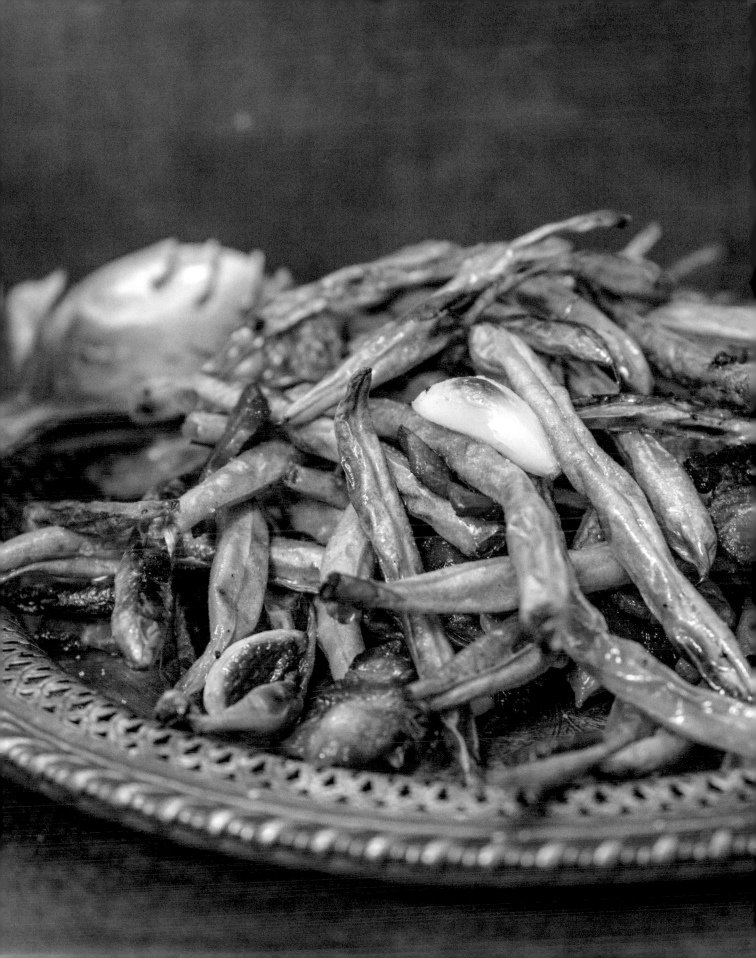

nut-free keto bread

It's interesting how we cling to certain foods. Bread and bread-like recipes will always be something we seek. No matter how far our habits and diets have come, there is always that moment when we just want something warm, toasted, and fluffy. It could be the weather or being under the weather, the moon or nostalgia, but when a craving for bread hits, this is a deliciously legit recipe that will leave you feeling great. There are just a few simple ingredients—nothing hard to find or hard to digest here. Just some real-food magic.

Makes one 8½ by 4½-inch loaf (12 slices)
PREP TIME: 15 minutes   COOK TIME: 50 minutes

6 large eggs, separated

⅓ cup coconut flour

1 teaspoon baking powder

½ teaspoon fine Himalayan salt

¼ cup flaxseed meal

½ cup filtered water

½ cup melted coconut oil

1 teaspoon poppy seeds, for garnish (optional)

∘ Preheat the oven to 350°F. Line an 8½ by 4½-inch loaf pan with parchment paper.

∘ Place the egg whites in the bowl of a stand mixer and beat on low until foamy, then bring up to medium speed and beat until soft peaks form. While the egg whites beat, prepare the rest of the recipe. (If you're using a handheld mixer instead of a stand mixer, beat the whites until soft peaks form, then set aside.)

∘ Sift the coconut flour, baking powder, and salt into a large bowl. Whisk in the flaxseed meal.

∘ In a small bowl, whisk together the egg yolks, water, and oil. Slowly pour the wet mixture into the dry mixture, whisking until fully combined. Use a spatula to fold in the beaten egg whites until you no longer see streaks of white.

∘ Pour the dough into the prepared loaf pan and sprinkle with the poppy seeds (if using). Bake on the middle rack of the oven for 50 to 60 minutes, until the bread is golden brown on the outside and firm to the touch.

∘ Remove the bread from the oven and let cool in the pan for an hour before unmolding and slicing. Store at room temperature in an airtight container or wrapped in plastic wrap for up to 5 days.

CHEF'S NOTES: Pair this bread with Hard Cheese (page 70), Pistou (page 74), and some veggies for a panini experience that is hard to forget. Or make a grilled cheese and dunk it in some Roasted Beet Marinara (page 78). With only 2½ grams of total carbs per slice, plenty of fiber, and lots of good fats, this is bread you can feel at ease about incorporating into your diet.

I like to use an 8½ by 4½-inch loaf pan, which results in a tall, conventionally shaped loaf, but you can use a larger loaf pan, too. If you use a larger loaf pan, cut the wide, short loaf in half vertically, as you would a baguette, then cut small sandwich-sized slices horizontally. This wider, shorter loaf will bake in less time; check it after 40 minutes.

SUBSTITUTIONS: You can use golden flaxseed meal for a lighter bread or brown flaxseed meal for a speckled look. Using baking soda instead of baking powder can give the bread a greenish tinge, but it won't affect the flavor. To make allergen-friendly baking powder, sift together equal parts baking soda, cream of tartar, and tapioca starch.

PER SLICE: Calories **142** · Fat **12.5g** · Total Carbohydrate **2.6g** · Dietary Fiber **2.5g** · Protein **4g**

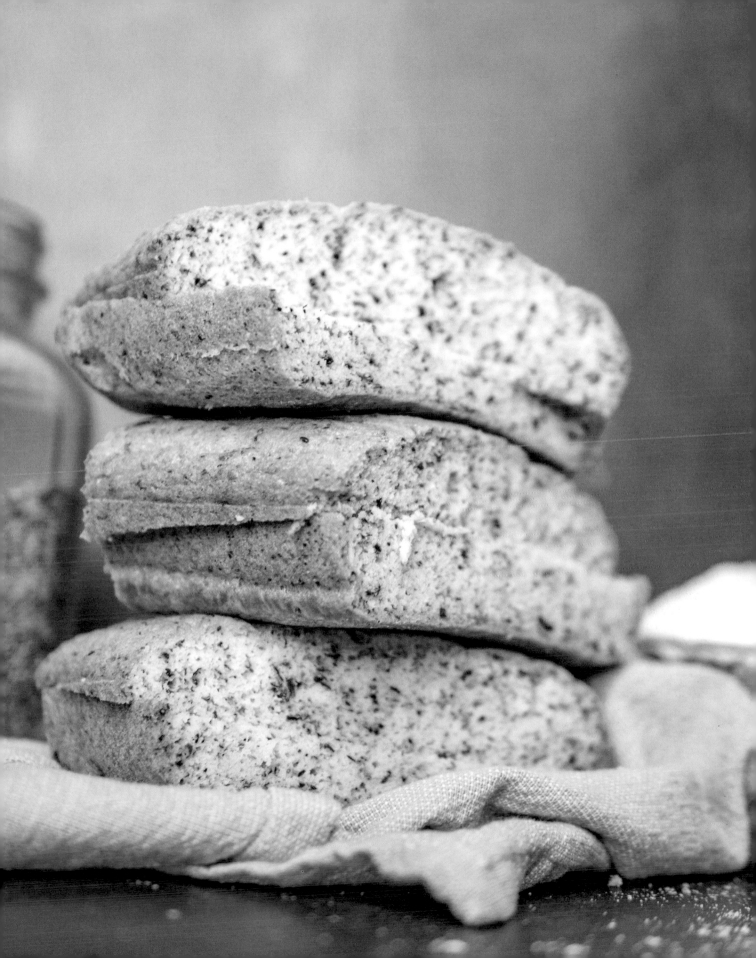

everything flaxseed meal crackers

Crunchy snacks are hard to come by when you're not eating carbs or nuts, but sometimes you just need that crunch and pork rinds aren't going to cut it. Enter this recipe. It's very easy to make, doesn't have flour or eggs, and really can be made with four ingredients if you leave out the seasonings—but don't leave out the seasonings. I like to make a batch of these every two weeks; they last a week or so and are perfect to top with deli meats or dip into soups. One of the awesome things about flaxseed meal is that it's almost all fiber, too!

2 cups flaxseed meal

1 cup water

½ cup apple cider vinegar or coconut vinegar

1 teaspoon dried dill weed

1 teaspoon dried rosemary needles

1 teaspoon fine Himalayan salt

1 teaspoon garlic powder

1 teaspoon ground black pepper

1 teaspoon poppy seeds

1 teaspoon sesame seeds

Makes 2 dozen crackers (4 per serving)
PREP TIME: 10 minutes   COOK TIME: 40 minutes

○ Preheat the oven to 350°F convection or 375°F bake. Line a baking sheet with parchment paper.

○ Place the flaxseed meal, water, and vinegar in a medium-sized bowl. Add the dill weed, rosemary, salt, garlic powder, pepper, and seeds and mix thoroughly until a thick paste forms.

○ Transfer the flaxseed meal paste to the prepared baking sheet and shape it into a square that's approximately 10 inches wide, ¼ inch thick, and smooth on top. Bake for 30 minutes, or until firm in the center. Remove from the oven, carefully cut the mass into squares, separate them a little bit, and bake for another 10 minutes. When they're done, the crackers will be dark brown, crispy, and hard to the touch.

○ Let the crackers cool to room temperature before storing in an airtight container in the pantry. They will keep for up to a week. If they soften, you can toast them at 400°F for 5 minutes before enjoying.

PER SERVING: Calories **154** · Fat **12.1g** · Total Carbohydrate **8.3g** · Dietary Fiber **10.3g** · Protein **5.3g**

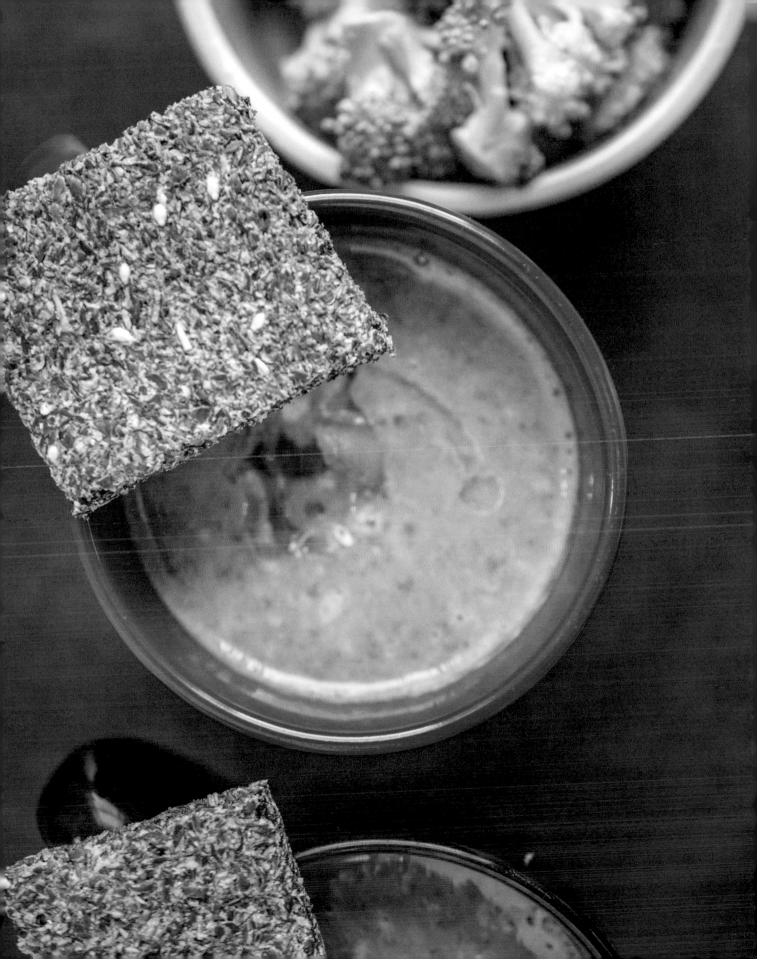

savory flax waffles

A super-easy, fiber-packed, bread-like food that comes together in minutes and with only a handful of ingredients. These waffles are crispy and light and don't taste like cardboard. I like to make a batch of these and keep them in the fridge. They're great topped with eggs or eaten alongside a salad, and for making quick meals like mini sandwiches. Or simply enjoy them with a pat of butter or a few slices of Hard Cheese (page 70) on top.

Makes 4 waffles (1 per serving)
PREP TIME: 5 minutes   COOK TIME: 20 minutes

4 large eggs

¼ cup coconut cream (see Note, page 144)

1 tablespoon coconut vinegar

1 cup flaxseed meal

½ teaspoon fine Himalayan salt

½ teaspoon garlic powder

½ teaspoon ground black pepper

½ teaspoon onion powder

○ In a large bowl, whisk together the eggs, coconut cream, and vinegar until well combined. Add the flaxseed meal, salt, garlic powder, pepper, and onion powder and mix until a thick batter forms.

○ Preheat a waffle iron per the manufacturer's instructions. When it's ready, pour in about ¼ cup of the batter. Cook until crispy, about 5 minutes, depending on your appliance. Repeat with the remaining batter.

○ Serve immediately. Store leftovers in an airtight container in the fridge for up to 1 week. To reheat, toast in a preheated 400°F oven for 4 minutes.

SUBSTITUTIONS: I have not tried making these waffles with a replacement for the eggs, but if you have an egg allergy, that could be a good option; however, please note that the macros will be different. If you want a flaxseed-free savory waffle, make the Mini Pumpkin Waffles (page 330) without the sweetener.

PER SERVING: Calories **249** · Fat **18.8g** · Total Carbohydrate **9.2g** · Dietary Fiber **8.2g** · Protein **11.6g**

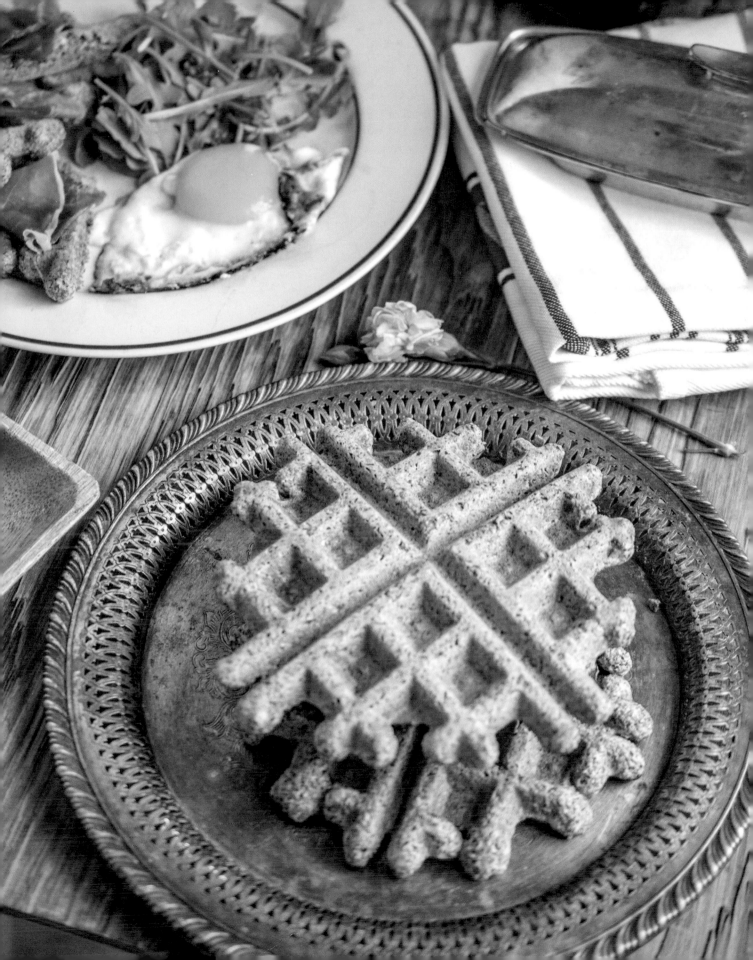

mini pumpkin waffles with blueberry compote

These lightly sweetened, fluffy waffles, served with a simple blueberry compote, are the perfect side to eggs and bacon. Who knew dairy-free keto waffles could be so good? I did. Just saying. (P.S. This batter makes killer pancakes, too!)

FOR THE COMPOTE:

½ cup frozen blueberries

2 tablespoons unsalted butter, ghee, or coconut oil

1 teaspoon granulated erythritol or other low-carb sweetener (see page 38)

FOR THE WAFFLES:

5 large eggs

3 tablespoons MCT oil or melted coconut oil

2 heaping tablespoons pumpkin puree

1 teaspoon pure vanilla extract

¼ cup coconut flour

2 tablespoons collagen peptides

Pinch of fine Himalayan salt

10 drops liquid stevia (optional)

Makes 4 waffles (1 per serving)
PREP TIME: 10 minutes   COOK TIME: 30 minutes

○ Preheat the oven to 400°F.

○ Make the compote: Combine the blueberries, butter, and erythritol in a small saucepan over medium heat. Cook until the blueberries thaw and their liquid begins to simmer, about 10 minutes, mashing them and stirring occasionally. Remove from the heat and set aside.

○ Make the waffles: In a large bowl, whisk together the eggs, oil, pumpkin puree, and vanilla extract. Add the coconut flour, collagen, salt, and stevia (if using). Whisk until well combined and mostly smooth.

○ Preheat a waffle iron per the manufacturer's instructions. When it's ready, pour in about ¼ cup of the batter. Cook until crispy, roughly 3 to 4 minutes, depending on your appliance. Repeat with the remaining batter.

○ Cut each waffle along the seams into four segments. Place the waffle wedges in the oven and toast, as the first waffle will be cold by the time the last one is done. Toast for 2 to 3 minutes. Serve with blueberry compote spooned on top.

○ You can make these waffles ahead of time so they're ready to go for the week. Store in an airtight container in the fridge for up to 5 days and toast as directed above to reheat.

CHEF'S NOTE: I love these waffles extra toasted, at about 6 minutes. They're soft in the center and crispy on the outside, and with the juicy compote on top, it's such a lovely combination. This simple compote is also amazing with Spiced Pork Tenderloin (page 292)—remember that!

TIME-SAVING TIP: If you're not into pumpkin, leave it out and add an extra tablespoon of coconut flour to the batter. Whisk until smooth, then let it sit for 2 to 3 minutes, until it thickens. Whisk in ¼ cup sparkling water and then continue with the recipe as written.

PER SERVING (with compote): Calories **289** · Fat **24.5g** · Total Carbohydrate **10.3g** · Dietary Fiber **5.7g** · Protein **14.5g**

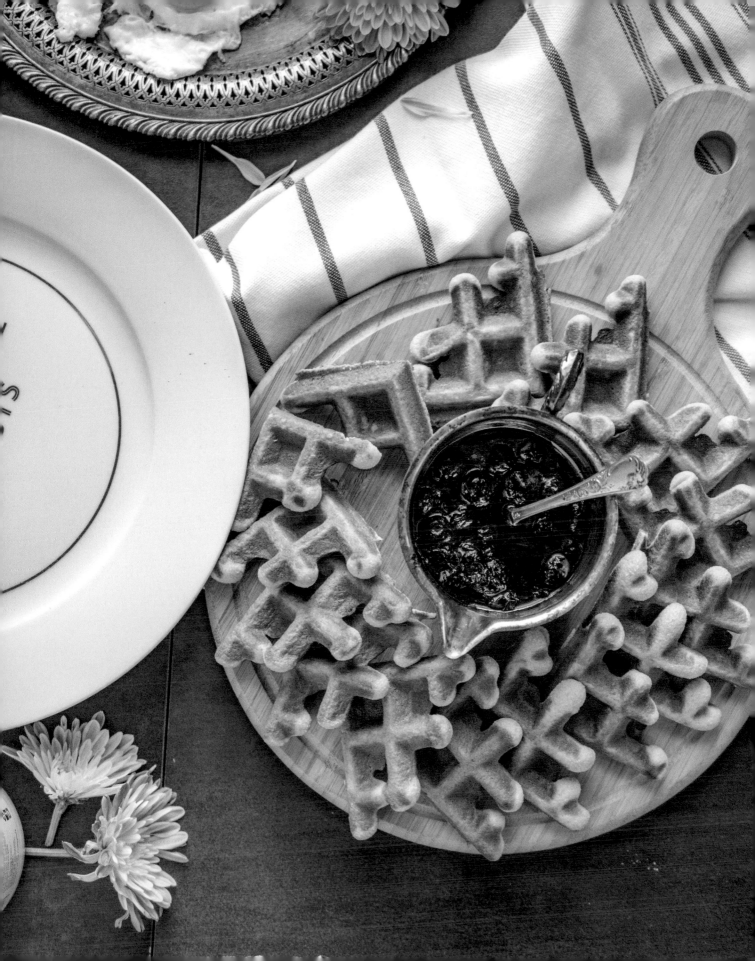

street taco tortillas

Full disclosure: This recipe almost drove me mad. In an effort to keep the ingredients easy to find and commonly used so that you aren't running out to buy specialty items, I limited myself to coconut flour, eggs, and flaxseed meal. I tried numerous ways to make a dough, a batter, and a paste from these, to bake, fry, or toast them, all to no avail. Then one fine day it hit me: I already had a fantastic low-carb dough recipe in my Savory Flax Waffles recipe (page 328). And just like that, with a few tweaks, I was able to make tortillas. These are not eggy or dry, and they hold up well. They are soft and savory, and I am quite proud of them.

Makes 6 tortillas (1 per serving)
PREP TIME: 20 minutes   COOK TIME: 18 minutes

2 cups riced cauliflower (see Note)

2 tablespoons flaxseed meal

1 teaspoon fine Himalayan salt

1 teaspoon garlic powder

1 teaspoon onion powder

Pinch of ground black pepper

1 tablespoon lime juice

2 large eggs

CHEF'S NOTE: I strongly suggest that you use fresh cauliflower for this recipe. (See the Note on page 140 for instructions.) While I love the convenience of frozen riced cauliflower, using it here will make the tortillas taste and smell very much like cauliflower. Also, frozen cauliflower doesn't hold up as well in this recipe; it will result in softer, weaker tortillas.

○ Preheat the oven to 375°F. Line a sheet pan with parchment paper.

○ Microwave the cauliflower on high for 2 minutes. Transfer it to a nut milk bag or clean kitchen towel and squeeze out the water. You should get about ¾ cup of water out of the cauliflower. This takes some elbow grease. Afterward, you will have a ball of paste-like cauliflower mush.

○ Place the cauliflower mush in a large bowl. Add the flaxseed meal, salt, garlic powder, onion powder, and pepper. Mix to combine, then stir in the lime juice.

○ Make a well in the cauliflower mixture. Crack the eggs into the well and use a fork to whisk the eggs, then slowly incorporate them into the mixture until a soft dough forms.

○ Spoon about 2 tablespoons of the dough on the lined sheet pan. Gently flatten it with the palm of your hand and use your fingers to gently mold it into a tortilla that's 3 to 4 inches across and ⅛ inch thick. (If you make the tortillas too thin, they will rip apart when loaded up with toppings.) Repeat with the rest of the dough to make a total of six tortillas.

○ Bake for 10 minutes, then gently flip the tortillas and bake for another 6 to 8 minutes, until the edges have browned and the tortillas look golden and glossy. Remove from the oven and let cool on the pan for 5 minutes before removing.

○ These tortillas can be made ahead and stored in an airtight container for up to 5 days. They're best warmed up in a hot, dry skillet. It really brings home the toasty tortilla flavor!

PER SERVING: Calories **41** · Fat **3g** · Total Carbohydrate **2.1g** · Dietary Fiber **1g** · Protein **3g**

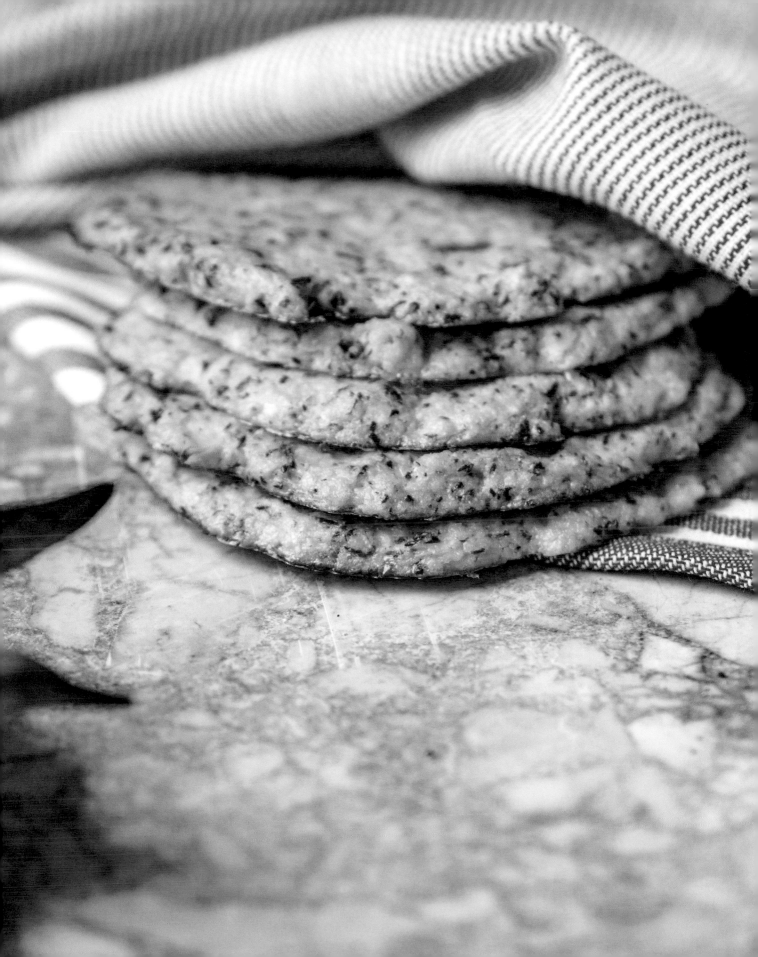

loaded roasted carrots

I love carrots when they're roasted but pretty much despise them raw. There, I said it. I'm an adult, and raw carrots taste like medicine to me. But these beauties are soft on the inside, with a wrinkled crispy skin that is studded with seeds and herbs, topped off with Ginger Sauce (page 102). I daresay you'll have a hard time sticking to just one serving. They're locked, loaded, and ready to deliver a delicious dose of vitamin C!

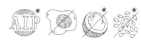

8 medium carrots with greens

2 tablespoons unsalted butter, ghee, or lard

1 teaspoon poppy seeds

1 teaspoon sesame seeds

1 teaspoon dried cilantro or thyme leaves

½ teaspoon fine Himalayan salt

¼ cup Ginger Sauce (page 102)

Makes 4 servings
PREP TIME: 5 minutes   COOK TIME: 40 minutes

◦ Preheat the oven to 400°F.

◦ Trim the carrot greens so there are about 3 inches left. Cut the carrots in half lengthwise and rub them with the butter. Lay them out evenly on a sheet pan. Sprinkle the seeds, cilantro, and salt all over the carrots.

◦ Roast for 40 to 45 minutes. Remove from the oven and drizzle the sauce over the carrots. Serve immediately. Store leftover carrots in separate airtight containers for up to 4 days. Reheat in a preheated 350°F oven for 8 minutes.

CHEF'S NOTE: The ginger sauce is amazing on these carrots (and on anything, really), but I love them without sauce as well. I like to add a scoop of Carne Molida (page 244) over them, too.

SUBSTITUTIONS: To make these carrots AIP-compliant, use coconut oil instead of butter, omit the seeds, and add 1 teaspoon onion powder. Serve with Toum (page 72) instead of ginger sauce—which will also make it coconut-free.

PER SERVING: Calories **120** · Fat **6.3g** · Total Carbohydrate **11.4g** · Dietary Fiber **3.3g** · Protein **2.1g**

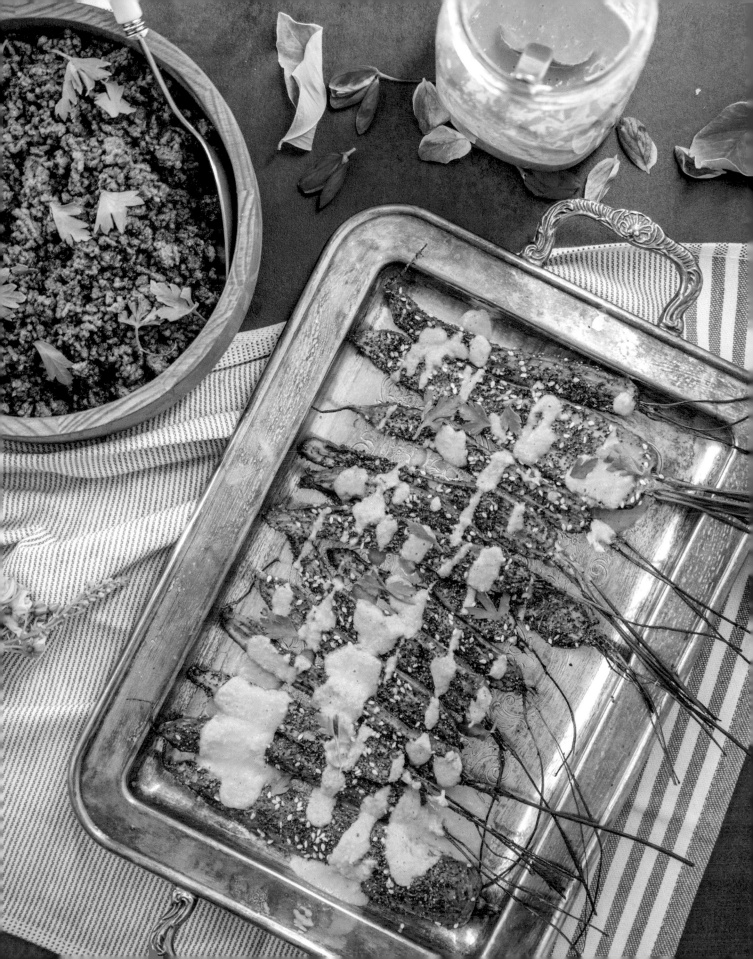

spiced broccolini with cool cilantro sauce

Crispy cruciferous vegetables are where it's at! I like to roast mine at a high temperature to get some dark-brown crispy bits. And when coated with a good amount of fat, roasted veggies go from okay to amazing. With warm garam masala and anti-inflammatory turmeric, you have a spicy, warm tray of crunchy broccolini. The super-cool cilantro sauce plays off the warm spices to deliver the most interesting broccoli dish in the world. (Yes, if you don't have broccolini, broccoli florets will work, too!)

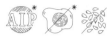

18 ounces broccolini, trimmed (about 4 cups)

3 tablespoons salted butter or bacon grease, melted

1 teaspoon garam masala

1 teaspoon turmeric powder

½ teaspoon fine Himalayan salt

FOR THE CILANTRO SAUCE:

⅔ cup Coconut Yogurt (page 96)

⅔ cup Homemade Mayo (page 82)

1 cup chopped fresh cilantro

Juice of 2 lemons

Makes 4 servings
PREP TIME: 10 minutes   COOK TIME: 40 minutes

○ Preheat the oven to 400°F.

○ Trim the broccolini about 3 inches below the florets. In a large bowl, toss the broccolini with the butter, garam masala, turmeric, and salt until all of it is evenly coated.

○ Spread the broccolini on a sheet pan so the florets are lying flat. Roast for 40 minutes. When the broccolini is ready, the tips will be crispy and brown and the stalks dark green.

○ While the broccolini roasts, make the sauce: Place the yogurt, mayo, cilantro, and lemon juice in a blender and pulse to combine. You want the cilantro minced but not pureed. The sauce should be white with green leaves, not completely green.

○ Remove the broccolini from the oven and use a spatula to scrape it off the sheet pan. Serve the broccolini with the sauce on the side or drizzled on top.

○ You will have extra sauce; store it in a jar in the refrigerator for up to 10 days. Shake to combine before using. Store leftover broccolini in an airtight container in the refrigerator for up to 5 days.

SUBSTITUTION: To make this dish AIP-compliant, replace the garam masala with ½ teaspoon each ginger powder and ground cinnamon. For the sauce, omit the mayo and double the yogurt.

PER SERVING (broccolini): Calories **143** · Fat **8.7g** · Total Carbohydrate **7.1g** · Dietary Fiber **7.3g** · Protein **6.6g**
PER 2 TABLESPOONS of cilantro sauce: Calories **137** · Fat **14g** · Total Carbohydrate **1g** · Dietary Fiber **0g** · Protein **7g**

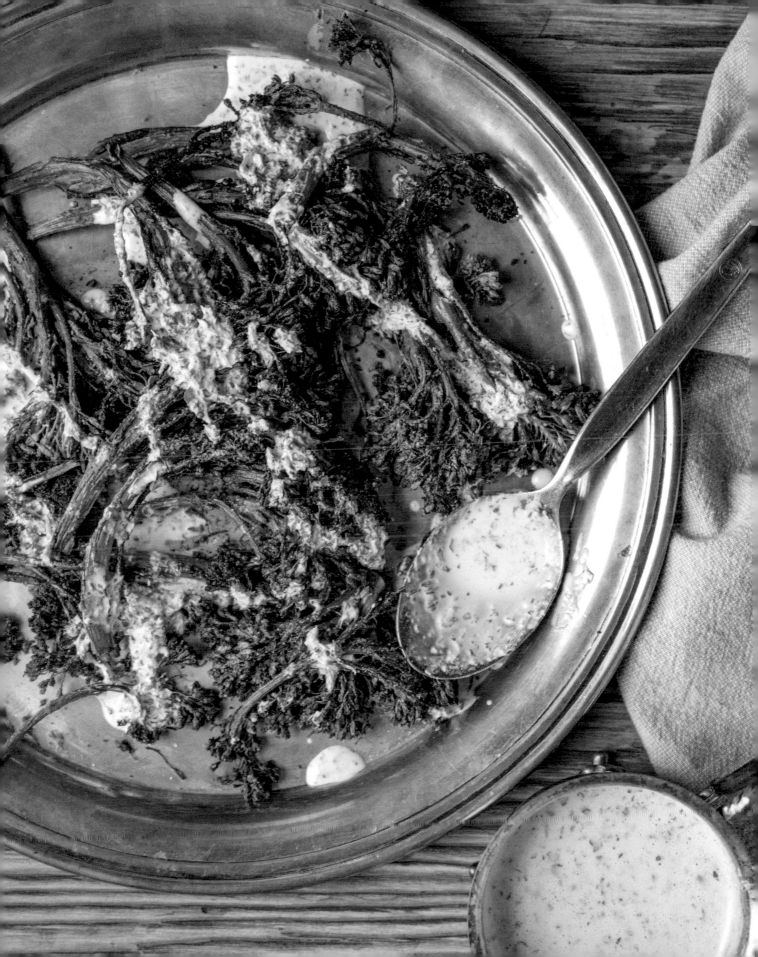

curried vegetable salad

Who loves mayo? I know I do. (I'm sure you could tell by the three recipes on page 82.) Mayo takes my favorite crispy curried vegetables and transforms them into a side dish that doesn't need to be heated, goes well with everything, and has plenty of satiating fats. Forget potato salad; this is your new potluck go-to!

3 cups halved Brussels sprouts

2 cups broccoli florets

5 cloves garlic, sliced

3 tablespoons avocado oil

1 teaspoon fish sauce

1 teaspoon fine Himalayan salt

1 teaspoon ground black pepper

1 teaspoon ground cumin

1 teaspoon turmeric powder

½ teaspoon ginger powder

¼ cup Homemade Mayo (page 82)

Makes 6 servings
PREP TIME: 10 minutes   COOK TIME: 45 minutes

◦ Preheat the oven to 400°F.

◦ Spread the Brussels sprouts, broccoli, and garlic evenly on a sheet pan. Drizzle with the avocado oil and fish sauce and sprinkle the salt, pepper, cumin, turmeric, and ginger powder over them. Toss to combine, massaging the oil and seasonings into the Brussels and broccoli. Then spread them out again on the sheet pan. Wash your yellow hands so the turmeric doesn't stain them!

◦ Roast the vegetables on the middle rack of the oven for 40 minutes. Remove from the oven and let cool to room temperature.

◦ Transfer the roasted vegetables to a bowl. Add the mayo and stir to combine. Store in the fridge for up to 5 days, until ready to serve or for meal prep.

VARIATIONS: Use 3 cups cauliflower florets and/or 2 cups halved radishes instead of the Brussels and broccoli. This variation makes a great "no-tato" salad!

PER SERVING: Calories **176** · Fat **16.6g** · Total Carbohydrate **6.6g** · Dietary Fiber **2.6g** · Protein **2.5g**

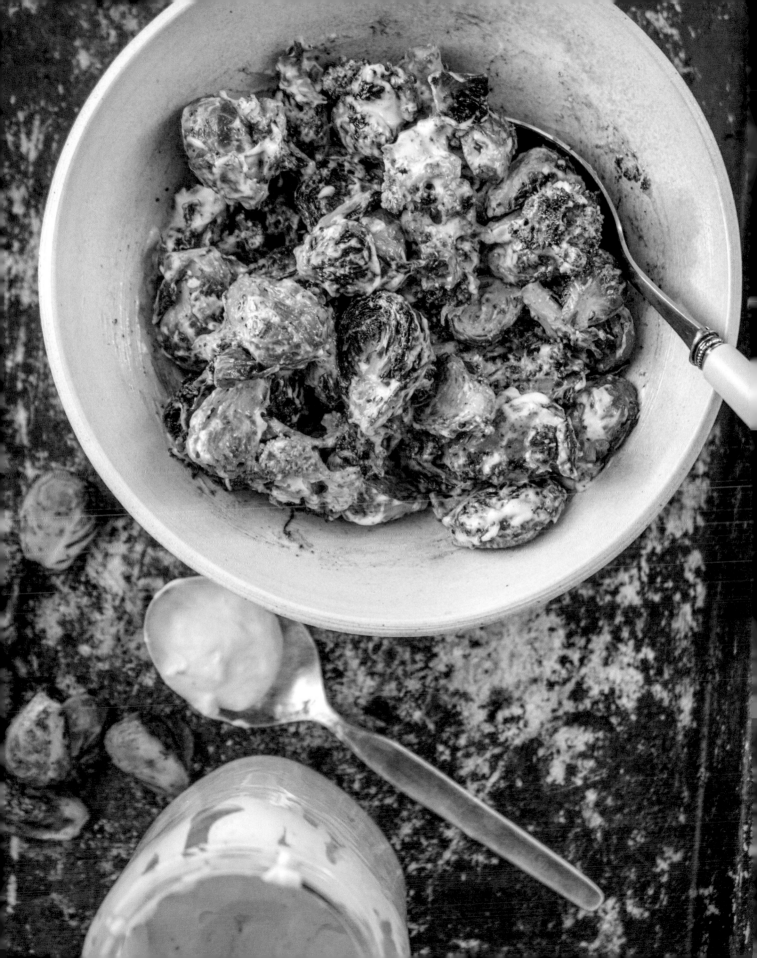

half-sour pickled salad

The first time I had half-sour pickles, I was in love. They're more cucumber than pickle: bright, crispy, and green. Keeping Pickled Red Onions (page 88) in the fridge makes short work of them, too; I just slice up the cucumbers and throw them into the jar with the onions for a day or two. Slice up some avocado and roll up my favorite deli meats, and voilà! A beautiful and simple salad that comes together effortlessly. I love serving this salad alongside kebabs or with grilled steaks.

1 large cucumber, cut into 4-inch spears

FOR THE BRINE:

2 cups water

1 cup apple cider vinegar

½ teaspoon fine Himalayan salt

1 whole clove

1 bay leaf

½ medium Hass avocado, peeled, pitted, and sliced

¼ cup Pickled Red Onions (page 88)

2 or 3 slices Genoa salami

2 or 3 slices soppressata or smoked turkey

¼ teaspoon fine Himalayan salt

1 tablespoon avocado oil

Makes 2 servings
PREP TIME: 10 minutes, plus at least 3 hours to marinate

○ Place the cucumber spears in a clean glass container. (If you have pickled red onions on hand, place the cucumbers in the pickled onions jar instead and skip the next step.)

○ In a saucepan over medium heat, bring the water, vinegar, salt, and clove to a light simmer. Add the bay leaf to the cucumbers and pour the brine over them.

○ Cover and refrigerate for at least 3 hours or up to overnight. To serve, arrange the pickled cucumbers on a plate with the avocado slices and pickled onions. Roll up the deli meats and place them around the spears. Sprinkle everything with the salt and drizzle with the avocado oil.

○ Store leftovers in an airtight container in the fridge for up to 2 days.

CHEF'S NOTE: This salad is extremely versatile. You can leave out the deli meat to keep it vegetarian. You can serve it as is or over lettuce. You can plate it as is or shave the pickles for a whole different look.

PER SERVING: Calories **236** · Fat **20.1g** · Total Carbohydrate **11.4g** · Dietary Fiber **4.1g** · Protein **6g**

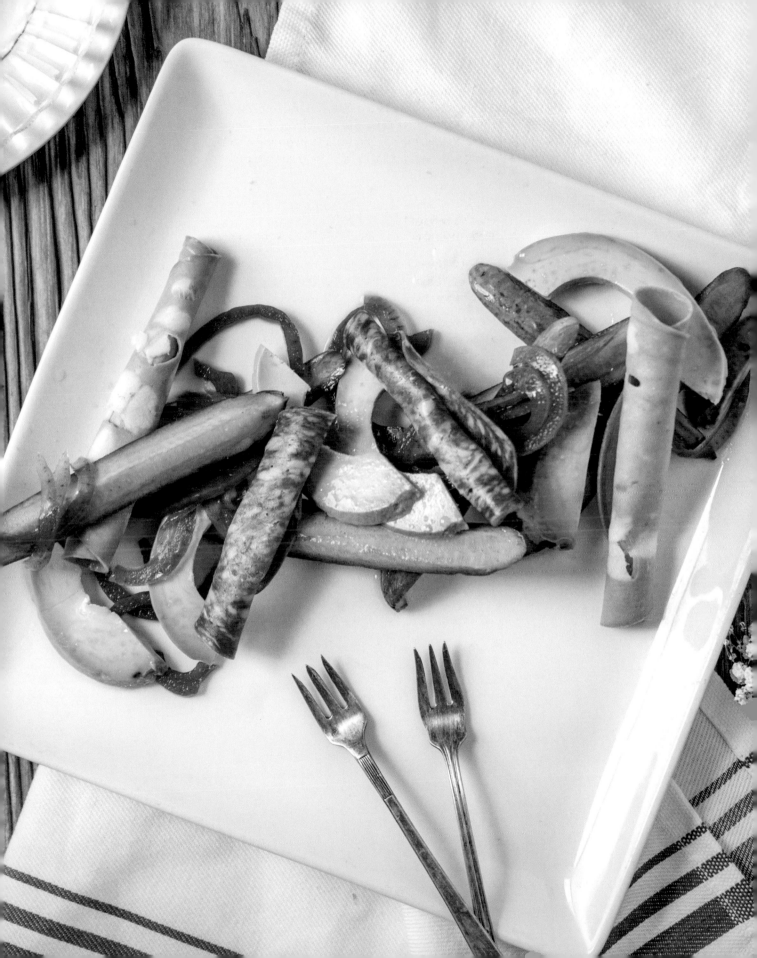

creamy cilantro rice

I just love a good creamy side dish. The perfect accompaniment to any protein, this cauliflower rice maintains a fresh and light flavor while delivering fantastic texture and plenty of good fats without an overpowering coconut flavor. The cool and tangy combination is perfection when paired with spiced dishes like Shredded Jerk Chicken (page 218), Chicken Kofta Kebabs (page 206), or Slow Cooker Shawarma (page 270)!

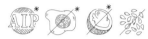

Makes 6 servings
PREP TIME: 10 minutes   COOK TIME: 10 minutes

2 tablespoons cooking fat (see page 53)

5 cloves garlic, minced

1 teaspoon grated lemon zest

4 cups riced cauliflower (see Note, page 140)

1 teaspoon fine Himalayan salt

½ cup full-fat coconut milk

Juice of 1 lemon

½ cup minced fresh cilantro, plus more for garnish

1 tablespoon Homemade Mayo (page 82)

Lemon wedges, for serving

○ Heat a large skillet over medium-high heat. When it's hot, melt the cooking fat, then add the garlic and lemon zest. Sauté, stirring constantly, for 1 to 2 minutes, until lightly browned and fragrant.

○ Add the riced cauliflower and salt. Stir and cook for 5 to 8 minutes, until lightly browned. If the cauliflower is frozen, cook until it has thawed and any liquid has boiled away.

○ Stir in the coconut milk and lemon juice and bring to a quick simmer. Simmer for 2 to 3 minutes, then stir in the cilantro and mayo and remove from the heat.

○ Garnish with more fresh cilantro and serve with lemon wedges. Store leftovers in an airtight container in the refrigerator for up to 5 days.

SUBSTITUTIONS: To make this dish AIP-compliant, omit the mayo. For a coconut-free version, omit the coconut milk and use ¼ cup bone broth (page 100) and 2 tablespoons mayo instead.

PER SERVING: Calories **130** · Fat **12.3g** · Total Carbohydrate **4.5g** · Dietary Fiber **1.3g** · Protein **1.6g**

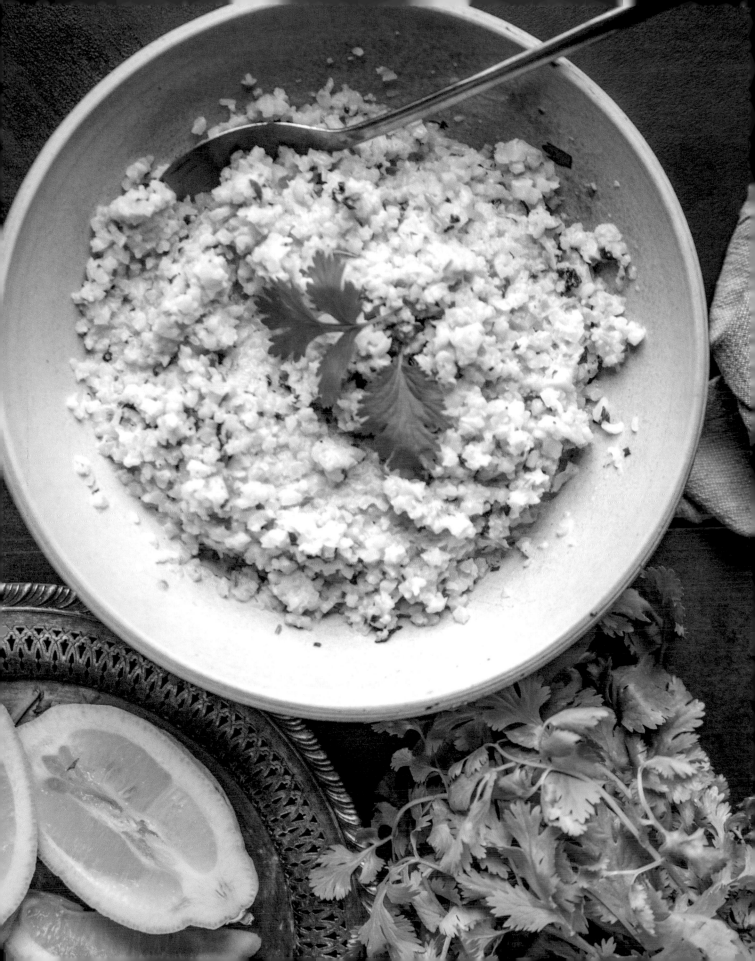

tender kale salad

Kale is one those greens that I used to eat only when it was cooked. The tough, bitter leaves did nothing for me raw; I felt like an animal out to pasture chewing on them. Then I had a massaged kale salad, and it was a whole other experience. Who knew all that kale needed was a little trip to the spa? A little salt and some magic fingers, and tough old kale turns into a soft, delicious green that pairs well with citrus, garlic, and other bold flavors. The best part is that this salad doesn't wilt. Make a big batch and keep it in the fridge for up to four days, ready to go as a side for Saucy Seasoned Liver (page 258) or Vietnamese Crispy Chicken (page 214).

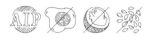

1 pound dinosaur or curly kale

1 teaspoon fine Himalayan salt

¼ cup ripe green olives, pitted

2 tablespoons Garlic Confit (page 76)

2 tablespoons Toum (page 72) or Homemade Mayo (page 82)

Juice of 1 lemon

Makes 4 servings
PREP TIME: 10 minutes

○ Tear the kale leaves into 1- to 2-inch pieces and place in a bowl with the salt. With your hands, massage the salt into the kale for 2 minutes, or until the kale begins to release some liquid and has become very tender.

○ Add the olives, garlic confit, toum, and lemon juice. Toss to combine and serve, or store in a quart-sized jar in the fridge for up to 4 days.

CHEF'S NOTE: This salad also works well with a creamy dressing like Ranch Dressing (page 94) or Tzatziki (page 98). You can omit the olives or serve them on the side if not everyone likes them, like my husband. Pickled Red Onions (page 88) are a welcome addition as well.

SUBSTITUTIONS: If you do not have any toum or mayo at the ready, use the juice of 1 lemon and add 1 tablespoon of oil from the garlic confit.

PER SERVING: Calories **87** · Fat **2g** · Total Carbohydrate **13g** · Dietary Fiber **2g** · Protein **3g**

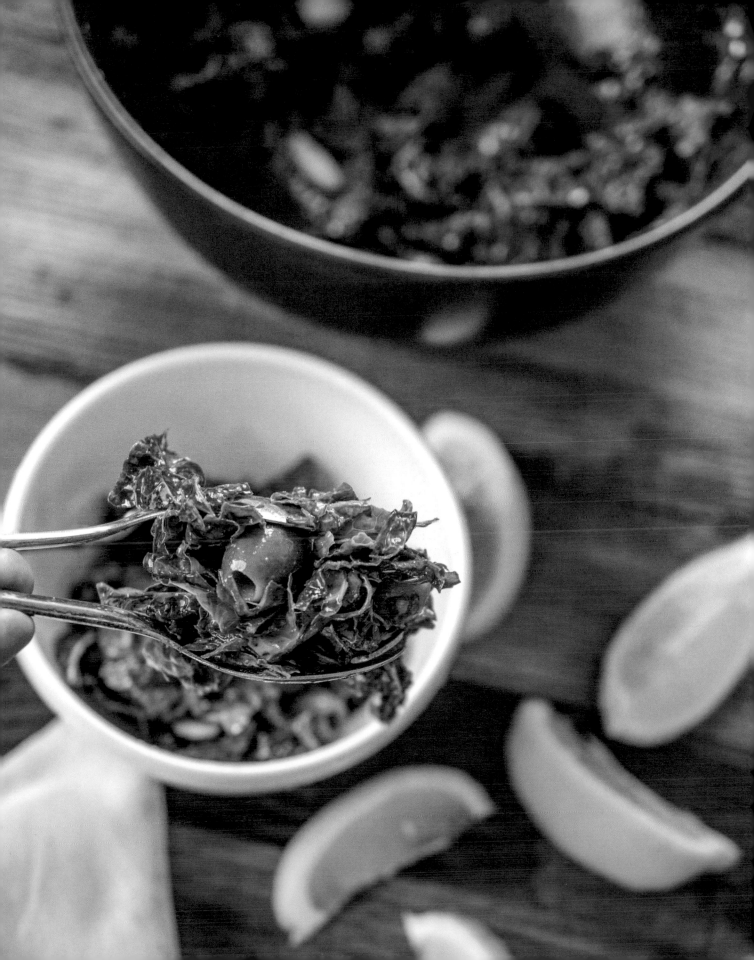

crunchy asian salad

This slaw-like salad is perfect for making in advance! I like to make a big batch and keep in the fridge, with the dressing on the side. Cabbage is pretty dense, so a little goes a long way. Grab a handful and toss it with some dressing, top with shredded chicken or a fried egg, and call it lunch. If eating raw cabbage doesn't agree with you, throw it in a skillet and make a stir-fry. Add any protein you like to make this an entrée salad; I'm partial to shredded chicken. You can also change up the dressing for fun variations. Try using ¼ cup Ginger Sauce (page 102) or Lemon Tahini Sauce (page 224). Versatile, colorful, and nutrient dense, this rainbow salad is a great way to get your veggies!

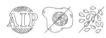

¼ medium head red cabbage

¼ medium head green cabbage

2 green onions, minced

Leaves from 2 sprigs fresh basil, minced

Leaves from 4 sprigs fresh cilantro, minced

1 teaspoon fine Himalayan salt

FOR THE DRESSING:

Juice of 4 limes

3 tablespoons avocado oil

2 tablespoons coconut aminos

4 cloves garlic, minced

1 (1-inch) piece ginger, peeled and minced

Makes 6 servings
PREP TIME: 20 minutes

⊙ Lay one of the cabbage wedges on the cutting board and use a sharp knife to trim off the core on the diagonal. Then slice the cabbage as thinly as possible. Repeat with the second wedge. Combine the shredded red and green cabbage in a large bowl.

⊙ Add the green onions, basil, and cilantro and toss with the cabbage. Sprinkle in the salt and toss to combine.

⊙ Make the dressing: Place the lime juice, avocado oil, and coconut aminos in a small bowl. Add the garlic and ginger and whisk to combine.

⊙ If you're serving the salad right away, pour the dressing over the cabbage and toss to thoroughly distribute the dressing.

⊙ If you're not serving the salad right away, store the salad in an airtight container in the fridge with a folded paper towel to absorb moisture. Store the dressing in a separate airtight container in the fridge. Both the salad and the dressing will keep for up to 5 days.

VARIATIONS: This salad can be made with as many or as few ingredients as you want—this recipe is really a base model. Matchstick carrots, zucchini, and beets are welcome additions. Toasted sesame seeds or hemp seeds can be used for garnish. If you don't have green onions, you can use shaved red onions or even Pickled Red Onions (page 88).

PER SERVING: Calories **103** · Fat **7.1g** · Total Carbohydrate **7g** · Dietary Fiber **2g** · Protein **0.9g**

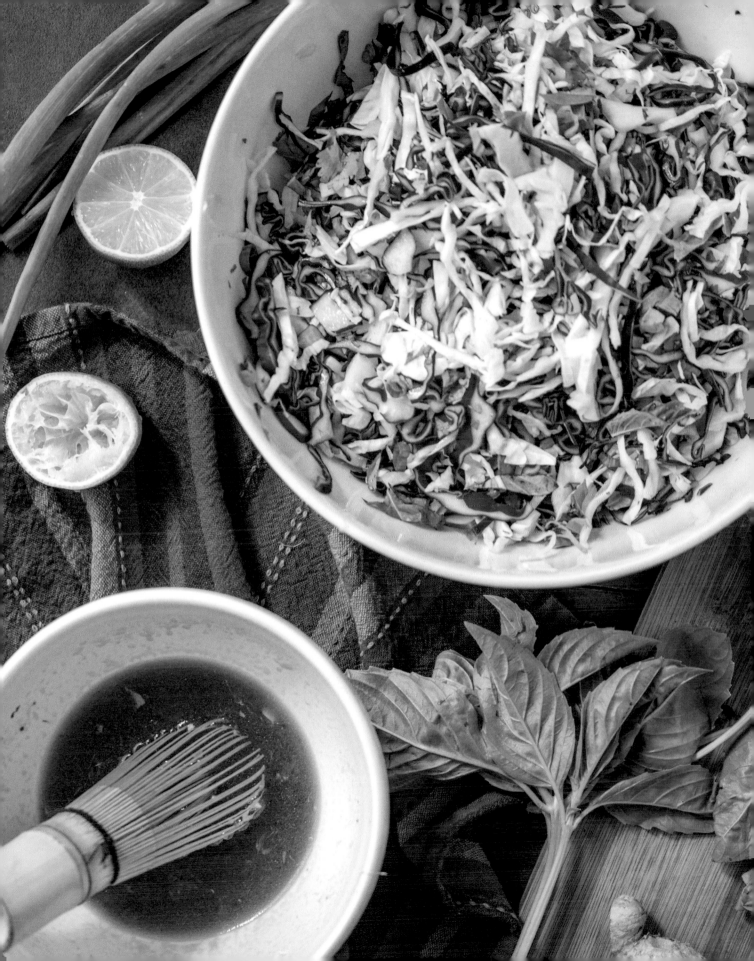

spinach salad

As simple as it gets—throw these four ingredients on a plate, top with a protein, and call it a day. Spinach, green onions, and avocado are a classic and refreshing combination that goes well with anything. It lends itself particularly well to being snuggled up to something hot: the spinach wilts a little and the avocado adds creaminess, but that green onion keeps its crunch! The perfect side salad indeed. Salty and savory pistou is my first pick for a dressing.

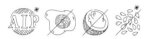

½ pound baby spinach

2 green onions, minced

1 small Hass avocado, peeled, pitted, and sliced

3 tablespoons Pistou (page 74)

Makes 4 servings
PREP TIME: 10 minutes

Toss all of the ingredients together in a medium-sized bowl. Serve right away.

VARIATIONS: Add sesame seeds and a scoop of warm cauliflower rice and replace the pistou with Ginger Sauce (page 102) for a quick Asian-inspired salad.

Use 2 tablespoons Pickled Red Onions (page 88) instead of the green onions, add ¼ cup olives and chopped fresh parsley, and use Greek Marinade + Dressing (page 108) for a Mediterranean salad.

SUBSTITUTIONS: To make this dish AIP-compliant, use the AIP-compliant version of pistou.

PER SERVING: Calories **314** · Fat **35g** · Total Carbohydrate **12.1g** · Dietary Fiber **8g** · Protein **11.1g**

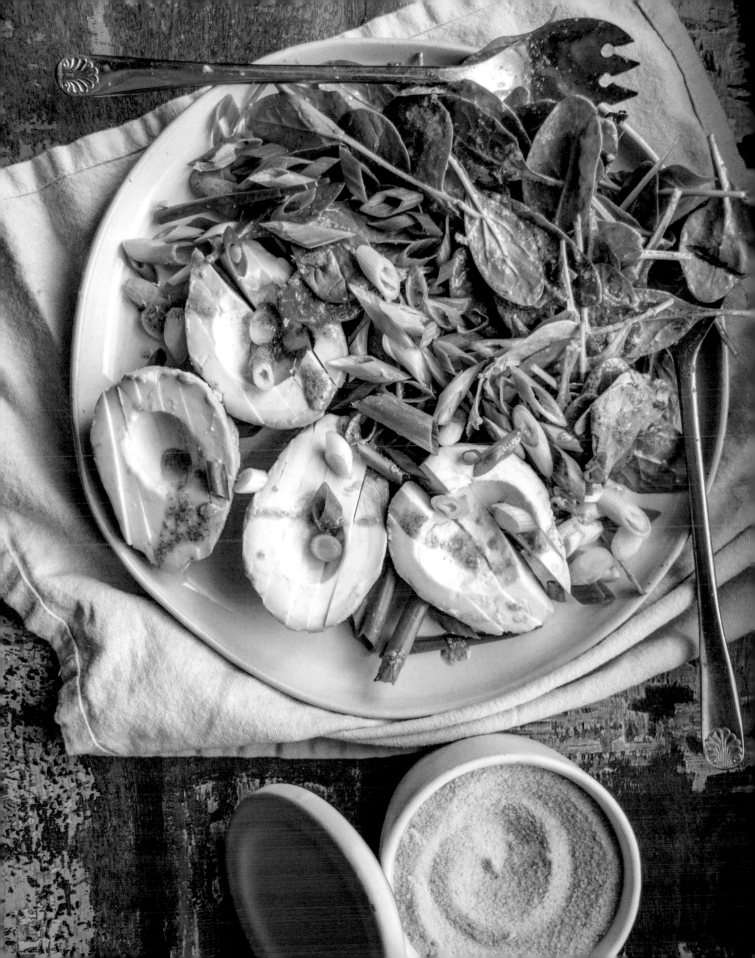

garlicky golden cauliflower

A side dish that is as delicious as it is beautiful. A new holiday staple. The perfect side dish to go with that good steak. You get the point. It's pretty, it's tasty. Serve this when you want to make an impression.

1 medium head cauliflower

½ cup Garlic Confit (page 76)

1 tablespoon fish sauce

1 teaspoon dried rosemary needles

1 teaspoon fine Himalayan salt

1½ cups bone broth (page 100)

1 teaspoon turmeric powder

½ teaspoon ground black pepper

Makes 4 servings
PREP TIME: 5 minutes   COOK TIME: 1 hour

- Preheat the oven to 400°F.

- Trim the leaves and stem off the head of cauliflower. Then use a paring knife to pierce it all over, a few stabs around the side and a cross on the top. Set on a sheet pan.

- Place the garlic confit, fish sauce, rosemary, and salt in a blender and blend until a chunky paste forms. (When you measure the confit, make sure you pour out some oil as well!) Use a spatula to scrape it out of the blender and smear it all over the cauliflower.

- Roast the cauliflower for 1 hour. Meanwhile, in a small bowl, combine the broth, turmeric, and pepper. Every 20 minutes, baste the cauliflower with ¼ cup of the broth mixture.

- Remove the cauliflower from the oven and serve warm. Slice it up like pie! Store leftovers in an airtight container in the fridge for up to 5 days. To reheat, pan-sear in a hot skillet for 4 to 5 minutes.

SUBSTITUTIONS: To make this dish AIP-compliant, omit the pepper. If you don't have garlic confit on hand, use ¼ cup minced garlic with ¼ cup avocado oil and add 1 teaspoon garlic powder.

PER SERVING: Calories **186** · Fat **9g** · Total Carbohydrate **13g** · Dietary Fiber **4g** · Protein **13g**

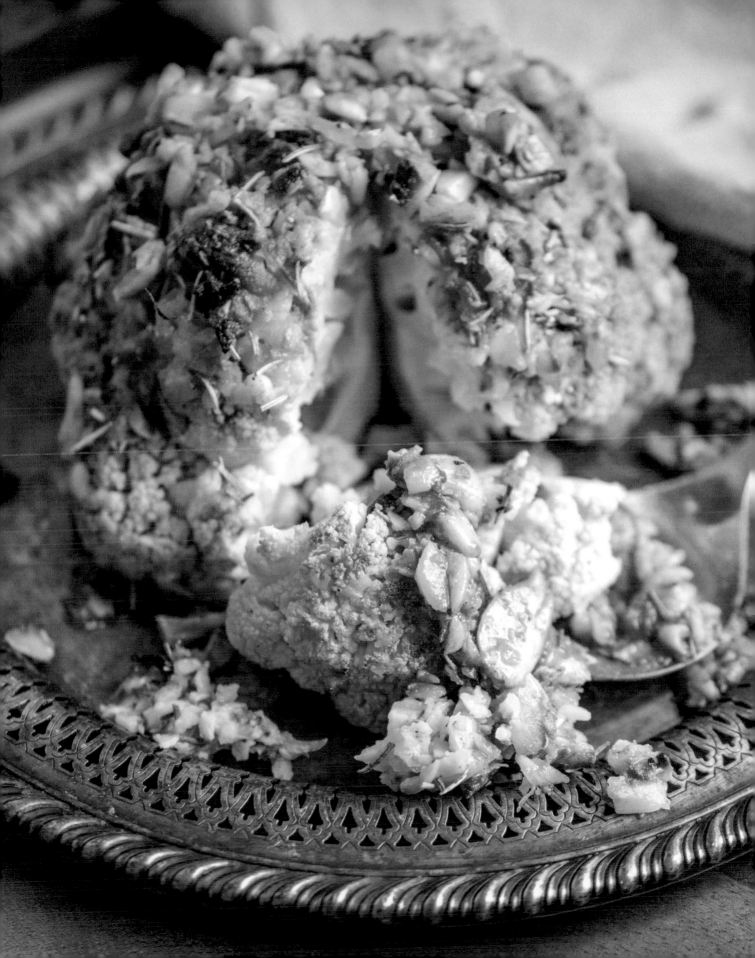

butter coffee

This is my cup of joe. It's what I drink every morning, usually slowly between the hours of 6 a.m. and 8 a.m., before I take Jack to preschool and head to the gym. I practice intermittent fasting with this fatty coffee (see page 34 for more on fasting). It keeps me focused, sated, and feeling amazing until my tummy tells me it's time for food. The ingredients here are combined for maximum deliciousness and health benefits. I am partial to light-roast coffee beans; I feel they have a much milder flavor, and since I don't sweeten my coffee, smooth is the name of the game. I do not recommend espresso for this recipe; it's too strong.

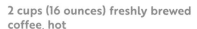

2 cups (16 ounces) freshly brewed coffee, hot

2 tablespoons unsalted butter, ghee, or coconut oil

1 tablespoon MCT oil or coconut oil

1 tablespoon ground cinnamon

1 scoop unflavored grass-fed beef gelatin (optional)

Makes two 8-ounce servings
PREP TIME: 5 minutes

○ Place the coffee, butter, MCT oil, and cinnamon in a blender. Make sure the lid is on tight and the vent is closed. Turn the blender on low and gradually bring the power up to high until the coffee goes from dark to light brown and frothy, about 30 seconds.

○ If you're using gelatin, lower the speed of the blender, add the gelatin via the lid vent, and pulse briefly to combine.

○ This recipe makes two cups of coffee. If you're like me and drink them both yourself, do as I do and keep the second cup hot in an insulated container until you're ready for it.

VARIATIONS: You can substitute raw cacao butter for the butter; it gives the coffee the most decadent mocha flavor! You can also use decaf coffee or black tea instead of regular coffee.

SUBSTITUTIONS: Using tea and 2 tablespoons coconut butter or cream instead of butter will make this delicious beverage AIP-compliant. If you can't do butter, ghee, or coconut and you don't have MCT oil, put the coffee and cinnamon in a blender, blend on high, and add two raw egg yolks while it blends.

PER SERVING: Calories **245** · Fat **22.1g** · Total Carbohydrate **2.7g** · Dietary Fiber **2g** · Protein **8.6g**

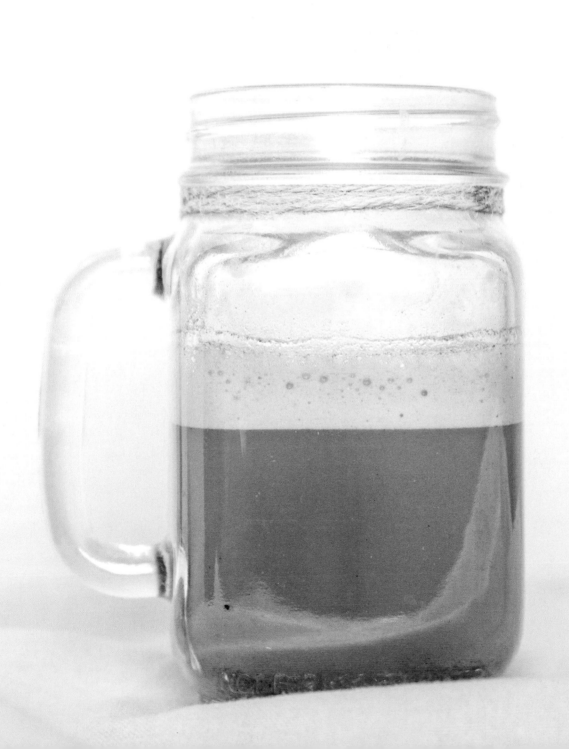

golden milk

It's more than just a buzzword or that hipster thing you saw on Instagram; golden milk has been used for centuries in Ayurvedic medicine. The healing properties of turmeric are miraculous. The big one is its powerful anti-inflammatory properties, activated when paired with warm coconut milk and a pinch of pepper. This creamy, sweet, and lightly spiced beverage is the perfect vessel to deliver all the benefits of this magical root. Bonus: It tastes amazing! If you like chai lattes, you're going to love this drink.

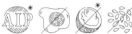

½ cup bone broth (page 100)

½ cup full-fat coconut milk

1 (1-inch) piece lemon zest

1 teaspoon granulated erythritol or other low-carb sweetener (see page 38)

1 scant teaspoon turmeric powder

½ teaspoon ground cinnamon

Pinch of ground black pepper

Pinch of ground cardamom (optional)

1 teaspoon unflavored grass-fed beef gelatin or collagen peptides

Makes one 8-ounce serving
PREP TIME: 10 minutes   COOK TIME: 5 minutes

○ Combine the broth, coconut milk, and lemon zest in a small saucepan over medium heat. When the mixture comes to a simmer, stir in the erythritol, turmeric, cinnamon, pepper, and cardamom (if using).

○ Remove the lemon zest. Using an immersion blender, blend the milk mixture until the spices are completely mixed in. Alternatively, you can transfer the mixture to a blender or whisk the mixture until frothy, but it might splatter a bit. Add the gelatin and blend to dissolve.

○ Serve immediately. Enjoy!

SUBSTITUTIONS: For a coconut-free version, omit the coconut milk and add 2 tablespoons unsalted butter or ghee and ¼ cup water. For an AIP-compliant version, replace the cardamom and pepper with ½ teaspoon ginger powder and omit the sweetener.

PER SERVING: Calories **289** · Fat **23g** · Total Carbohydrate **4g** · Dietary Fiber **4.4g** · Protein **12g**

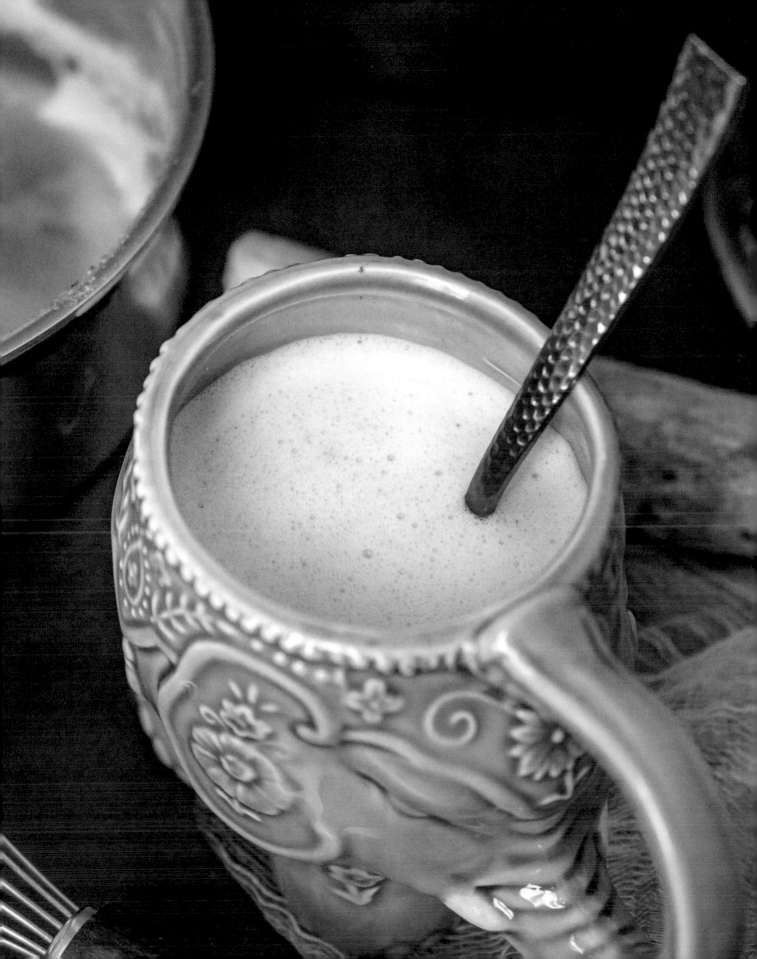

korean cinnamon tea

When we lived in San Diego, we would often head to Convoy Street for Korean barbecue. Prior to that, I wasn't very familiar with Korean cuisine. My friend Lisa had taught English in Seoul, and she used her cultural insight to navigate us through the meal with respect and delight, always ordering for the table and explaining all the amazing dishes that passed through. I loved the cinnamon tea that they served at the end of the meal. Here, I have re-created it with much less sweetener and a little twist, because I just can't help myself. I like to use Ceylon cinnamon for its healing properties (see page 51).

6 cups filtered water

6 cinnamon sticks

1 star anise (optional)

3 tablespoons granulated erythritol or other low-carb sweetener (see page 38)

10 drops liquid stevia

Makes six 8-ounce servings
COOK TIME: 30 minutes

◦ In a large pot over medium-high heat, combine the water, cinnamon sticks, and star anise (if using). When it begins to steam, stir in the erythritol. Bring to a simmer, then cover and let it steep for 20 minutes.

◦ Remove from the heat, add the stevia, discard the cinnamon sticks and star anise, and transfer to a large pitcher. Set in the fridge to chill.

◦ Serve cold after meals.

CHEF'S NOTE: Sometimes, when I need a little extra protein, I stir some collagen peptides into this tea. You can also stir in some MCT oil powder and sip on it for an afternoon pick-me-up.

SUBSTITUTIONS: For an AIP-compliant version, omit the sweetener.

PER SERVING: Calories **5** · Fat **0g** · Total Carbohydrate **5g** · Dietary Fiber **0g** · Protein **0g**

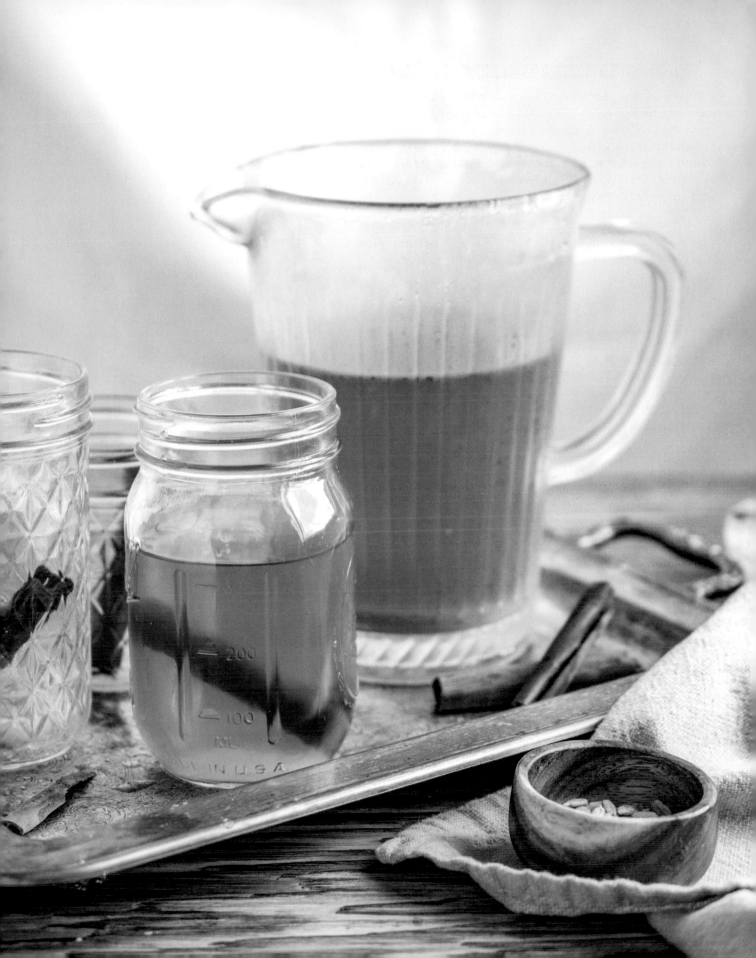

coconut butter matcha latte

Soothing, relaxing, and just the right amount of pick-me-up, matcha is a great option for those who don't drink coffee (and those who do). It gives you a nice caffeine boost with powerful antioxidants and a lovely earthy flavor that makes you feel all healthy and tingly inside.

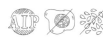

Makes one 8-ounce serving
PREP TIME: 10 minutes

1½ cups filtered water

2 tablespoons coconut butter

1 teaspoon ground cinnamon

1 teaspoon matcha tea powder

1 teaspoon pure vanilla extract

1 tablespoon unflavored grass-fed beef gelatin (optional)

○ Warm the water in a small saucepan over medium heat until it begins to steam; do not let it boil.

○ Place the coconut butter, cinnamon, matcha, and vanilla extract in a blender. Add the water and blend on high until frothy.

○ If you're using gelatin, lower the speed, add the gelatin, and blend until just combined.

○ Pour into your favorite mug and enjoy right away!

PER SERVING: Calories **224** · Fat **11.7g** · Total Carbohydrate **8.5g** · Dietary Fiber **7.2g** · Protein **2.8g**

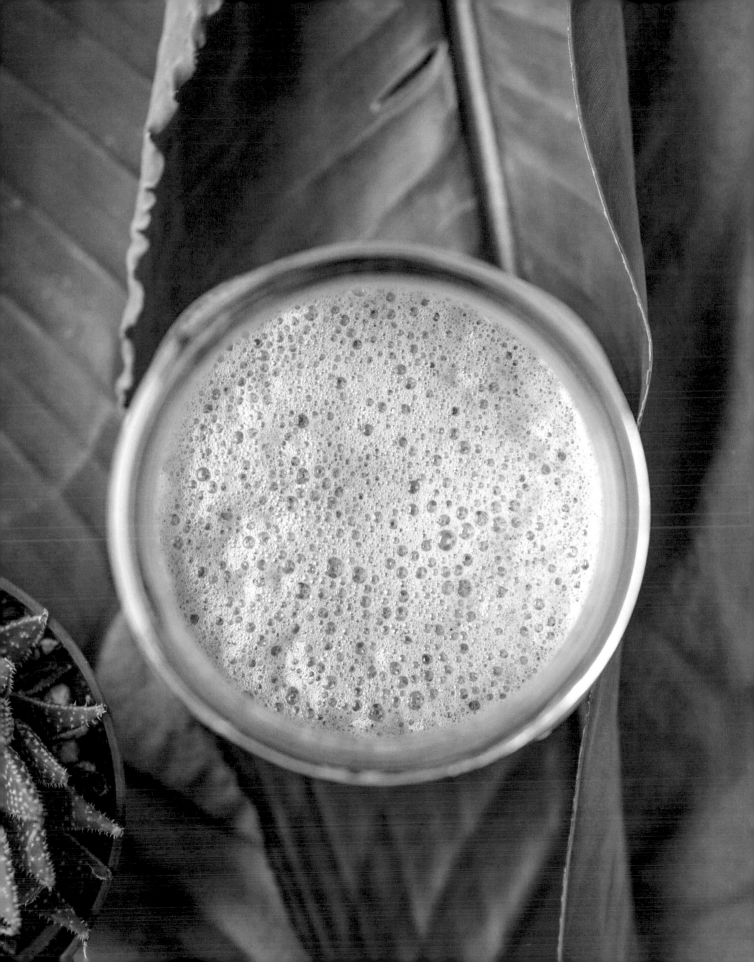

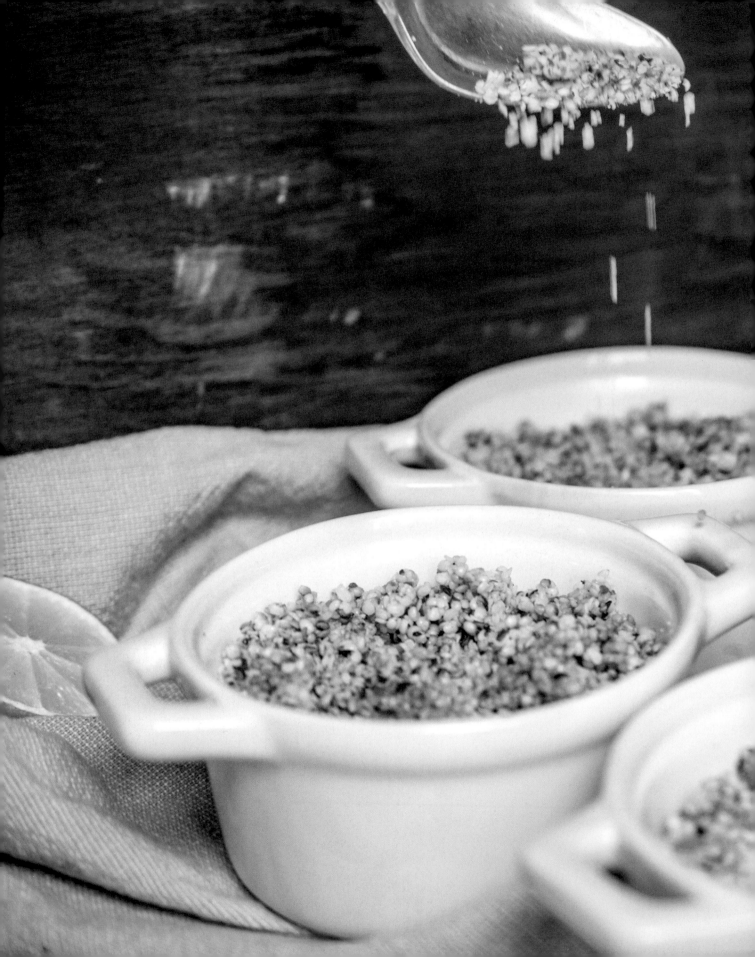

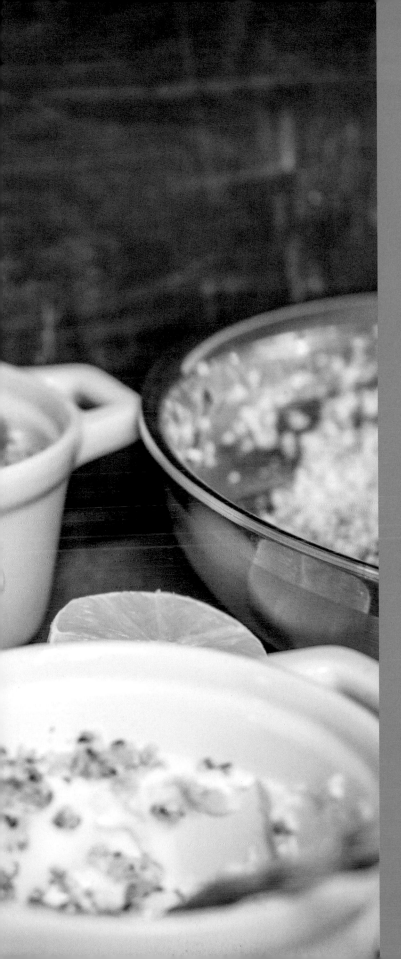

TREATS

Sweet endings to your meals and decadent desserts to share. Treats are best enjoyed when shared with loved ones. These delectable treats are drool-worthy and will win over even the keto naysayers! Friendly reminder: I count total carbs, so the sugar alcohols have not been subtracted from the nutritional information for these recipes. You can review my reason why on page 35.

chewy chocolate chip cookies

I know I'm not alone in this, but chocolate chip cookies are my all-time favorite treat. It's part melty, chewy chocolate goodness and part nostalgia—there's something about mixing and shaping the cookies, something about the smell of them baking in the oven, something about the pools of warm chocolate. It's all so comforting. These cookies remind me of Saturday nights when I was growing up, wearing thick socks and watching movies with the biggest chocolate lover I know, my sister. Wouldn't you know it—I also developed this recipe while visiting her. I wanted to make a clean treat that we could share with our kids and indulge in after a day of play at the beach, something that would hit the ol' chocoholic spot and still be totally worth it for me. Yup, these are it: my all-time, real-deal, Saturday-night-baking chocolate chip cookies.

2 large eggs

⅓ cup granulated erythritol or other low-carb sweetener (see page 38)

¼ cup (½ stick) unsalted butter, ghee, or coconut oil, softened

1 teaspoon pure vanilla extract

⅓ cup plus 1 tablespoon coconut flour

1 tablespoon unflavored grass-fed beef gelatin

½ teaspoon baking soda

Pinch of fine Himalayan salt

1 (4-ounce) bar stevia-sweetened semisweet baking chocolate, finely chopped, or ½ cup stevia-sweetened semisweet chocolate chips

Makes 1 dozen cookies
PREP TIME: 10 minutes   COOK TIME: 8 to 10 minutes

⚬ Preheat the oven to 350°F. Line a baking sheet with parchment paper.

⚬ In a large bowl, whisk the eggs with a fork or wire whisk until frothy. Add the erythritol, butter, and vanilla extract and whisk until well combined.

⚬ Add the coconut flour, gelatin, baking soda, and salt to the wet ingredients. Using a rubber spatula, mix the ingredients together until a dough forms.

⚬ Fold the chopped chocolate into the dough.

⚬ Using a medium-sized cookie scoop or a tablespoon, scoop up a mounded tablespoon of the dough and shape it into a 1-inch ball. Repeat with the rest of dough, spacing the dough balls 2 inches apart on the lined baking sheet. (You should have a total of twelve.)

⚬ Using the palm of your hand, gently flatten the balls so they are about ½ inch thick. Bake the cookies for 8 to 10 minutes, until the edges are lightly browned.

⚬ Remove the cookies from the oven and let cool to room temperature on the baking sheet before handling. The more they cool, the chewier they will be. Store in an airtight container at room temperature for up to 5 days.

CHEF'S NOTE: Although I always recommend letting cookies cool for structural integrity, there is nothing better than a warm cookie in some cold coconut milk. You may burn your fingers or the roof of your mouth, but if melted, doughy cookies are your thing, I give you permission to sneak one fresh out of the oven.

SUBSTITUTIONS: An equal amount of bacon fat can be used in place of the butter, ghee, or coconut oil. If you do not have gelatin on hand, you can use unflavored collagen peptides or hydrolysate for the added nutritional benefit. The cookies will turn out perfect, though not quite as chewy as when made with gelatin. If you want to use a nut-based flour, try version 1.0 of this cookie, which is made with almond meal. Search for "Keto Chewy Chocolate Chip Cookies" on my website, thecastawaykitchen.com.

PER COOKIE: Calories **63** · Fat **4.3g** · Total Carbohydrate **9.9g** · Dietary Fiber **4.3g** · Protein **2.9g**

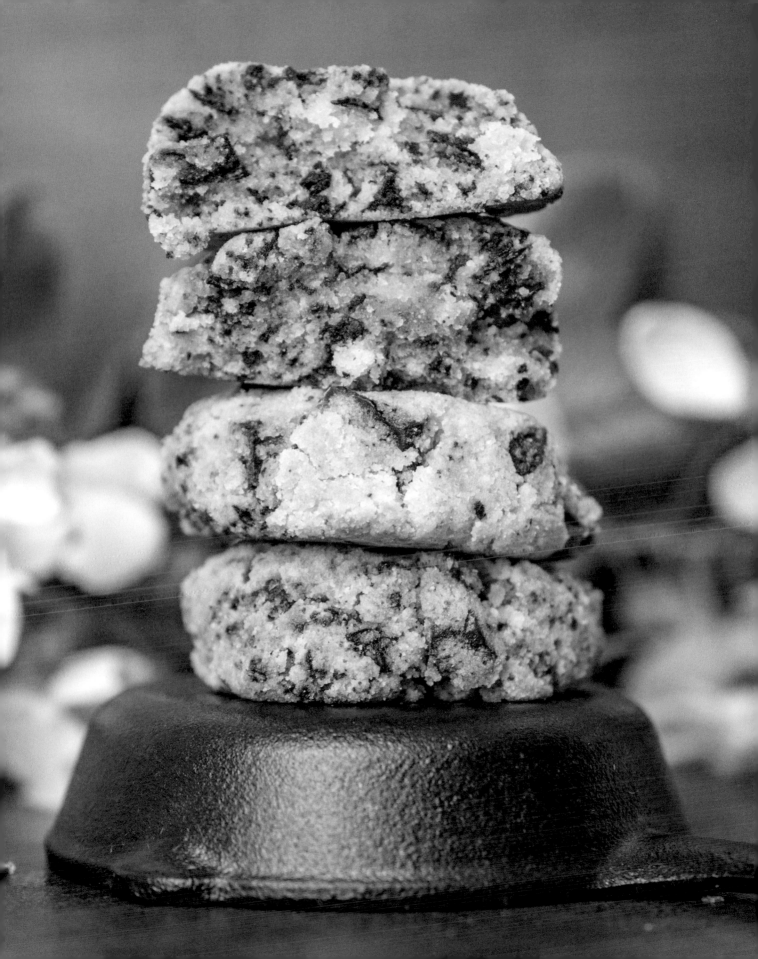

key lime pie pots de crème

These might sound fancy, but they're quite possibly the simplest dessert ever. Creamy and delicate, with a little added crunch, these pie-inspired pots are the perfect treat. I love serving this kind of dessert when entertaining. They look lovely and are easily thrown together while talking to guests. You can even make them ahead of time; just remember not to leave them in the fridge too long or they will be more jiggly than creamy. Once they're set up, you can leave them on the kitchen counter to enjoy after dinner.

Want to know a little secret? I just use regular limes for this. They are easier to source and less expensive. Plus, the added lemongrass really gives it an extra-special flavor!

Makes 3 servings
PREP TIME: 15 minutes, plus at least 30 minutes to set   **COOK TIME:** 15 minutes

FOR THE FILLING:

1 (13.5-ounce) can full-fat coconut milk

2 teaspoons pure vanilla extract

1 teaspoon grated lime zest

Juice of 2 limes

20 drops liquid stevia, or 2 tablespoons granulated erythritol

Pinch of fine Himalayan salt

1 stalk lemongrass, cut into 3 pieces

1 heaping tablespoon unflavored grass-fed beef gelatin

FOR THE HEMP SEED CRUMBLE:

½ cup shelled hemp seeds (aka hemp hearts)

1 tablespoon granulated erythritol or other low-carb sweetener (see page 38)

1 teaspoon grated lime zest

Pinch of fine Himalayan salt

○ Make the filling: Combine the coconut milk, vanilla extract, lime zest, lime juice, stevia, salt, and lemongrass in a small saucepan over medium-low heat. Cook, stirring occasionally, for 5 minutes, or until the milk begins to steam. It will become aromatic and begin to bubble a little on the edges. Use tongs or a slotted spoon to remove the pieces of lemongrass.

○ As you whisk the coconut milk mixture, sprinkle in the gelatin until it is fully dissolved. Remove the pan from the heat. Pour the mixture through a fine-mesh sieve into three 4-ounce ramekins.

○ Refrigerate for 30 to 45 minutes, until set. Place the ramekins in the coldest part of the refrigerator, usually the back of the top shelf.

○ Make the hemp seed crumble: Combine the hemp seeds, erythritol, lime zest, and salt in a small skillet over medium heat. Cook, stirring slowly, for 5 to 6 minutes. The seeds will begin to toast and the mixture will smell sweet and popcorn-like. When most of the seeds are browned, remove the pan from the heat. Use a spoon to flatten the mixture and set it under a fan to cool while the pots de crème finish setting.

○ When the pots de crème are ready, remove them from the refrigerator. Use a spoon to break up the candied hemp seeds and sprinkle them over the pots de crème for a crunchy, toasty, sweet crust.

○ These are best enjoyed right away. The creamy pots will turn full-on firm if they set any longer. However, you can keep them in the fridge for up to 5 days.

SUBSTITUTIONS: If you can't find lemongrass, a big chunk of lime zest will do the trick.

CHEF'S NOTE: Not a citrus person? You can omit the lime and lemongrass. Instead, stir ½ cup dark chocolate chips into the coconut milk mixture until smooth. Then add the gelatin and continue with the recipe as written. Now you have chocolate pots de crème!

PER SERVING: Calories **368** · Fat **32.7g** · Total Carbohydrate **10.6g** · Dietary Fiber **5.5g** · Protein **11.1g**

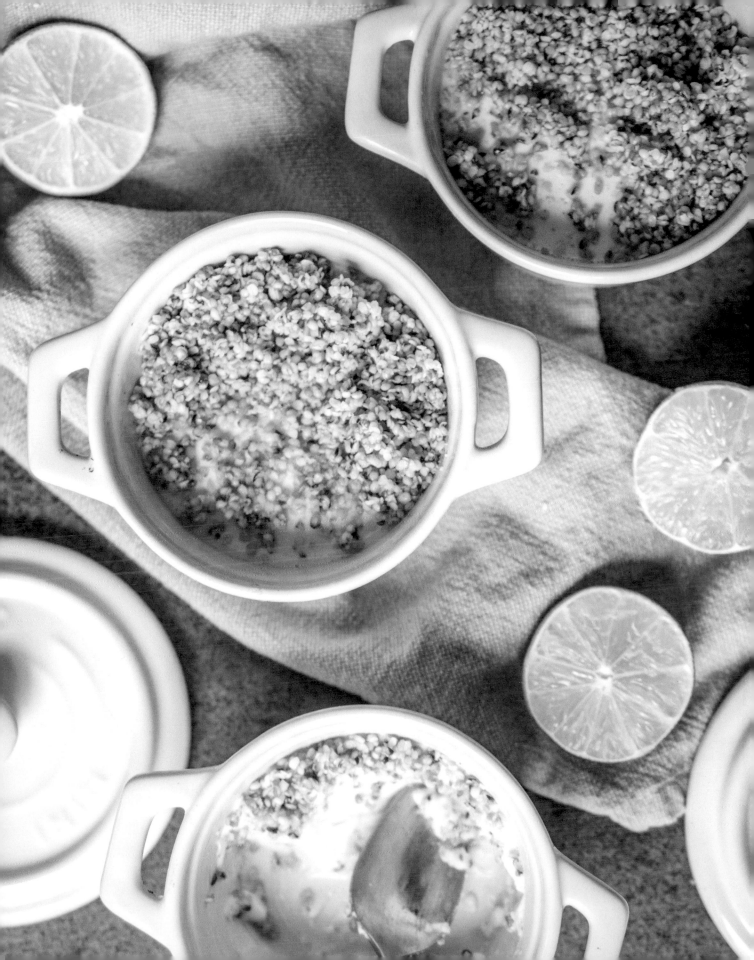

coconut citrus tart

My sweet tooth has two modes: death by chocolate and fresh and light. This recipe definitely falls in the fresh-and-light category. This coconut custard tart with hints of citrus and vanilla is beautiful, delicate, and pretty darn easy to make. Nice and firm when properly chilled, it's the perfect dessert for parties—it can easily be sliced into up to sixteen pieces, because sharing is caring. (Although once you taste it, you might not be so keen on sharing it!)

2 tablespoons ghee, unsalted butter, or lard

2 tablespoons granulated erythritol or other low-carb sweetener (see page 38)

1 (13.5-ounce) can full-fat coconut milk

1 teaspoon pure vanilla extract

Grated zest of 1 lime or lemon, plus more for garnish

Pinch of fine Himalayan salt

1 tablespoon unflavored grass-fed beef gelatin

1 Pie Crust (page 92), baked in an 8-inch springform pan

2 tablespoons unsweetened shredded coconut, for garnish

Makes one 8-inch tart (16 servings)
PREP TIME: 10 minutes, plus 4 hours to chill   COOK TIME: 15 minutes

○ In a small saucepan over medium heat, melt the ghee. Add the erythritol and let it simmer, stirring occasionally, until it melts into a syrup, about 10 minutes.

○ While the ghee mixture simmers, in a small bowl, whisk together the coconut milk, vanilla extract, citrus zest, and salt.

○ Quickly stir the coconut milk mixture into the syrup. Cook for 5 to 8 minutes, until the mixture is steaming, almost at a simmer. As you whisk vigorously, sprinkle in the gelatin. Stir until it's fully dissolved.

○ Slowly pour the coconut milk mixture into the prepared crust. Place the tart on a plate or tray in case anything seeps from the springform pan. Chill in the fridge for 4 hours, or until the center is completely set.

○ Garnish with more grated citrus zest and shredded coconut and serve. Wrap the leftovers in plastic wrap and store in the fridge for up to 3 days.

CHEF'S NOTE: If the gelatin doesn't completely dissolve in the coconut milk, you can pour the coconut milk mixture into a blender and blend until smooth, then pour it through a fine-mesh sieve into the pie crust.

VARIATION: To make this tart vegetarian, you can use agar agar powder instead of gelatin. Use 1 tablespoon and bring the coconut milk mixture to a rapid simmer before mixing it in.

PER SERVING: Calories **142** · Fat **13.5g** · Total Carbohydrate **4.4g** · Dietary Fiber **1.4g** · Protein **2.4g**

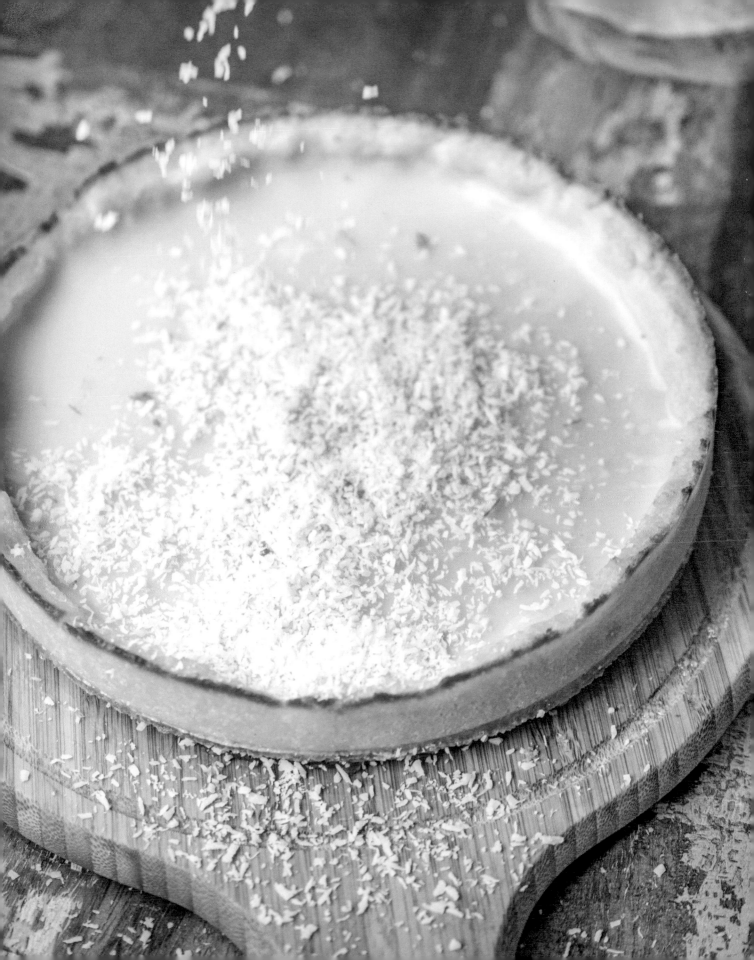

cortado panna cotta

A cortado is the Cuban version of a macchiato: potent and sweetened coffee cut ("cortado") with milk. Traditionally, evaporated milk is used, which makes canned coconut milk the perfect replacement! Like croquetas, this shot of caffeine is available at nearly any street corner in Miami. It's the perfect afternoon pick-me-up or ending to a meal. I've made a keto-fied cortadito here and mixed it with grass-fed beef gelatin for a boosted treat that will satisfy your cravings for coffee and sweets with each creamy spoonful.

Espresso-grind dark-roast coffee

½ cup full-fat coconut milk

1 tablespoon granulated erythritol or other low-carb sweetener (see page 38)

1 tablespoon unflavored grass-fed beef gelatin

Coconut Yogurt (page 96), for serving (optional)

Special equipment:

Moka pot or French press

Makes 4 servings
PREP TIME: 5 minutes, plus 2 hours to set   COOK TIME: 10 minutes

◦ Prepare your stovetop espresso using a moka pot or French press: Fill the bottom chamber with water up to the bolt or knob. Fill the basket with the ground coffee, full but not too packed. Place that over the chamber, then screw on the top. Place the moka pot on a burner over medium-high heat. The espresso will take a few minutes to brew, but keep your ears listening for the sound of rising water, when the pressure begins to build.

◦ Heat the coconut milk in a small saucepan over medium heat. Have the erythritol ready in a 2-cup glass measuring cup next to the stove, along with a teaspoon measuring spoon.

◦ When the first drops of coffee come through the spout of the moka pot, measure 4 teaspoons into the measuring cup containing the sweetener. Place the moka pot back on the stove to finish brewing.

◦ Vigorously mix the sweetener and coffee into a sugary paste or syrup. Once the coffee has finished brewing, the moka pot will be full; continue to beat the syrup as you pour the remaining coffee from the moka pot into the measuring cup. Stir until fully combined. Add the steamed coconut milk and then sprinkle in the gelatin as you continue to whisk the coffee mixture.

◦ Set four 6-ounce glasses on a small tray and divide the coffee mixture equally among them. Place in the fridge to cool and firm up for at least 2 hours.

◦ Serve chilled with a dollop of coconut yogurt on top, if desired.

CHEF'S NOTE: If you're serving this treat at night, I recommend using decaf coffee. It packs as much caffeine as a *colada*, and as any Latino will tell you, those will keep you up a while!

PER SERVING (without yogurt): Calories 75 · Fat **7.2g** · Total Carbohydrate **1.7g** · Dietary Fiber **0.7g** · Protein **2.3g**

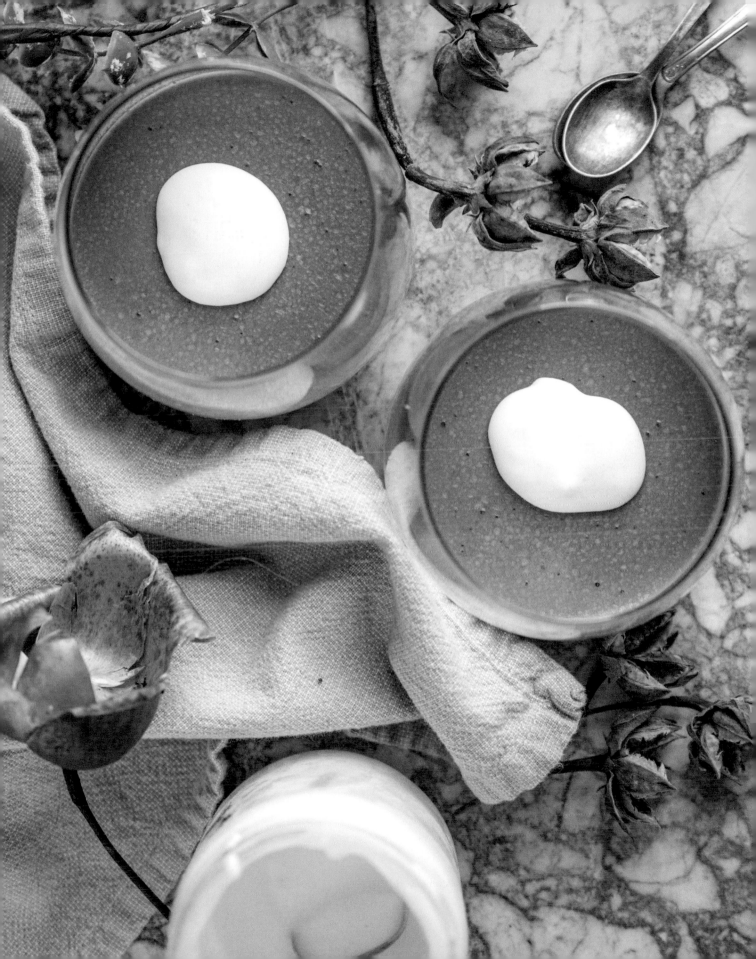

chocolate pudding mug cake

I won't lie to you, the first time I heard of mug cakes I was aghast, deeply disturbed that anyone would cook anything with eggs in the microwave. Then these little coffee-cup concoctions began to fill my social media feeds, made by some of my blogging heroes, and when I gave them a try, I was hooked. What a perfect indulgence. Fast. Easy. Single serving. Mug cakes are the answer to all your craving emergencies. Made with wholesome ingredients and plenty of good fats, there is no guilt here. And this one is cooked up in a 16-ounce mug, so there's plenty for sharing—snuggle up and grab a pair of spoons.

Makes 2 servings
PREP TIME: 5 minutes   COOK TIME: 2 minutes

1 large egg

¼ cup coconut cream (see Note, page 144)

2 tablespoons sunflower seed butter

2 tablespoons granulated erythritol or other low-carb sweetener (see page 38)

Pinch of fine Himalayan salt

¼ teaspoon pure vanilla extract (optional)

3 tablespoons cacao powder

○ Place the egg, coconut cream, and sunflower seed butter in a large mug and use a fork to whisk until smooth.

○ Add the erythritol, salt, and vanilla extract (if using) and stir to combine. Add the cacao powder and mix again until the batter is silky smooth and even in color.

○ Microwave on high for 90 seconds. The edges will be done and the center will be warm, saucy, and pudding-like. Microwave for another 30 seconds if you would like to make the cake drier.

PER SERVING: Calories **244** · Fat **18g** · Total Carbohydrate **20.8g** · Dietary Fiber **15.6g** · Protein **9.8g**

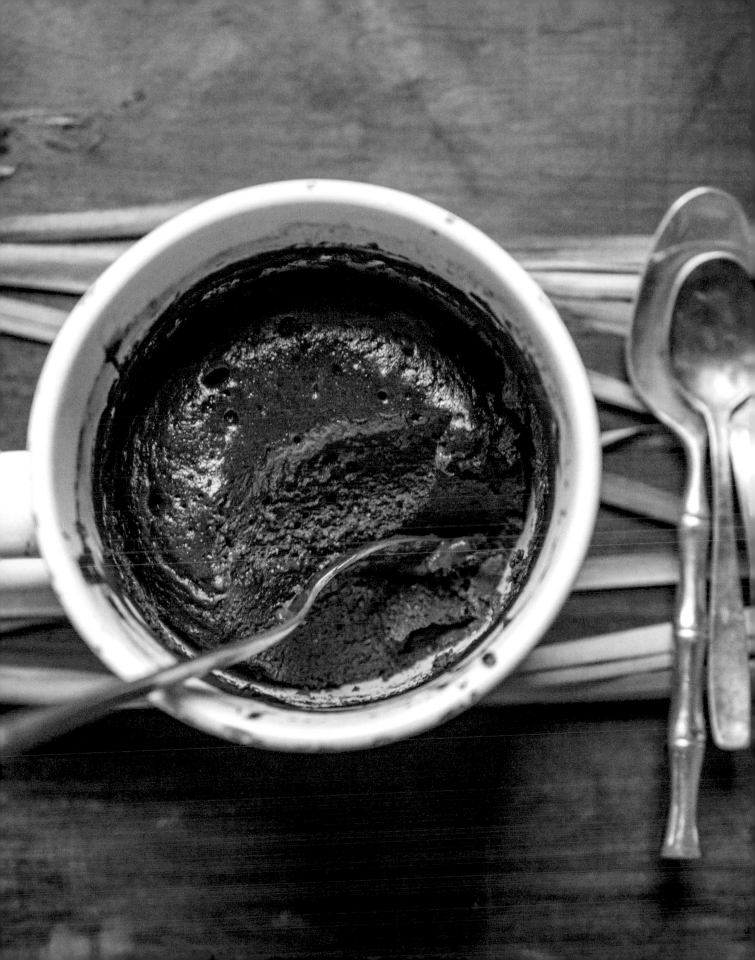

flourless brownies

These flourless brownies were my first recipe to go viral. It's a magical mix that bakes up into delicious, chocolaty perfection. You can make these with avocado (a popular pick) or pumpkin (my favorite). Either way, you can't go wrong. These have been made and loved by thousands of readers since April 2017!

1½ cups unsweetened pumpkin puree or mashed avocado (about 2 small avocados)

1 heaping cup cacao powder

⅔ cup coconut oil, softened

⅔ cup granulated erythritol or other low-carb sweetener (see page 38)

¼ cup plus 2 tablespoons sunflower seed butter

2 teaspoons baking soda

2 teaspoons pure vanilla extract or peppermint extract

½ teaspoon fine Himalayan salt

4 large eggs

TOPPINGS (OPTIONAL):

Coconut butter

Shelled hemp seeds (aka hemp hearts)

Stevia-sweetened semisweet chocolate chips

Makes sixteen 2-inch brownies
PREP TIME: 10 minutes   COOK TIME: 40 minutes

○ Preheat the oven to 350°F. Lightly grease an 8-inch square baking pan.

○ In a blender, combine everything but the eggs. Blend on high until a thick batter forms. You may need to stop and scrape down the sides with a spatula.

○ Add the eggs and blend again until fully combined and smooth.

○ Use the spatula to scrape the batter into the prepared pan. Spread out the batter. If you're using toppings, add them now.

○ Bake the brownies on the middle rack of the oven for 35 to 40 minutes. When the sides are dry and risen and the center is firm to the touch and doesn't look wet (darker than the rest), they're ready. You can also go by the toothpick test. While it won't come out totally clean, when you insert a toothpick in the center of the brownies, it should come out streaked and crumbly, not totally brown and moist.

○ Remove the brownies from the oven and let cool for 20 minutes before cutting. Store in an airtight container at room temperature for up to 3 days.

SUBSTITUTIONS: In place of coconut oil, ⅔ cup softened butter or ghee works well. You may use any nut or seed butter you like as long as it is 100% nuts or seeds, without added fats or fillers.

PER BROWNIE: Calories **172** · Fat **13.6g** · Total Carbohydrate **11.4g** · Dietary Fiber **5g** · Protein **5.2g**

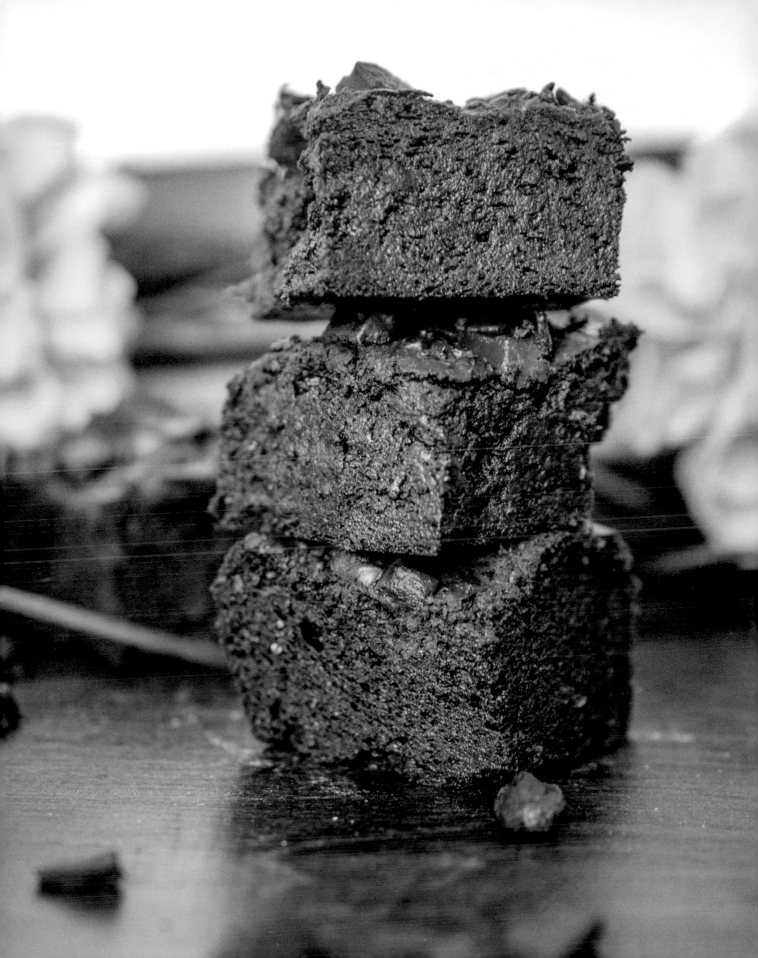

dark chocolate muffins with chocolate ganache

The perfect recipe for all your celebratory needs—rich and decadent, but really quite wholesome. These lightly sweetened muffins are packed with good fats and fiber and topped with a simple creamy chocolate ganache that doubles as an excellent dairy-free buttercream.

Makes 1 dozen muffins
PREP TIME: 10 minutes   COOK TIME: 25 minutes

FOR THE MUFFINS:

1 cup cacao powder

⅔ cup coconut flour

½ cup granulated erythritol or other low-carb sweetener (see page 38)

1 teaspoon baking soda

¼ teaspoon fine Himalayan salt

3 large eggs

½ cup full-fat coconut milk

¼ cup olive oil or avocado oil

1 teaspoon pure vanilla extract

20 drops liquid stevia

1 cup boiling water

FOR THE GANACHE:

4 ounces stevia-sweetened semisweet baking chocolate, chopped

½ cup coconut cream (see Note, page 144)

○ Preheat the oven to 350°F. Line a standard-size 12-cup muffin tin with baking cups, if desired, and lightly grease.

○ Make the muffins: In a large bowl, whisk together the cacao powder, coconut flour, erythritol, baking soda, and salt.

○ In a small bowl, whisk together the eggs, coconut milk, oil, vanilla extract, and stevia. Add the wet ingredients to the dry ingredients and whisk until a thick batter forms. Slowly add the boiling water and stir until the mixture softens and smooths out.

○ Use a ¼-cup measuring cup to scoop the batter into the prepared muffin tin, filling each cup to the top. Bake for 20 to 25 minutes, until the muffins are rounded and firm to the touch.

○ Remove from the oven and let the muffins cool in the pan before removing. If you didn't use baking cups, run a small rubber spatula around the edge of each muffin before carefully unpanning. Let the muffins cool completely before icing.

○ Make the ganache: Put the chocolate in a large microwave-safe bowl. Microwave for 30 to 40 seconds, until soft and melting. Whisk vigorously until smooth. Slowly pour in the coconut cream and whisk until cool, smooth, and glossy.

○ Use a rubber spatula to spread the ganache on top of the muffins, 1 to 2 tablespoons per muffin.

○ Store in an airtight container at room temperature for up to 2 days or in the fridge for up to a week. If stored in the fridge, let the muffins come to room temperature before enjoying.

VARIATIONS: Garnish your muffins with flake salt, pork rind dust (shown at right), sugar-free sprinkles, powdered freeze-dried berries, or chocolate chips!

To make a cake, pour the batter into two lightly greased 6-inch cake pans and bake for 30 minutes. Use the ganache as icing.

SUBSTITUTIONS: For a coconut-free version, replace the coconut flour with 1 cup flaxseed meal and follow the recipe as written. Use your preferred nondairy milk instead of coconut milk. In the ganache, use a nondairy alternative to coconut cream, such as cashew cream or almond milk.

PER MUFFIN (with ganache): Calories **182** · Fat **13.8g** · Total Carbohydrate **20.6g** · Dietary Fiber **14g** · Protein **4.7g**

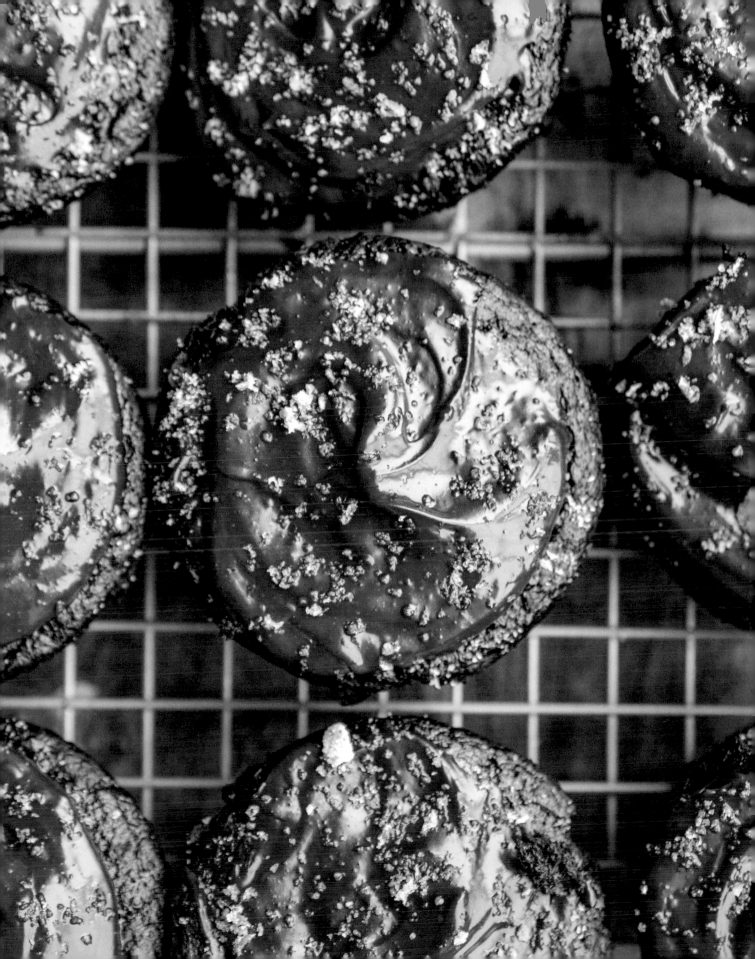

egg-free vanilla spice cookies

I call these my period cookies. For those who practice seed cycling—taking certain seeds during specific times of your menstrual cycle to balance hormones and mitigate PMS symptoms—flax seeds and pumpkin seeds are recommended during the follicular phase to boost estrogen and provide healthy fats and proteins to help stabilize mood and energy. These cookies fit the bill. Made from superfood seeds, lightly sweetened, and packed with vanilla, cinnamon, and cardamom, these cookies are tea party–worthy: big, fluffy, and chewy. These green-hued beauties are made with a home-ground pumpkin seed flour blend. I use my Vitamix, but you can throw the seeds into a coffee grinder or food processor. This green-pepita-and-coconut-flour blend bakes up so well and complements the flax egg perfectly!

Makes 10 cookies
PREP TIME: 15 minutes   COOK TIME: 15 minutes

1½ cups raw pumpkin seeds

2 tablespoons coconut flour

1 tablespoon flaxseed meal

1 tablespoon water

⅓ cup granulated erythritol or other low-carb sweetener (see page 38)

3 tablespoons coconut oil or lard, softened

2 teaspoons pure vanilla extract

2 tablespoons unflavored grass-fed beef gelatin (optional)

1 teaspoon ground cinnamon

½ teaspoon fine Himalayan salt

¼ to ½ teaspoon ground cardamom

⅓ cup full-fat coconut milk

○ Preheat the oven to 350°F. Line a baking sheet with parchment paper.

○ Combine the pumpkin seeds and coconut flour in a high-powered blender, food processor, or coffee grinder. Process until ground to a fine crumb. Set aside.

○ In a large bowl, combine the flaxseed meal and water and let sit for 2 minutes. Add the erythritol, coconut oil, and vanilla extract and mix until well combined. Add the pumpkin-seed-and-coconut-flour mixture, gelatin (if using), cinnamon, salt, and cardamom. Whisk until a dry dough forms. Add the coconut milk and use a rubber spatula to mix until the dough is moist and uniform.

○ Using a tablespoon, shape 2 tablespoons of the dough into a ball and place it on the prepared baking sheet, then gently flatten. Repeat until all the dough is used, spacing the cookies 2 inches apart. You should get about ten cookies.

○ Bake for 15 minutes, or until the edges are lightly browned. Remove from the oven and let cool to room temperature before handling.

○ Store in an airtight container at room temperature for up to 4 days.

VARIATION: These have an addictive texture and make great chocolate chip cookies, too! Feel free to mix in 1 cup stevia-sweetened semisweet chocolate chips for ooey-gooey egg-free chocolate chip cookies.

PER COOKIE: Calories **193** · Fat **16.4g** · Total Carbohydrate **6.6g** · Dietary Fiber **2.5g** · Protein **7.2g**

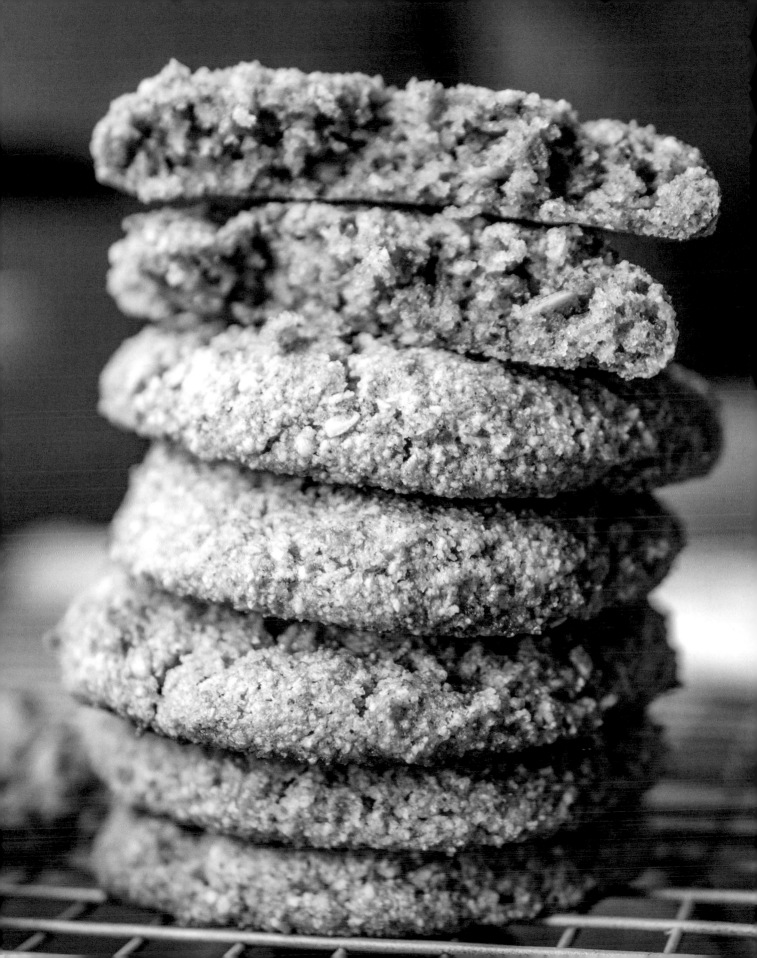

super seed slice

This is the perfect freezer stash, emergency dessert, or snack. It's like a peanut butter cup melted in your pocket and then you threw it in the freezer—nutty, chocolaty, and crunchy. Don't hold these slices too long or they will melt in your fingers.

¼ cup coconut oil

3 tablespoons granulated erythritol or other low-carb sweetener (see page 38)

¼ cup sunflower seed butter

1 teaspoon pure vanilla extract

½ teaspoon fine Himalayan salt (see Note)

½ cup raw pumpkin seeds

¼ cup stevia-sweetened semisweet chocolate chips

Makes one 8½ by 4½-inch loaf (10 slices)
PREP TIME: 15 minutes, plus 30 minutes to freeze

- Line an 8½ by 4½-inch loaf pan with parchment paper.

- Heat the coconut oil in a small saucepan over medium heat. Add the erythritol and stir until dissolved, about 10 minutes—it will look separated but no longer granular.

- Add the sunflower seed butter and vanilla extract and mix until smooth. Stir in the salt, then remove from the heat. Use a rubber spatula to scrape all of this smooth seed butter mixture into the prepared loaf pan and spread it out evenly.

- Sprinkle on the pumpkin seeds and chocolate chips. Use a small spoon to swirl them around as the chocolate chips melt.

- Set the loaf pan in the freezer on a flat surface to harden for 30 to 40 minutes.

- Once it is hard and the center is set, remove it from the freezer. Unpan it and use a sharp knife to cut it into ten even slices. A sharp knife is essential, as is cutting straight down to avoid shattering the slice. The longer you wait to unpan it, the harder it will be to cut!

- Store the slices in an airtight container in the freezer for up to a month.

CHEF'S NOTE: If you're using salted sunflower seed butter, use only ¼ teaspoon fine Himalayan salt. I love to sprinkle some flake salt over the slices before eating!

VARIATION: If you want the chocolate to be more pronounced in this recipe, mix the pumpkin seeds into the seed butter mixture and freeze it for 10 minutes while you melt the chocolate gently in 10-second increments in the microwave. Mix in 2 tablespoons coconut oil to stretch it out. Pour that over the slightly cooled sunflower seed butter mixture and then set it back in the freezer.

PER SLICE: Calories **144** · Fat **12.6g** · Total Carbohydrate **6.1g** · Dietary Fiber **1.9g** · Protein **3.9g**

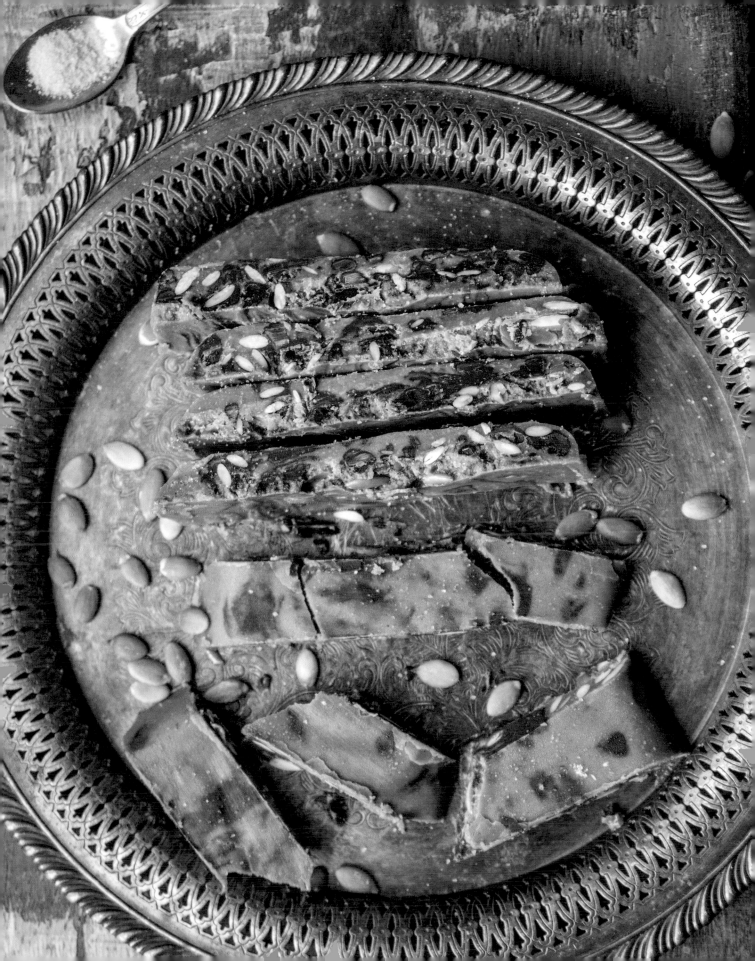

coconut caramel slice

This candy-like treat is so easy to make and has just a handful of ingredients. It also brings a healthy dose of nostalgia. From Almond Roca to the UK candy Bounty, this recipe always gets an "Oh my gosh, it tastes like [insert favorite treat here]." It's already egg-free, but check the substitution notes for how to make this treat dairy-free and AIP-friendly!

¼ cup salted butter or ghee

3 tablespoons granulated erythritol or other low-carb sweetener (see page 38)

1 cup unsweetened shredded coconut

3 to 4 ounces stevia-sweetened semisweet baking chocolate, chopped

1 tablespoon coconut oil

Makes one 8½ by 4½-inch loaf (10 slices)
PREP TIME: 15 minutes, plus 40 minutes to chill   COOK TIME: 10 minutes

◦ Melt the butter in a small saucepan over medium heat, then add the erythritol. Cook, stirring occasionally, for 8 to 10 minutes, until the mixture is smooth and as thick as syrup. You want the butter to simmer and brown just a little; the mixture should smell like candy.

◦ Once the butter is golden brown and the erythritol has dissolved into the butter, remove the saucepan from the heat and quickly stir in the shredded coconut. Stir until well combined.

◦ Transfer the coconut mixture to an 8½ by 4½-inch loaf pan and flatten to the bottom. Set aside.

◦ Place the chopped chocolate in a microwave-safe bowl, add the coconut oil, and microwave in 20-second increments until the mixture is mostly liquid. Stir to smooth it out, then pour it over the top of the coconut mixture, spreading it evenly. Set the pan in the freezer to harden for 30 to 40 minutes.

◦ Use a knife or spatula to lift the hard coconut loaf out of the pan. Place it chocolate side up on a cutting board and use a sharp knife to cut it into ten even slices. It will be very hard! Use both hands to cut straight down, applying some body weight. Keep your fingers up and out!

◦ Store the slices in an airtight container in the fridge or freezer for up to 10 days.

SUBSTITUTIONS: To make this treat dairy-free, use ¼ cup coconut cream (see Note, page 144) instead of butter or ghee to make the caramel. You will need to cook it down with the sweetener for about 15 minutes, until you can see the melted sweetener on a spoon when you stir. Continue with the recipe as written.

To make this treat AIP-compliant, make the dairy-free caramel as instructed above and use an AIP-compliant granulated sweetener. Omit the chocolate; instead, combine ¼ cup coconut oil with 3 tablespoons carob powder for the chocolate layer. No need to melt it; just mix, pour, spread, and set.

PER SLICE: Calories **165** · Fat **16.2g** · Total Carbohydrate **10g** · Dietary Fiber **2.2g** · Protein **1.3g**

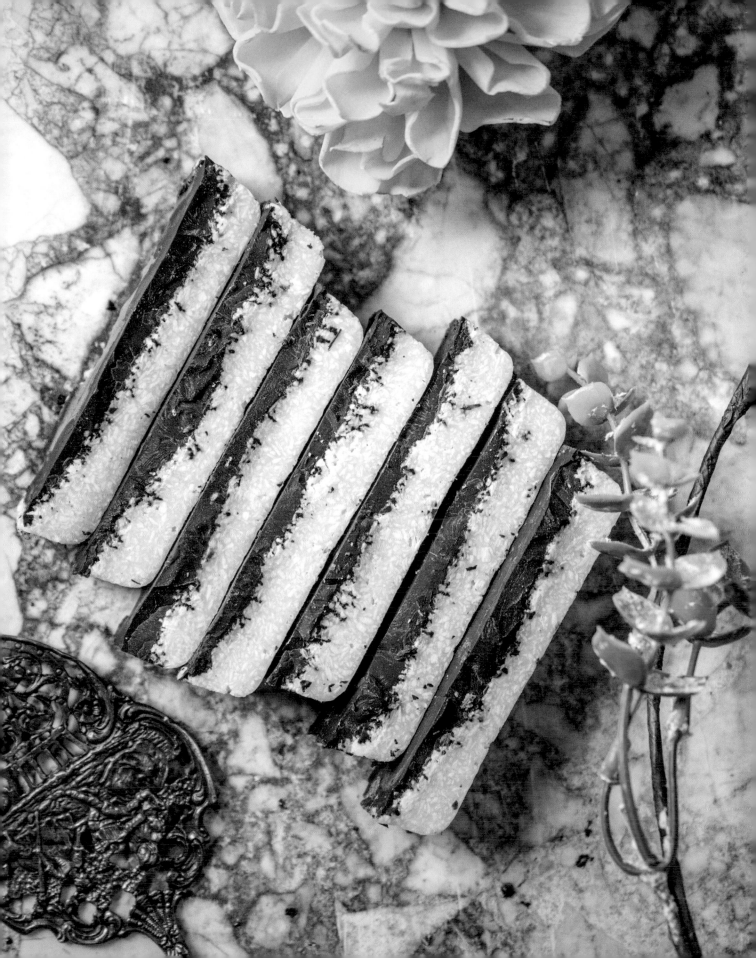

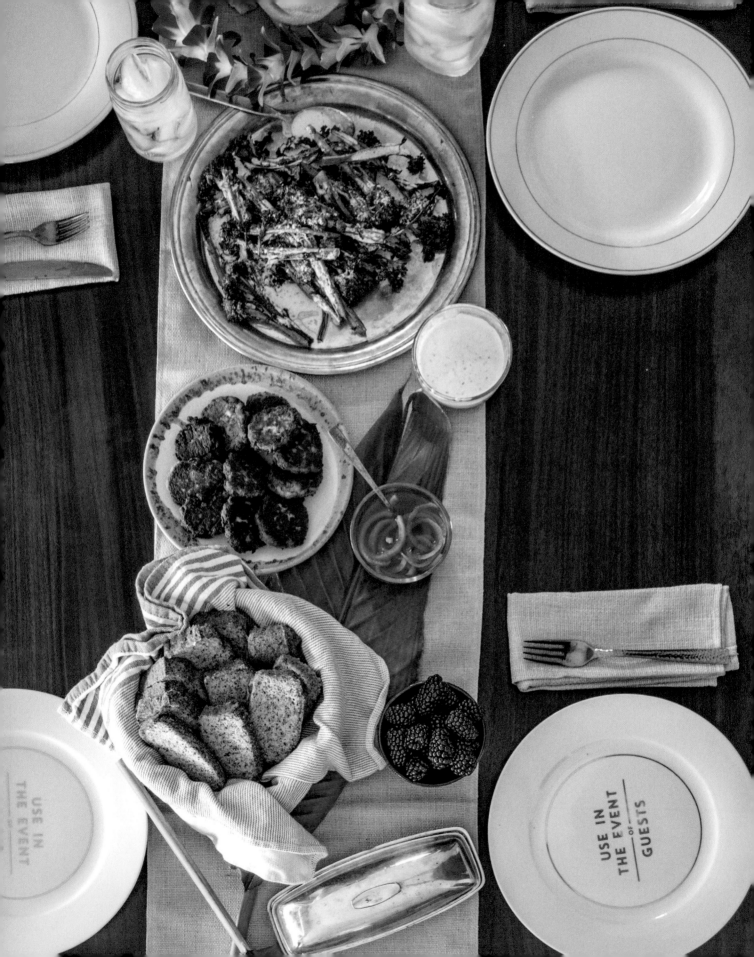

Two-Week Meal Plans

The following meal plans are all designed to feed two people for two weeks. If you'll be cooking for more people, make double batches as needed. Leftovers not used in the plan can be frozen to eat later or eaten as snacks.

Please keep in mind that these meal plans are intended as templates; you may need more or fewer calories. Make sure you're eating until you feel satisfied—this way of eating is not about deprivation! Easy ways to tweak the macros are to double or cut portion sizes or to add a drizzle of olive oil to your plate.

The shopping lists are designed for the recipes as written, so if you're modifying dishes to accommodate restrictions, please check the recipes for necessary substitutions. (The exception to this is the shopping list for the AIP meal plan, which takes into account any modifications needed to make a recipe AIP-friendly.)

Salt, pepper, and items listed as "optional" in a recipe's ingredients list are not included in the shopping lists. When a recipe lists multiple ingredients as options, only the first ingredient listed is included in the shopping list. For example, if a recipe calls for "4 cups chopped watercress, ong choy, or broccoli florets," the shopping list will include only watercress.

The shopping lists include everything called for in the recipes, so be sure to check your pantry and refrigerator to see if you already have enough of an item on hand.

kid-friendly keto

Cooking for your family when you're trying to stick to clean foods that work best for you can be a challenge. These tasty creations are kid approved, and my five-year-old isn't some foodie prodigy. He's the kid who picks the onion out of the ground beef. I've learned to make fun, tasty, uncomplicated meals he can thrive on while keeping it all Paleo and keto. After all, the whole family deserves to eat healthy, nutritious food!

Week 1 — meal plan

Monday

BREAKFAST

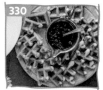
330
Mini Pumpkin Waffles with Blueberry Compote

84
8 slices Everything Bacon *(4 per person)*

LUNCH

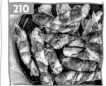
210
Prosciutto-Wrapped Chicken Tenders

322
Crispy Bacon Green Beans

DINNER

220
Chicken Katsu

230
2 servings Crispy Broccoli

82
Homemade Mayo

Fat **70%** · Carbohydrate **11%** · Protein **19%**

Tuesday

BREAKFAST

124
Smooth Chia Pudding

LUNCH

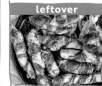
leftover
Prosciutto-Wrapped Chicken Tenders

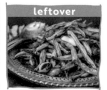
leftover
Crispy Bacon Green Beans

DINNER

246
Beef Carnitas

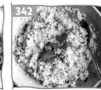
342
Creamy Cilantro Rice

2 Hass avocados *(1 per person)*

Fat **65%** · Carbohydrate **13%** · Protein **21%**

Wednesday

BREAKFAST

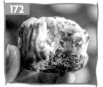
172
Mini Quiche Muffins *(2 per person)*

LUNCH

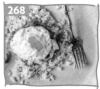
268
Lazy Moco

DINNER

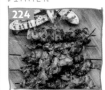
224
Chicken Satay + Grilled Zucchini with Lemon Tahini Sauce

Fat **66%** · Carbohydrate **8%** · Protein **26%**

Thursday

BREAKFAST

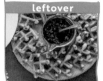

Mini Pumpkin Waffles with Blueberry Compote

4 scrambled eggs cooked in avocado oil *(2 per person)*

LUNCH

Turkey Cheeseburgers with Crispy Rainbow Slaw

DINNER

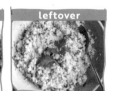

Beef Carnitas

Creamy Cilantro Rice

Fat **62%** · Carbohydrate **10%** · Protein **29%**

Friday

BREAKFAST

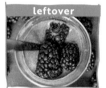

Smooth Chia Pudding

2 hard-boiled eggs *(1 per person)*

LUNCH

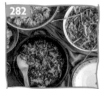

Crispy Kalua Pork + Korean Vegetable Salad

DINNER

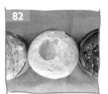

Sheet Pan Dinner: Chicken

Homemade Mayo

Fat **65%** · Carbohydrate **9%** · Protein **26%**

Saturday

BREAKFAST

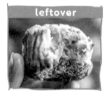

Mini Quiche Muffins *(2 per person)*

LUNCH

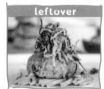

Turkey Cheeseburgers with Crispy Rainbow Slaw

2 Hass avocados *(1 per person)*

DINNER

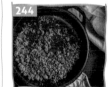

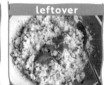

Carne Molida

Hard Cheese

Creamy Cilantro Rice

Fat **66%** · Carbohydrate **12%** · Protein **22%**

Sunday

BREAKFAST

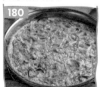

Brussels + Bacon Frittata *(2 pieces per person)*

LUNCH

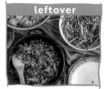

Crispy Kalua Pork + Korean Vegetable Salad

DINNER

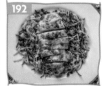

Sheet Pan Dinner: Pad Thai

2 Hass avocados *(1 per person)*

Fat **63%** · Carbohydrate **11%** · Protein **26%**

PRODUCE

blueberries, frozen, ½ cup

broccoli, 2 crowns

Brussels sprouts, 1 ⅓ pounds

cauliflower, 1 pound

cilantro, ½ cup minced

garlic, 20 cloves (about 2 heads)

ginger, 1 (½-inch) piece

green beans, 1 pound

Hass avocados, 6

lemons, 5

limes, 5

onions, 2½ large

rainbow slaw, 10 cups

riced cauliflower: 4 large heads for homemade or 5 (10-ounce) packages for store-bought

salad greens, for serving

sweet onion, 1

thyme, 3 sprigs

watercress, 4 cups chopped

zucchini, 3 small

PANTRY

bone broth, homemade (page 100) or store-bought, 3 cups

chia seeds, 3 tablespoons

cocoa powder, ¼ cup

coconut aminos, ½ cup + 1 tablespoon

coconut flour, 1 cup + 2 tablespoons

coconut milk, full-fat, 3 cups

coconut vinegar, ¼ cup + 3 tablespoons

collagen peptides, 2 tablespoons

Dijon mustard, 3 tablespoons

fish sauce, 1½ teaspoons

flaxseed meal, ¼ cup + 2 tablespoons

granulated erythritol, ¼ cup + 1 teaspoon

liquid smoke, 2 tablespoons

mayo, homemade (page 82) or store-bought, ¾ cup + 1 tablespoon

nutritional yeast, ¾ cup

poppy seeds, 1 teaspoon

pumpkin puree, 2 heaping tablespoons

pure vanilla extract, 1 teaspoon

shredded coconut, unsweetened, 1 cup + 2 tablespoons

sunflower seed butter, 2 tablespoons

tahini, 2 tablespoons

toasted sesame seeds, 1 teaspoon

unflavored grass-fed beef gelatin, 2 tablespoons

PROTEIN

bacon, 32 slices

chicken breasts, boneless, skinless, 4 pounds

chicken thighs, boneless, skinless, 3 pounds

chuck shoulder roast, 3 to 4 pounds

eggs, large, 3 dozen

ground beef, 85% lean, 3 pounds

ground turkey, 93% lean, 2 pounds

pork shoulder, bone-in, 3 pounds

prosciutto di Parma, 8 slices

DRIED HERBS + SPICES

bay leaves, 2

Chinese five-spice powder, ¼ teaspoon

dried dill weed, 1 tablespoon + 1 teaspoon

dried Italian herb blend, ½ teaspoon

dried oregano, 2 teaspoons

dried parsley, 2 teaspoons

dried thyme leaves, 1 teaspoon

garlic powder, 2 tablespoons + 1 teaspoon

ginger powder, 1 tablespoon

granulated garlic, 1 tablespoon

ground cumin, 1 tablespoon

Italian herb blend, 2 tablespoons

onion powder, 1 tablespoon + 1 teaspoon

turmeric powder, 2 teaspoons

COOKING FATS + OILS

avocado oil, ¾ cup + 1 tablespoon

bacon fat, 2 tablespoons

butter, unsalted, 3 tablespoons

coconut oil, ¾ cup + 1 tablespoon

cooking fat (any), ¼ cup + 1 tablespoon

ghee, 3 tablespoons

lard, ¼ cup + 2 tablespoons

MCT oil, 3 tablespoons

sesame oil, 1 tablespoon

toasted sesame oil, 1 tablespoon

STAPLES FROM THE BOOK

Fiesta Guacamole (page 90), for serving

Pickled Red Onions (page 88), for serving

Week's snack

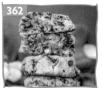

362

Chewy Chocolate Chip Cookies

Monday

BREAKFAST

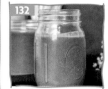

132

Chocolate Shake

LUNCH

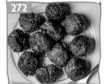

272

Sticky Pistou Meatballs

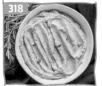

318

Creamy Cauliflower Mash

DINNER

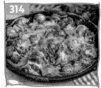

314

Little Lobster Mac Skillet

326

Everything Flaxseed Meal Crackers

Fat 61% · Carbohydrate 12% · Protein 27%   **WITH SNACK:** Fat 60% · Carbohydrate 14% · Protein 26%

Tuesday

BREAKFAST

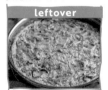

leftover

Brussels + Bacon Frittata *(2 pieces per person)*

LUNCH

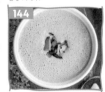

144

Creamy Broccoli Soup

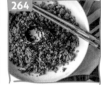

326

Everything Flaxseed Meal Crackers

DINNER

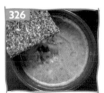

264

Protein Fried Rice

2 fried eggs *(1 per person)*

1 Hass avocado *(½ per person)*

Fat 70% · Carbohydrate 11% · Protein 19%   **WITH SNACK:** Fat 68% · Carbohydrate 13% · Protein 19%

Wednesday

BREAKFAST

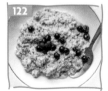

122

Protein Porridge

LUNCH

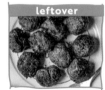

leftover

Sticky Pistou Meatballs

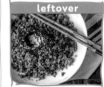

leftover

Creamy Cauliflower Mash

DINNER

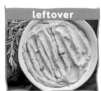

leftover

Protein Fried Rice

2 fried eggs *(1 per person)*

Fat 68% · Carbohydrate 9% · Protein 23%   **WITH SNACK:** Fat 67% · Carbohydrate 11% · Protein 23%

Thursday

BREAKFAST

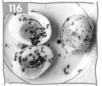

116

4 Fried Hard-Boiled Eggs *(2 per person)*

LUNCH

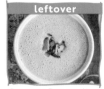

leftover

Creamy Broccoli Soup

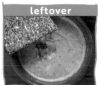

leftover

Everything Flaxseed Meal Crackers

DINNER

196

Crispy Chicken Milanese with Hollandaise

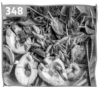

348

Spinach Salad

Fat 73% · Carbohydrate 11% · Protein 16%   **WITH SNACK:** Fat 72% · Carbohydrate 12% · Protein 16%

Friday

BREAKFAST

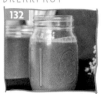

Chocolate Shake

LUNCH

Deli Skewers

Ranch Dressing

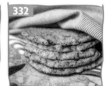

Street Taco Tortillas
(3 per person)

DINNER

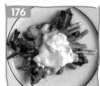

Eggs Benny

Fat 66% · Carbohydrate 12% · Protein 22%   WITH SNACK: Fat 65% · Carbohydrate 14% · Protein 21%

Saturday

BREAKFAST

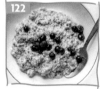

Protein Porridge

LUNCH

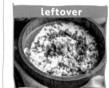

Fricase de Pollo

DINNER

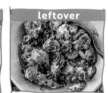

Pumpkin Chili

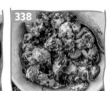

Curried Vegetable Salad

Fat 66% · Carbohydrate 10% · Protein 24%   WITH SNACK: Fat 64% · Carbohydrate 12% · Protein 23%

Sunday

BREAKFAST

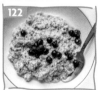

Protein Porridge

LUNCH

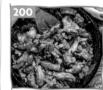

Pumpkin Chili

DINNER

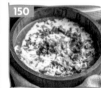

Crispy Chicken Milanese with Hollandaise

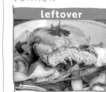

Curried Vegetable Salad

Fat 67% · Carbohydrate 11% · Protein 22%   WITH SNACK: Fat 65% · Carbohydrate 13% · Protein 22%

PRODUCE

asparagus spears, 1 pound

baby spinach, ½ pound

broccoli, 4 pounds

Brussels sprouts, ½ pound

carrots, 2 large + 2 medium

cauliflower, 2 medium heads

celery, 11 ribs (about 1½ bunches)

cilantro, ¼ cup minced

cucumber, 1 large

garlic, 27 cloves (about 2 heads)

ginger, 1 (1-inch) piece

green onions, 4

Hass avocados, 2½

lemon, 1

lime, 1

onions, 1 large + 1 medium

oregano, 2 sprigs

parsley, for garnish

radishes, 3

red onion, ½

riced cauliflower: 1 large head for homemade or 2 (10-ounce) packages for store-bought

rosemary, 2 sprigs

zucchini, 2 medium

PANTRY

apple cider vinegar, ½ cup

baking soda, ½ teaspoon

black sesame seeds, 1 teaspoon

bone broth, homemade (page 100) or store-bought, 6½ cups (52 fluid ounces)

cacao powder, ¼ cup

chia seeds, 2 tablespoons

coconut aminos, 3 tablespoons

coconut butter, 2 tablespoons

coconut cream, ½ cup + 2 tablespoons

coconut flour, 1 cup

coconut milk, full-fat, 1 cup (8 fluid ounces)

coconut vinegar, 1 tablespoon

collagen peptides, ½ cup

Dijon mustard, 1 teaspoon

fish sauce, 1 tablespoon + 1 teaspoon

flaxseed meal, 3¼ cups

granulated erythritol, ⅓ cup + 3 tablespoons + 1 teaspoon

mayo, homemade (page 82) or store-bought, ½ cup + 3 tablespoons

nutritional yeast, ¼ cup + 2 tablespoons

poppy seeds, 1 teaspoon

pumpkin puree, unsweetened, ½ cup

pure vanilla extract, 1 tablespoon

ranch dressing, homemade (page 94) or store-bought, ½ cup

red wine vinegar, 1 tablespoon

sesame seeds, 1 teaspoon

shelled hemp seeds (aka hemp hearts), ½ cup

stevia-sweetened semisweet baking chocolate, 1 (4-ounce) bar

unflavored grass-fed beef gelatin, 3 tablespoons

white vinegar, 1 tablespoon

PROTEIN

bacon, 17 slices

chicken breasts, boneless, skinless, 2 (about 1 pound)

chicken thighs, boneless, skinless, 2 pounds

eggs, 3 dozen

Genoa salami, 12 slices

ground beef, 85% lean, 3⅓ pounds

ground pork, 1 pound

precooked langostino tails, 1 pound

smoked turkey breast, 4 slices

DRIED HERBS + SPICES

bay leaves, 2

dried dill weed, 2 teaspoons

dried rosemary needles, 1 teaspoon

dry mustard, 1 teaspoon

garam masala, 1 teaspoon

garlic powder, 1 tablespoon

ginger powder, ½ teaspoon

ground cinnamon, 2 tablespoons + 2 teaspoons

ground cumin, 1 tablespoon

ground nutmeg, ¼ teaspoon

onion powder, 1 tablespoon + ½ teaspoon

turmeric powder, 1 teaspoon

COOKING FATS + OILS

avocado oil, 1 cup + 1 tablespoon

bacon fat, 2 tablespoons

butter, unsalted, ¼ cup (½ stick) + 1 tablespoon

coconut oil, 1 tablespoon

ghee, 1 cup

sesame oil, 3 tablespoons

STAPLES FROM THE BOOK

Green Goddess Dressing (page 106), ½ cup

Hollandaise (page 196), ¼ to ½ cup

Pickled Red Onions (page 88), ¼ cup

Pistou (page 74), ¼ cup + 3 tablespoons

keto reset

This meal plan is lean and mean—not for the keto newbie. I recommend trying this only after you are fat adapted because ideally you will skip breakfast or start your day with a fat-rich, satiating beverage. (The daily calories and macros include a morning beverage.) Either option will work great once you're fat adapted and your body is efficiently burning fat for energy, but until then, you might need something more substantial in the morning. These two weeks are great if you're looking to clean up your keto: no treats, no shenanigans, just serious low-carb, high-fat goodness to break a stall, quickly shed some water weight, and get the most of the fat-burning zone.

Week 1 · meal plan

Monday

BREAKFAST

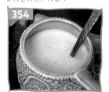
354

Fast /
Double batch
Golden Milk

LUNCH

164

Castaway Chicken
Salad

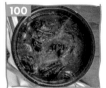
100

4 cups Bone Broth
(2 per person)

DINNER

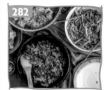
282

Crispy Kalua
Pork + Korean
Vegetable Salad

4 fried eggs
(2 per person)

Fat **65%** · Carbohydrate **5%** · Protein **30%**

Tuesday

BREAKFAST

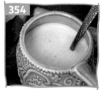
354

Fast /
Double batch
Golden Milk

LUNCH

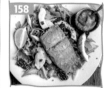
158

Broiled Salmon
Salad

DINNER

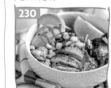
230

Chicken +
Broccoli Bowls

OIL

2 tablespoons
sesame oil
(1 per person)

Fat **68%** · Carbohydrate **6%** · Protein **26%**

Wednesday

BREAKFAST

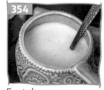
354

Fast /
Double batch
Golden Milk

LUNCH

leftover

Castaway Chicken
Salad

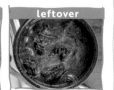
leftover

2 cups Bone Broth
(1 per person)

DINNER

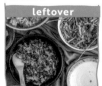
leftover

Crispy Kalua
Pork + Korean
Vegetable Salad

4 fried eggs
(2 per person)

Fat **65%** · Carbohydrate **5%** · Protein **30%**

Thursday

BREAKFAST

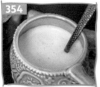
354

Fast /
Double batch
Golden Milk

LUNCH

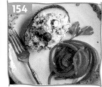
154

Salmon Salad
Avocado Boats

DINNER

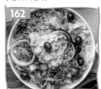
162

Taco Salad

Fat 73% · Carbohydrate 9% · Protein 18%

Friday

BREAKFAST

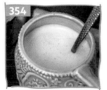
354

Fast /
Double batch
Golden Milk

LUNCH

278

Berry Bliss
Slow Cooker Pork

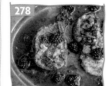
318

Creamy
Cauliflower Mash

DINNER

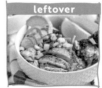
leftover

Chicken +
Broccoli Bowls

OIL

2 tablespoons sesame
oil (1 per person)

Fat 65% · Carbohydrate 7% · Protein 28%

Saturday

BREAKFAST

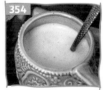
354

Fast /
Double batch
Golden Milk

LUNCH

222

Sheet Pan Dinner:
Chicken

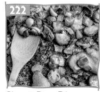
348

Spinach
Salad

DINNER

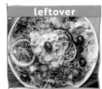
leftover

Taco Salad

Fat 66% · Carbohydrate 10% · Protein 24%

Sunday

BREAKFAST

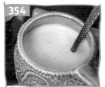
354

Fast /
Double batch
Golden Milk

LUNCH

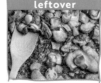
leftover

Sheet Pan Dinner:
Chicken

DINNER

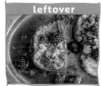
leftover

Berry Bliss
Slow Cooker Pork

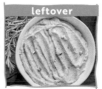
leftover

Creamy
Cauliflower Mash

OIL

1 tablespoon olive
oil (½ per person)

Fat 62% · Carbohydrate 10% · Protein 29%

Week 1

 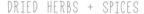

PRODUCE

arugula, ⅓ pound

baby spinach, 1½ pounds

blueberries, ¼ cup

broccoli, 2 crowns

Brussels sprouts, 1 pound

cauliflower, 1 medium head

celery, 4 ribs

garlic, 11 cloves (about 1 head)

ginger, 1 (1-inch) piece

green onions, 7

Hass avocados, 2 medium + 1 small

hearts of romaine, 4

lemons, 3

limes, 5

onion, 1 large

parsley, ¼ cup + 2 tablespoons minced

radishes, 2 ounces

raspberries, 2 cups

red onion, 1

rosemary, 2 sprigs

strawberries, 2 cups

sweet onion, 1

watercress, ⅔ pound

PANTRY

black olives, pitted, ½ cup

bone broth, homemade (page 100) or store-bought, 16 cups (128 fluid ounces)

coconut aminos, 2 tablespoons

coconut cream, ¼ cup

coconut milk, full-fat, 7 cups (56 fluid ounces)

coconut vinegar, 1 tablespoon

Dijon mustard, 2 tablespoons

fish sauce, 1 teaspoon

granulated erythritol, ¼ cup + 1 tablespoon

liquid smoke, 2 tablespoons

mayo, homemade (page 82) or store-bought, ½ cup + 3 tablespoons

nutritional yeast, ¼ cup

red wine vinegar, ¼ cup

unflavored grass-fed beef gelatin or collagen peptides, ¼ cup + 2 teaspoons

PROTEIN

bacon, 14 slices

chicken cutlets, 4

chicken thighs, boneless, skinless, 4 pounds

eggs, large, 1 dozen

ground beef, 85% lean, 2 pounds

pork chops, boneless, thick-cut, 1 pound

pork shoulder, bone-in, 3 pounds

salmon steaks, 2 (3 ounces each)

wild-caught salmon, 1 (6-ounce) can

DRIED HERBS + SPICES

dried dill weed, 1 teaspoon

dried parsley, 2 teaspoons

dried thyme leaves, 1 teaspoon

garlic powder, 1 teaspoon

granulated garlic, 1 tablespoon

ground cinnamon, 2 tablespoons + 1 teaspoon + 1 dash

ground cumin, 1 teaspoon

ground nutmeg, pinch

onion powder, 2 teaspoons

turmeric powder, ¼ cup + 1 tablespoon

COOKING FATS + OILS

avocado oil, ½ cup

bacon fat, 2 tablespoons

cooking fat (any), ¼ cup

lard, 2 tablespoons

olive oil, 1 tablespoon

sesame oil, ¼ cup + 1 tablespoon

STAPLES FROM THE BOOK

Everything Bacon (page 84), 6 slices

Fiesta Guacamole (page 90), 2 cups

Pickled Red Onions (page 88), ¼ cup

Pistou (page 74), 3 tablespoons

Raspberry Vinaigrette (page 104), ¼ cup

Monday

BREAKFAST

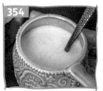

354

Fast /
Double batch
Golden Milk

LUNCH

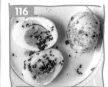

116

4 Fried Hard-Boiled
Eggs *(2 per person)*

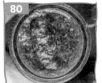

80

Chimichurri

DINNER

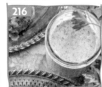

216

4 Turkey Falafel
(2 per person)

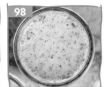

98

Tzatziki

2 cups chopped
romaine lettuce
(1 per person)

Fat **77%** · Carbohydrate **6%** · Protein **16%**

Tuesday

BREAKFAST

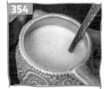

354

Fast /
Double batch
Golden Milk

LUNCH

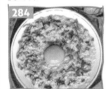

leftover

4 Turkey Falafel
(2 per person)

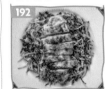

leftover

Tzatziki

2 cups chopped
romaine lettuce
(1 per person)

DINNER

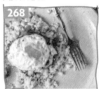

268

Lazy Moco

Fat **70%** · Carbohydrate **7%** · Protein **22%**

Wednesday

BREAKFAST

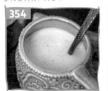

354

Fast /
Double batch
Golden Milk

LUNCH

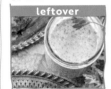

284

Cauliflower
Carbonara

DINNER

192

Sheet Pan Dinner:
Pad Thai

2 Hass avocados
(1 per person)

Fat **62%** · Carbohydrate **14%** · Protein **24%**

Thursday

BREAKFAST

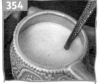

354

Fast /
Double batch
Golden Milk

LUNCH

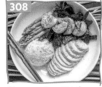

308

Deconstructed
Dragon Roll

DINNER

312

Toasted Coconut
Salmon

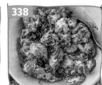

338

Curried Vegetable
Salad

Fat **70%** · Carbohydrate **10%** · Protein **20%**

Friday

BREAKFAST

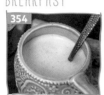

Fast /
Double batch
Golden Milk

LUNCH

128

Double batch
Cold Soup
Smoothie (with
2 tablespoons
MCT oil)

leftover

4 Turkey Falafel
(2 per person)

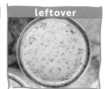
leftover

Tzatziki

DINNER

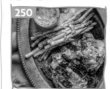
250

Churrasco +
Chimichurri

Fat **65%** · Carbohydrate **8%** · Protein **28%**

Saturday

BREAKFAST

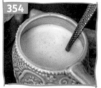
354

Fast /
Double batch
Golden Milk

LUNCH

198

Orange Chicken
Skewers

342

Creamy Cilantro
Rice

2 Hass avocados
(1 per person)

DINNER

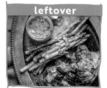
leftover

Churrasco +
Chimichurri

Fat **63%** · Carbohydrate **8%** · Protein **29%**

Sunday

BREAKFAST

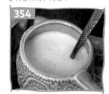
354

Fast /
Double batch
Golden Milk

LUNCH

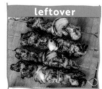
leftover

Orange Chicken
Skewers

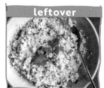
leftover

Creamy Cilantro
Rice

2 Hass avocados
(1 per person)

DINNER

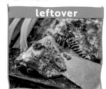
leftover

Toasted Coconut
Salmon

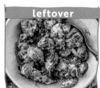
leftover

Curried Vegetable
Salad

Fat **66%** · Carbohydrate **9%** · Protein **25%**

PRODUCE

asparagus, 2½ pounds

broccoli, 1½ pounds

Brussels sprouts, ½ pound

butternut squash, 1 pound

cilantro, ½ cup minced

garlic, 24 cloves (about 2 heads)

green onion, 1

Hass avocados, 7

lemons, 8

navel orange, 1

onions, 2 large

parsley, ½ cup + 2 tablespoons minced

rainbow slaw, 4 cups

riced cauliflower: 5 large heads cauliflower for homemade or 7 (10-ounce) packages for store-bought

romaine lettuce, ½ pound

thyme, 3 sprigs

DRIED HERBS + SPICES

dried thyme leaves, 1 tablespoon

garlic powder, 1½ teaspoons

ginger powder, 1 tablespoon

ground cinnamon, 2 tablespoons + 1 teaspoon

ground cumin, 1 tablespoon + 2 teaspoons

onion powder, 1 teaspoon

turmeric powder, ¼ cup + 1 tablespoon

PANTRY

apple cider vinegar, 2 tablespoons + 2 teaspoons

black sesame seeds, 1 teaspoon

bone broth, homemade (page 100) or store-bought, 10 cups (80 fluid ounces)

coconut aminos, ½ cup

coconut butter, ¼ cup

coconut cream, ½ cup

coconut flour, ⅓ cup + 2 tablespoons

coconut milk, full-fat, 8¼ cups (66 fluid ounces)

coconut vinegar, 1 tablespoon

Dijon mustard, 2 tablespoons + 1 teaspoon

fish sauce, 1 teaspoon

granulated erythritol, ¼ cup + 1 tablespoon

mayo, homemade (page 82) or store-bought, ¼ cup + 1 tablespoon

MCT oil, 2 tablespoons

nori, 2 sheets

nutritional yeast, 1 tablespoon

sesame seeds, 1 tablespoon + 1 teaspoon

shelled hemp seeds (aka hemp hearts), ⅓ cup

shredded coconut, unsweetened, 2 tablespoons

sunflower seed butter, 2 tablespoons

tahini, 1 tablespoon

unflavored grass-fed beef gelatin, ¼ cup + 1 teaspoon

COOKING FATS + OILS

avocado oil, 10 tablespoons

bacon fat, 2 tablespoons

butter, unsalted, 2 tablespoons

coconut oil, ⅔ cup

cooking fat (any), 2 tablespoons

ghee, 3 tablespoons

olive oil, ¼ cup + 1 tablespoon

STAPLES FROM THE BOOK

Chimichurri (page 80), 1¼ cups

Tzatziki (page 98), 4 cups

PROTEIN

chicken breasts, boneless, skinless, 1 pound

chicken thighs, boneless, skinless, 2 pounds

eggs, large, 2 dozen

ground beef, 85% lean, 1 pound

ground turkey, 93% lean, 2 pounds

ham steak, boneless, ½ pound

jumbo shrimp, 8

salmon fillet, 1 large (about 1½ pounds)

skirt steak, 2 pounds

AIP

The autoimmune protocol can be daunting. Reading that long list of foods to be eliminated can often instill doubt. This meal plan takes the guesswork out of it: just follow along and before you know it, you're halfway through a month of the best elimination diet around! Rinse and repeat for a full thirty days of gut-healing, anti-inflammatory meals. Remember to add foods back in one at a time after an elimination diet. Reintroduction is where the magic happens. (See page 23 for more on AIP.)

Week 1 — meal plan

Week's snack

132

Chocolate Shake, made with carob powder

Monday

BREAKFAST

358

Double batch Coconut Butter Matcha Latte

LUNCH

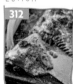

138

Roasted Vegetable Soup

2 tablespoons olive oil *(1 per person)*

DINNER

230

Chicken + Broccoli Bowls

72

Toum

Fat 73% · Carbohydrate 10% · Protein 17%   WITH SNACK: Fat 69% · Carbohydrate 13% · Protein 18%

Tuesday

BREAKFAST

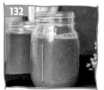

280

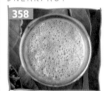

70

Double batch Pork Sausage *with substitutions (save half the mix for Thursday dinner)*

8 slices Hard Cheese *with substitutions (4 per person)*

LUNCH

312

334

Toasted Coconut Salmon

Loaded Roasted Carrots *with substitutions*

DINNER

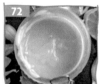

244

Double batch Carne Molida *with substitutions*

342

Creamy Cilantro Rice *with substitutions*

1 Hass avocado *(½ per person)*

Fat 63% · Carbohydrate 13% · Protein 24%   WITH SNACK: Fat 60% · Carbohydrate 16% · Protein 25%

Wednesday

BREAKFAST

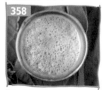

358

Double batch Coconut Butter Matcha Latte

LUNCH

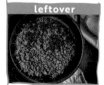

leftover

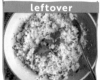

leftover

Carne Molida

Creamy Cilantro Rice

2 Hass avocados *(1 per person)*

DINNER

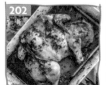

202

Cristina's Roast Chicken *with substitutions*

250

Seared Asparagus

Fat 71% · Carbohydrate 11% · Protein 18%   WITH SNACK: Fat 67% · Carbohydrate 13% · Protein 20%

Thursday

BREAKFAST

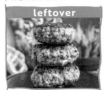

Pork Sausage

2 Hass avocados, mashed *(1 per person)*

LUNCH

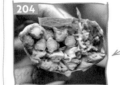

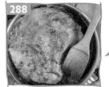

Collard Chicken Wraps *with substitutions, made with leftover* Cristina's Roast Chicken

DINNER

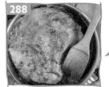

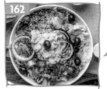

Cabbage + Sausage Casserole *with substitutions, made with leftover* Pork Sausage

Fat **69%** · Carbohydrate **8%** · Protein **24%**　　WITH SNACK: Fat **65%** · Carbohydrate **11%** · Protein **25%**

Friday

BREAKFAST

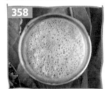

Double batch Coconut Butter Matcha Latte

LUNCH

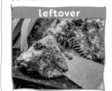

Toasted Coconut Salmon

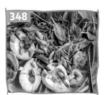

Loaded Roasted Carrots *with substitutions*

Spinach Salad

DINNER

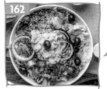

Taco Salad *with substitutions, made with leftover* Carne Molida

Fat **69%** · Carbohydrate **13%** · Protein **18%**　　WITH SNACK: Fat **65%** · Carbohydrate **15%** · Protein **20%**

Saturday

BREAKFAST

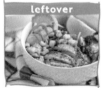

Chicken + Broccoli Bowls

LUNCH

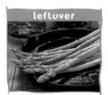

Cristina's Roast Chicken

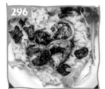

Seared Asparagus

DINNER

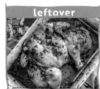

Shrimp + Grits *with substitutions*

2 Hass avocados *(1 per person)*

Fat **64%** · Carbohydrate **9%** · Protein **27%**　　WITH SNACK: Fat **61%** · Carbohydrate **12%** · Protein **27%**

Sunday

BREAKFAST

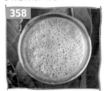

Double batch Coconut Butter Matcha Latte

LUNCH

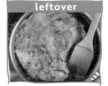

Cabbage + Sausage Casserole

DINNER

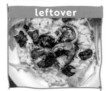

Shrimp + Grits

¼ cup avocado oil *(2 tablespoons per person)*

Fat **73%** · Carbohydrate **8%** · Protein **19%**　　WITH SNACK: Fat **68%** · Carbohydrate **11%** · Protein **21%**

Week 1

PRODUCE

arugula, for garnish

asparagus, 2 pounds

baby Brussels sprouts, 3 ounces

baby spinach, 1 pound

broccoli, 18 ounces

cabbage, ¼ medium head

carrots, 10 medium (8 with greens)

cauliflower, 2 large heads

celery, 5 ribs

cilantro, 1 cup

collard leaves, 4 large

garlic, 35 cloves (about 2½ heads)

ginger, 1 (2-inch) piece

green onions, 4

Hass avocados, 9

hearts of romaine, 4

lemongrass, 4 stalks

lemons, 8

limes, 4

radish sprouts

red onion, ½

riced cauliflower: 3 large heads for homemade or 3 (10-ounce) packages for store-bought

rosemary, 1 teaspoon minced

savoy cabbage, 1 large head

PANTRY

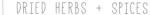

AIP-compliant sweetener (see page 23), ¼ cup + 2 teaspoons

black olives, pitted, ½ cup

bone broth, homemade (page 100) or store-bought, 3 cups (24 fluid ounces)

carob powder, ¾ cup + 2 tablespoons

coconut aminos, 3 tablespoons

coconut butter, 1¼ cups + 3 tablespoons

coconut milk, full-fat, ½ cup

collagen peptides, 1¾ cups

fish sauce, 2 tablespoons

matcha tea powder, 2 tablespoons + 2 teaspoons

nutritional yeast, ¼ cup + 1 tablespoon

pure vanilla extract, 2 tablespoons + 2 teaspoons

PROTEIN

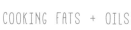

bacon, 5 slices

chicken, 1 whole (4 to 5 pounds)

chicken thighs, boneless, skinless, 8 (about 2 pounds)

ground beef, 85% lean, 4 pounds

ground pork, 4 pounds

salmon fillet, 1 large (about 1½ pounds)

shrimp, 1 pound (preferably tail-on)

DRIED HERBS + SPICES

dried cilantro, 1 teaspoon

dried dill weed, 1 teaspoon

dried parsley, 1 tablespoon + 1 teaspoon

dried thyme leaves, 1 tablespoon + 1 teaspoon

ginger powder, 1 teaspoon

granulated garlic, 2 tablespoons

ground cinnamon, ½ cup + 2 tablespoons

onion powder, 1 tablespoons + 2 teaspoons

COOKING FATS + OILS

avocado oil, ¾ cup

coconut oil, ¼ cup + 3 tablespoons

cooking fat (any), 2 tablespoons

extra-virgin olive oil, 2 cups

lard, ¼ cup + 2 tablespoons

olive oil, ¼ cup + 2 tablespoons

STAPLES FROM THE BOOK

Chimichurri (page 80), ¼ cup

Fiesta Guacamole (page 90), 2 cups

Hard Cheese (page 70), 8 slices

Pistou, AIP-compliant version (page 74), 3 tablespoons

Toum (page 72), ¼ cup

Week's snack

380

Double batch Coconut Caramel Slice *with substitutions*

Monday

BREAKFAST

96

Coconut Yogurt

1 cup fresh blueberries *(½ cup per person)*

LUNCH

222

Sheet Pan Dinner: Chicken *with substitutions*

1 Hass avocado *(½ per person)* with 2 tablespoons olive oil *(1 per person)*

DINNER

262

Gyro Skillet Sausages *with substitutions*

98

Tzatziki *with substitutions*

2 cups chopped romaine lettuce *(1 per person)*

Fat **64%** · Carbohydrate **12%** · Protein **25%**   WITH SNACK: Fat **65%** · Carbohydrate **13%** · Protein **22%**

Tuesday

BREAKFAST

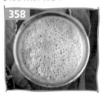

358

Double batch Coconut Butter Matcha Latte

LUNCH

264

Protein Fried Rice *with substitutions*

DINNER

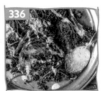

214

Vietnamese Crispy Chicken *with substitutions*

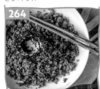

336

Spiced Broccolini with Cool Cilantro Sauce *with substitutions*

Fat **68%** · Carbohydrate **8%** · Protein **24%**   WITH SNACK: Fat **69%** · Carbohydrate **10%** · Protein **21%**

Wednesday

BREAKFAST

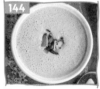

144

Creamy Broccoli Soup *with substitutions*

2 tablespoons olive oil *(1 per person)*

LUNCH

leftover

Sheet Pan Dinner: Chicken

DINNER

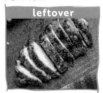

leftover

Vietnamese Crispy Chicken

leftover

Spiced Broccolini with Cool Cilantro Sauce

Fat **64%** · Carbohydrate **9%** · Protein **27%**   WITH SNACK: Fat **65%** · Carbohydrate **10%** · Protein **25%**

Thursday

BREAKFAST

leftover

Coconut Yogurt

1 cup fresh blueberries *(½ cup per person)*

LUNCH

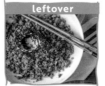

leftover

Protein Fried Rice

2 Hass avocados *(1 per person)*

DINNER

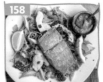

158

Broiled Salmon Salad *with substitutions*

leftover

Tzatziki *with substitutions*

Fat **73%** · Carbohydrate **12%** · Protein **15%**   WITH SNACK: Fat **74%** · Carbohydrate **13%** · Protein **14%**

Friday

BREAKFAST

Gyro Skillet
Sausages

Tzatziki *with substitutions*

1 Hass avocado
(½ per person)

LUNCH

Double batch
Cold Soup
Smoothie

8 slices
Everything
Bacon
(4 per person)

DINNER

Churrasco +
Chimichurri

1 Hass avocado
(½ per person)

Fat **65**% · Carbohydrate **7**% · Protein **27**%   WITH SNACK: Fat **67**% · Carbohydrate **9**% · Protein **25**%

Saturday

BREAKFAST

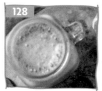 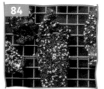

Double batch
Cold Soup
Smoothie

8 slices Everything
Bacon
(4 per person)

LUNCH

 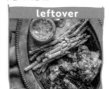

Pan-Seared
Cod *(cook only
2 fillets, halve
seasonings)*

Spinach
Salad

DINNER

Churrasco +
Chimichurri

Fat **64**% · Carbohydrate **7**% · Protein **29**%   WITH SNACK: Fat **65**% · Carbohydrate **8**% · Protein **26**%

Sunday

BREAKFAST

Creamy Broccoli
Soup

¼ cup olive oil
*(2 tablespoons
per person)*

LUNCH

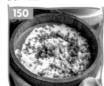

Pumpkin Chili
with substitutions

DINNER

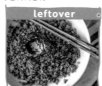

Protein Fried Rice

Spinach
Salad

Fat **73**% · Carbohydrate **8**% · Protein **20**%   WITH SNACK: Fat **73**% · Carbohydrate **9**% · Protein **18**%

PRODUCE

arugula, ⅓ pound

asparagus, 1¼ pounds

baby spinach, ½ pound

blueberries, 1 pint

broccoli, 2½ pounds

broccolini, 1 pound 2 ounces (about 4 cups)

Brussels sprouts, 1 pound

butternut squash, 1 pound

celery, 7 ribs

cilantro, 1¼ cups chopped

garlic, 14 cloves (about 1 head)

ginger, 1 (1-inch) piece

green onions, 6

Hass avocados, 7

lemongrass, 4 stalks

lemons, 4

limes, 2

onions, 2 large + 1 medium + 1 small

parsley, ½ cup chopped + 1 sprig

radishes, 3

riced cauliflower: ½ large head cauliflower for homemade or 1 (10-ounce) package for store-bought

romaine lettuce, ⅓ pound

PANTRY

AIP-compliant sweetener (see page 23), ¼ cup + 2 tablespoons

apple cider vinegar, 2 tablespoons + 2 teaspoons

bone broth, homemade (page 100) or store-bought, 11 cups (88 fluid ounces)

carob powder, ¼ cup + 2 tablespoons

coconut aminos, ¼ cup + 2 tablespoons

coconut butter, ¼ cup

coconut cream, 1 cup + 1 tablespoon

coconut flour, 2 tablespoons

coconut milk, full-fat, additive-free, 3 cups

fish sauce, 2 tablespoons + 1 teaspoon

live-culture probiotics, dairy-free, 2 capsules

matcha tea powder, 2 teaspoons

nutritional yeast, ¼ cup

pumpkin puree, unsweetened, ½ cup

pure vanilla extract, 2 teaspoons

shredded coconut, unsweetened, 2 cups

unflavored grass-fed beef gelatin, 1 tablespoon + 2 teaspoons

PROTEIN

bacon, 10 slices

chicken thighs, bone-in, with skin, 8

chicken thighs, boneless, skinless, 2 pounds

cod fillets, boneless, skinless, 2 (6 ounces each)

ground beef, 85% lean, 3 pounds

ground lamb, 1 pound

ground pork, 1 pound

salmon steaks, 2 (3 ounces each)

skirt steak, 1 pound

DRIED HERBS + SPICES

dried dill weed, 1 tablespoon + 1 teaspoon

dried oregano, 1 tablespoon

dried thyme leaves, 1 tablespoon

garlic powder, 1 teaspoon

ginger powder, 1 tablespoon + 1½ teaspoons

granulated garlic, 2 teaspoons

ground cinnamon, 1 tablespoon + ½ teaspoon

onion powder, 1 tablespoon + 1 teaspoon

turmeric powder, 1 tablespoon

COOKING FATS + OILS

avocado oil, ¼ cup

bacon fat, ¼ cup + 2 tablespoons

coconut oil, ½ cup + 3 tablespoons

cooking fat (any), ¼ cup + 1 tablespoon

garlic-infused avocado oil, 3 tablespoons

olive oil, 1 cup

STAPLES FROM THE BOOK

Chimichurri (page 80), ½ cup

Coconut Yogurt (page 96), 2 cups

Everything Bacon, AIP-compliant version (page 84), 22 slices

Garlic Confit (page 76), ½ tablespoon

Pistou, AIP-compliant version (page 74), 3 tablespoons

Raspberry Vinaigrette (page 104), ¼ cup

cook once, eat twice

This is for the busy home chef who still likes to cook, but not every night! This meal plan has you cooking larger batches of food every two days and enjoying leftovers in between. It's flexible enough that you can move things around easily to follow your heart (or stomach), but it has enough structure to keep you on plan without too much work!

Week 1 — meal plan

Monday

BREAKFAST

Butter Coffee
352

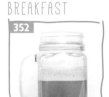
8 Baked Scotch Eggs *(1 per person; store remainder for leftovers)*
178

LUNCH

Multinational Beef + Rice
238

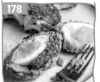
2 Hass avocados *(1 per person)*

DINNER

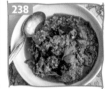
Salmon Zoodle Casserole
306

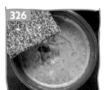
Everything Flaxseed Meal Crackers
326

Fat 69% · Carbohydrate 12% · Protein 19%

Tuesday

BREAKFAST

Butter Coffee
352

2 Baked Scotch Eggs *(1 per person)*
leftover

LUNCH

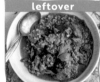
Multinational Beef + Rice
leftover

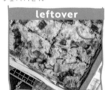
Everything Flaxseed Meal Crackers
leftover

DINNER

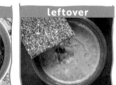
Salmon Zoodle Casserole
leftover

1 Hass avocado *(½ per person)*

Fat 68% · Carbohydrate 11% · Protein 20%

Wednesday

BREAKFAST

Butter Coffee
352

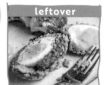
2 Baked Scotch Eggs *(1 per person)*
leftover

LUNCH

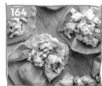
Castaway Chicken Salad
164

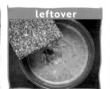
Everything Flaxseed Meal Crackers
leftover

DINNER

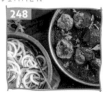
Spaghetti + Meatballs
248

1 Hass avocado *(½ per person)*

Fat 67% · Carbohydrate 9% · Protein 25%

Thursday

BREAKFAST

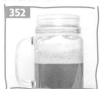

352

Butter Coffee

leftover

2 Baked Scotch Eggs *(1 per person)*

LUNCH

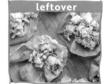

leftover

Castaway Chicken Salad

DINNER

leftover

Spaghetti + Meatballs

1 Hass avocado *(½ per person)*

Fat 67% · Carbohydrate 7% · Protein 26%

Friday

BREAKFAST

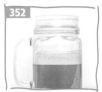

352

Butter Coffee

12 hard-boiled eggs *(2 per person; store remainder for leftovers)*

LUNCH

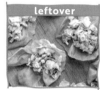

leftover

Castaway Chicken Salad

DINNER

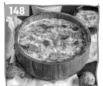

148

Thai Coconut Soup with 8 jumbo shrimp

Fat 71% · Carbohydrate 5% · Protein 24%

Saturday

BREAKFAST

352

Butter Coffee

4 hard-boiled eggs *(2 per person; use eggs cooked on Friday)*

LUNCH

leftover

Salmon Zoodle Casserole

DINNER

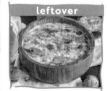

leftover

Thai Coconut Soup with shrimp

1 Hass avocado *(½ per person)*

Fat 73% · Carbohydrate 8% · Protein 19%

Sunday

BREAKFAST

352

Butter Coffee

4 hard-boiled eggs *(2 per person; use eggs cooked on Friday)*

LUNCH

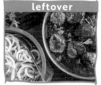

leftover

Spaghetti + Meatballs *(make additional zoodles if needed)*

DINNER

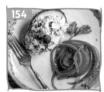

154

Double batch Salmon Salad Avocado Boats

Fat 70% · Carbohydrate 8% · Protein 22%

PRODUCE

baby bella mushrooms, 1 pound

basil, 3 to 4 sprigs

blueberries, ¼ cup

celery, 12 ribs

cilantro, ¼ cup minced

cremini mushrooms, 5

garlic, 16 cloves (about 1 head)

ginger, 1 (2-inch) piece

green onions, 4

Hass avocados, 7

lemongrass, 2 stalks

limes, 2

onion, 1 large

parsley, 2 tablespoons minced + more for garnish

radishes, 2 ounces

red onion, 1

riced cauliflower: 1 medium head cauliflower for homemade or 1 (10-ounce) package for store-bought

strawberries, 1 pint

thyme, 2 sprigs

zucchini, 2 large + 2 medium

PANTRY

apple cider vinegar, ½ cup

bone broth, homemade (page 100) or store-bought, 4 cups (32 fluid ounces)

coconut aminos, 2 tablespoons

coconut milk, full-fat, 2 (13.5-ounce) cans

Dijon mustard, ¼ cup

fish sauce, 2 tablespoons

flaxseed meal, 2 cups

ground coffee, 1¾ cups (for 14 cups brewed)

kelp noodles, 1 (12-ounce) package

mayo, homemade (page 82) or store-bought, ½ cup + 3 tablespoons

MCT oil, ¼ cup + 3 tablespoons

poppy seeds, 1 teaspoon

red wine vinegar, 2 tablespoons

sesame seeds, 1 teaspoon

shelled hemp seeds (aka hemp hearts), ¼ cup

sunflower seed butter, 2 tablespoons

PROTEIN

bacon, 18 slices

chicken cutlets, 4

eggs, large, 2 dozen

ground beef, 85% lean, 2 pounds

ground pork, 2 pounds

stew meat, 1 pound

wild-caught salmon, boneless, skinless, 4 (6-ounce) cans

DRIED HERBS + SPICES

celery salt, ¼ teaspoon

dried dill weed, 2 teaspoons

dried rosemary needles, 1 teaspoon

dried thyme leaves, 1 teaspoon

garam masala, 1½ teaspoons

garlic powder, 1 teaspoon

ginger powder, 1¼ teaspoons

ground cinnamon, ½ cup

ground nutmeg, ½ teaspoon + pinch

Italian herb blend, 2 tablespoons

COOKING FATS + OILS

avocado oil, 5 tablespoons

butter, unsalted, ¾ cup + 2 tablespoons

STAPLES FROM THE BOOK

Cauliflower Alfredo (page 86), 3 cups

Pickled Red Onions (page 88), for serving, ¼ cup

Roasted Beet Marinara (page 78), 3 cups

Monday

BREAKFAST

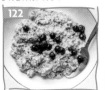

122

Double batch
Protein Porridge

LUNCH

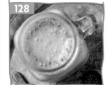

128

Double batch
Cold Soup
Smoothie

DINNER

260

Party Meatballs

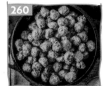

348

Spinach Salad

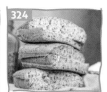

324

2 slices Nut-Free
Keto Bread
(1 per person)

Fat 71% · Carbohydrate 11% · Protein 18%

Tuesday

BREAKFAST

leftover

Protein Porridge

LUNCH

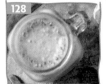

128

Double batch
Cold Soup
Smoothie

leftover

2 slices Nut-Free
Keto Bread
(1 per person)

DINNER

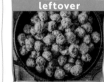

leftover

Party Meatballs

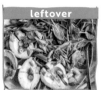

leftover

Spinach Salad

Fat 71% · Carbohydrate 11% · Protein 18%

Wednesday

BREAKFAST

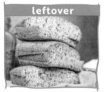

leftover

4 slices
Nut-Free Keto
Bread, toasted
(2 per person)

1 Hass avocado
(½ per person),
4 fried eggs
(2 per person)

LUNCH

114

Deli Skewers

DINNER

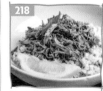

218

Shredded
Jerk Chicken

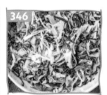

346

Crunchy Asian
Salad

Fat 69% · Carbohydrate 9% · Protein 22%

Thursday

BREAKFAST

352

Butter Coffee

4 fried eggs
(2 per person)

LUNCH

leftover

Party Meatballs

leftover

Crunchy Asian
Salad

DINNER

leftover

Shredded
Jerk Chicken

318

Creamy
Cauliflower
Mash

1 Hass
avocado
(½ per person)

Fat 68% · Carbohydrate 8% · Protein 24%

Friday

BREAKFAST

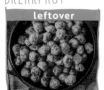
leftover

Party Meatballs

1 Hass avocado (½ per person), 4 fried eggs (2 per person)

LUNCH

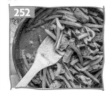
252

Suya Stir-Fry

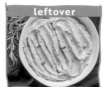
leftover

Creamy Cauliflower Mash

DINNER

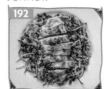
192

Sheet Pan Dinner: Pad Thai

Fat 62% · Carbohydrate 13% · Protein 26%

Saturday

BREAKFAST

352

Butter Coffee

4 fried eggs (2 per person)

LUNCH

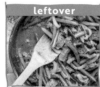
leftover

Sheet Pan Dinner: Pad Thai

DINNER

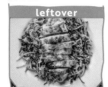
leftover

Suya Stir-Fry

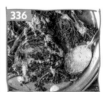
336

Spiced Broccolini with Cool Cilantro Sauce

Fat 63% · Carbohydrate 12% · Protein 26%

Sunday

BREAKFAST

352

Butter Coffee

4 fried eggs (2 per person)

LUNCH

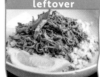
leftover

Shredded Jerk Chicken

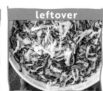
leftover

Crunchy Asian Salad

DINNER

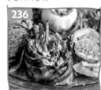
236

Flank Steak Pinwheels

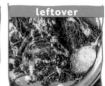
leftover

Spiced Broccolini with Cool Cilantro Sauce

Fat 64% · Carbohydrate 7% · Protein 29%

Week 2 shopping list

PRODUCE

baby spinach, ½ pound

basil, 2 sprigs

broccoli, ½ pound

broccolini, 1 pound 2 ounces (about 4 cups)

butternut squash, 1 pound

cauliflower, 1 medium head

cilantro, 1 cup chopped + 4 sprigs

cucumber, 1 large

garlic, 16 cloves (about 1 head)

ginger, 1 (1-inch) piece

green beans, 1 pound

green cabbage, ¼ medium head

green onions, 4

Hass avocados, 4 large

lemons, 3

limes, 4

onion, 1 large + 1 medium

oregano, 6 sprigs

rainbow slaw, 4 cups

red cabbage, ¼ medium head

rosemary, 2 sprigs

thyme, 3 sprigs

DRIED HERBS + SPICES

Chinese five-spice powder, 1 teaspoon

dried dill weed, 2 teaspoons

dried parsley, 2 teaspoons

dried thyme, 1 teaspoon

garam masala, 1 teaspoon

garlic powder, 2 tablespoons + ½ teaspoon

ginger powder, 1 tablespoon

ground cinnamon, ¼ cup

ground cloves, ¼ teaspoon

onion powder, 2 teaspoons

turmeric powder, 1 teaspoon

PANTRY

apple cider vinegar, 1 tablespoon + 1 teaspoon

baking powder, 1 teaspoon

bone broth, homemade (page 100) or store-bought, 3½ cups (28 fluid ounces)

chia seeds, 2 tablespoons

coconut aminos, ½ cup

coconut cream, ¼ cup

coconut flour, ⅓ cup

coconut milk, full-fat, 1 cup

Dijon mustard, 2 tablespoons

flaxseed meal, ¼ cup + 2 tablespoons

granulated erythritol, 2 tablespoons

ground coffee, ¾ cup (for 6 cups brewed)

mayo, homemade (page 82) or store-bought, ⅔ cup

MCT oil, 3 tablespoons

nutritional yeast, 1 tablespoon

pure vanilla extract, 2 teaspoons

raw pumpkin seeds, 2 tablespoons

red wine vinegar, 2 tablespoons

shelled hemp seeds (aka hemp hearts), ½ cup

shredded coconut, unsweetened, 2 tablespoons

sunflower seed butter, 2 tablespoons

whole flax seeds, 2 tablespoons

COOKING FATS + OILS

avocado oil, ¾ cup

bacon fat, 2 tablespoons

butter, salted, 3 tablespoons

butter, unsalted, ¼ cup + 2 tablespoons

coconut oil, 1½ cups

STAPLES FROM THE BOOK

Cheesy Yellow Sauce (page 68), ¼ cup

Coconut Yogurt (page 96), ⅔ cup

Green Goddess Dressing (page 106), ½ cup

Pistou (page 74), 3 tablespoons

PROTEIN

bacon, thick-cut, 6 to 8 slices

chicken breasts, boneless, skinless, 1 pound

chicken thighs, boneless, skinless, 2 pounds

eggs, large, 3 dozen

flank steak, 1 to 1½ pounds

Genoa salami, 12 slices

ground beef, 85% lean, 2 pounds

smoked turkey breast, 4 slices

tri-tip steak, 1 pound

Recommended Brands

APPLIANCES
Cuisinart, Breville, Vitamix

SKILLETS
Lodge (cast iron) and Cuisinart Multiclad

BUTTER

Kerrygold

CACAO POWDER, CHIA SEEDS, COLLAGEN, MATCHA, MCT OIL
Wild Foods

COCONUT FLOUR

Anthony's Goods, Bob's Red Mill

COCONUT MILK
365 Brand Organic, Thai Kitchen, Hawaiian Sun Frozen Additive-Free

COCONUT VINEGAR AND COCONUT AMINOS
Coconut Secret

CONDIMENTS, SALAD DRESSINGS, MARINADES, AND AVOCADO OIL

Primal Kitchen

DARK CHOCOLATE
Lily's, Alter Eco Dark Blackout

FISH SAUCE
Red Boat

GELATIN
Vital Proteins, Now Foods, Great Lakes

GHEE
Tin Star, 4th and Heart

MCT POWDER
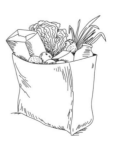
Perfect Keto

NUTRITIONAL YEAST
Braggs

OLIVE OIL

California Olive Ranch

RAINBOW SLAW
Mann's Veggies Made Easy

SHELLED HEMP SEEDS
Manitoba Harvest

SWEETENER (GRANULATED ERYTHRITOL)
Ketologie Sweet Like Sugar

Recommended Store

Barefoot Provisions is great for avocado oil, MCT powder, beef jerky, and more!

Special Thanks

Thank you to my amazing husband, Justin, who picked up all the slack as I cooked and typed away for hours on end and who is my number-one taste-tester and cheerleader. Your unwavering support and love mean everything to me.

To Kyndra Holley, who took a chance on an internet friend and made my dreams of writing a cookbook come true. Your support and guidance have been everything to me. You're an amazing person and friend.

To the amazing team at Victory Belt Publishing, for taking a chance on a first-time author. For everything you have taught me and for working with me to create the book of my dreams.

To my neighbor Darylin, who practically adopted Jack. I don't know how many hours Jack spent playing at your house. I'm so grateful for your friendship, and for the one our children share as well.

To my mother, who taught me how to cook and shared her contagious passion for life with me. You are my hero.

To my sisters, for inspiring me and pushing me to grow and evolve.

To all of my blog and social media followers, readers, and friends: Thank you for being the most caring, loving, and just sweetest community. I appreciate all of you so much.

About the Author

Cristina Curp is the one-woman show behind *The Castaway Kitchen*, a blog dedicated to delicious foods and healing diets. In the last few years, through dedicated self-experimentation, Cristina has healed her body from leaky gut, put her autoimmune disease into remission, and lost over 60 pounds.

Cristina holds a BA in anthropology from Florida International University and has over six years of commercial kitchen experience. Using her restaurant chef skills and love for food, she now creates recipes to help others find health and happiness through keto, Paleo, and AIP lifestyles!

Her mission is to spread the word that food is thy medicine, and it should taste damn good. As a military spouse and mom on the move, staying healthy is a must. From Hawaii to Washington, DC, you can find her in the kitchen, on a hike with her schnauzer, Bruce, or sipping butter coffee on her porch with her husband, Justin, and their son, Jack.

Staples Index

All the dishes in the Staples chapter are used in other recipes throughout the book. The lists below include all the recipes that have a particular staple in the ingredients list, but there are many more options! Check out the variations and substitution boxes for more ways you can use these essentials.

Cheesy Yellow Sauce

Creamy Kale Noodles (page 320)

Egg Tart (page 182)

Flank Steak Pinwheels (page 236)

Savory Meat Pie (page 234)

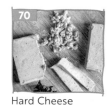

Hard Cheese

Turkey Cheeseburgers with Crispy Rainbow Slaw (page 212)

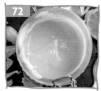

Toum

Chicken Kofta Kebabs (page 206)

Tender Kale Salad (page 344)

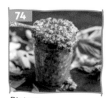

Pistou

Egg Roll-ups (page 186)

Spinach Salad (page 348)

Sticky Pistou Meatballs (page 272)

Zucchini Latkes (page 120)

Garlic Confit

Braised Pork Chops with Creamy Green Beans (page 290)

Camarones Enchilados (page 304)

Castaway Chicken Salad (page 164)

"Corn" Chowder (page 142)

Garlic Mayo (page 82)

Garlicky Golden Cauliflower (page 350)

Pan-Seared Cod (page 300)

Smoky Shrimp Omelet (page 184)

Tender Kale Salad (page 344)

Roasted Beet Marinara

Calamari Two Ways (page 298)

Camarones Enchilados (page 304)

Multinational Beef + Rice (page 238)

Prosciutto Chips (page 78)

Slow Cooker Arroz con Pollo (page 208)

Spaghetti + Meatballs (page 248)

Zucchini Latkes (page 120)

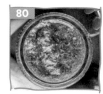

Chimichurri

Put it on everything!

Chicken Kofta Kebabs (page 206)

Churrasco + Chimichurri (page 250)

Herb Mayo (page 82)

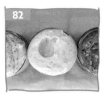

Homemade Mayo

Castaway Chicken Salad (page 164)

Collard Chicken Wraps (page 204) [Beet Mayo variation]

Creamy Broccoli Soup (page 144)

Creamy Cilantro Rice (page 342)

Curried Crab Cake Salad (page 156)

Curried Vegetable Salad (page 338)

Prosciutto-Wrapped Chicken Tenders (page 210)

Pumpkin Chili (page 150)

Salmon Salad Avocado Boats (page 154)

Spiced Broccolini with Cool Cilantro Sauce (page 336)

Tender Kale Salad (page 344)

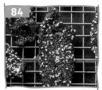

Everything Bacon

Eat them on their own as a snack or add to any dish!

Broiled Salmon Salad (page 158)

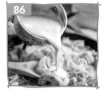

Cauliflower Alfredo

Egg Tart (page 182)

Salmon Zoodle Casserole (page 306)

Shrimp Linguine (page 310)

Spinach Alfredo Chicken Bake (page 194)

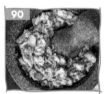

Pickled Red Onions

Beef Carnitas (page 246)

Camarones Enchilados (page 304)

Curried Crab Cake Salad (page 156)

Half-Sour Pickled Salad (page 340)

Kailua Breakfast Bowl (page 170)

Little Lobster Mac Skillet (page 314)

Salmon Salad Avocado Boats (page 154)

Taco Salad (page 162)

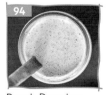

Fiesta Guacamole

Beef Carnitas (page 246)

Party Meatballs (page 260)

Taco Salad (page 162)

Pie Crust

Coconut Citrus Tart (page 366)

Egg Tart (page 182)

Savory Meat Pie (page 234)

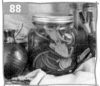

Ranch Dressing

Excellent on any salad!

Chicken Caesar Lettuce Cups (page 160)

Party Meatballs (page 260)

Coconut Yogurt

Cortado Panna Cotta (page 368)

Kailua Breakfast Bowl (page 170)

Multinational Beef + Rice (page 238)

Parfaits (page 130)

Spiced Broccolini with Cool Cilantro Sauce (page 336)

Tzatziki (page 98)

Zucchini Latkes (page 120)

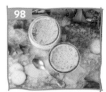

Tzatziki

Turkey Falafel (page 216)

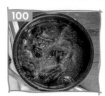
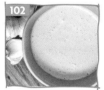

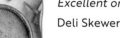
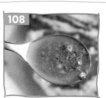

Recipe Index

Staples, Sauces + Dressings

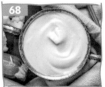
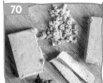

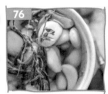

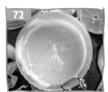
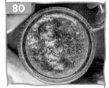
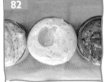
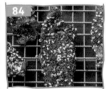
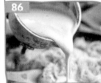
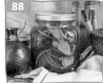
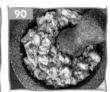
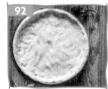
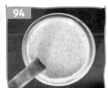
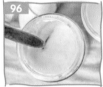
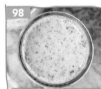
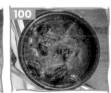
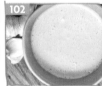
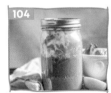
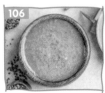
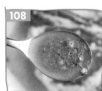

Snacks + Small Bites

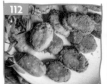
112 Croquetas de Jamón

114 Deli Skewers

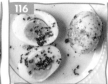
116 Fried Hard-Boiled Eggs

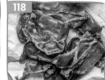
118 Prosciutto Chips

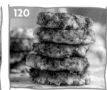
120 Zucchini Latkes

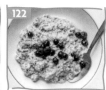
122 Protein Porridge

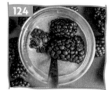
124 Smooth Chia Pudding

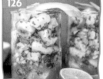
126 Ceviche

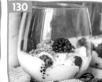
128 Cold Soup Smoothie

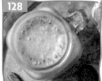
130 Parfaits

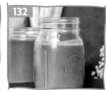
132 Chocolate Shake

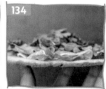
134 Crispy Thin Flatbread

Soups + Salads

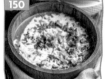
138 Roasted Vegetable Soup

140 Feel-Good Soup

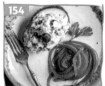
142 "Corn" Chowder

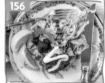
144 Creamy Broccoli Soup

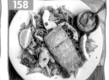
146 Egg Drop Soup

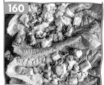
148 Thai Coconut Soup

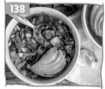
150 Pumpkin Chili

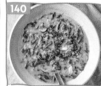
152 Chicken + Dumpling Soup

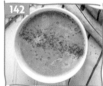
154 Salmon Salad Avocado Boats

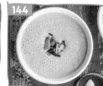
156 Curried Crab Cake Salad

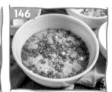
158 Broiled Salmon Salad

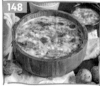
160 Chicken Caesar Lettuce Cups

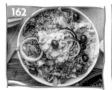
162 Taco Salad

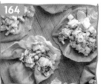
164 Castaway Chicken Salad

Mains

Eggs

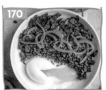
170 Kailua Breakfast Bowl

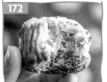
172 Mini Quiche Muffins

174 Crispy Eggs + Cabbage

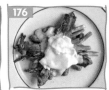
176 Eggs Benny

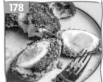
178 Baked Scotch Eggs

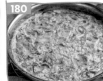
180 Brussels + Bacon Frittata

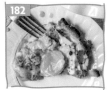
182 Egg Tart

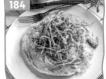
184 Smoky Shrimp Omelet

186 Egg Roll-ups

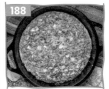
188 Persian Herb Frittata

Poultry

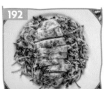
192 Sheet Pan Dinner: Pad Thai

194 Spinach Alfredo Chicken Bake

196 Crispy Chicken Milanese with Hollandaise

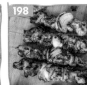
198 Orange Chicken Skewers

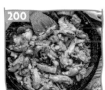
200 Fricase de Pollo

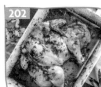
202 Cristina's Roast Chicken

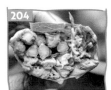
204 Collard Chicken Wraps

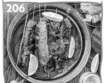
206 Chicken Kofta Kebabs

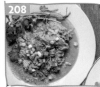
208 Slow Cooker Arroz con Pollo

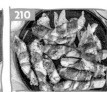
210 Prosciutto-Wrapped Chicken Tenders

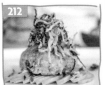
212 Turkey Cheeseburgers with Crispy Rainbow Slaw

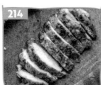
214 Vietnamese Crispy Chicken

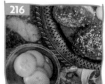 216
Turkey Falafel

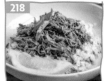 218
Shredded Jerk Chicken

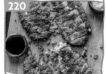 220
Chicken Katsu

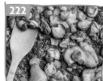 222
Sheet Pan Dinner: Chicken

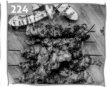 224
Chicken Satay + Grilled Zucchini with Lemon Tahini Sauce

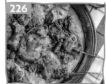 226
Coconut-Braised Curried Chicken

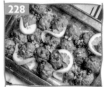 228
Herbed Turkey Meatballs with Lemon Caper Sauce

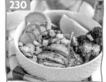 230
Chicken + Broccoli Bowls

Beef + Lamb

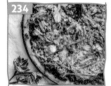 234
Savory Meat Pie

 236
Flank Steak Pinwheels

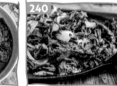 238
Multinational Beef + Rice

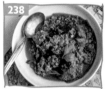 240
Vaca Frita

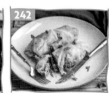 242
Stuffed Cabbage, Dolmas-Style

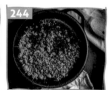 244
Carne Molida

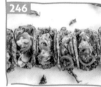 246
Beef Carnitas

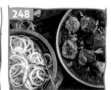 248
Spaghetti + Meatballs

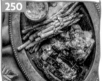 250
Churrasco + Chimichurri

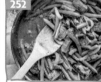 252
Suya Stir-Fry

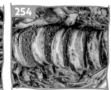 254
Bacon-Wrapped Meatloaf

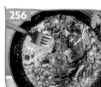 256
Braised Short Ribs

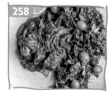 258
Saucy Seasoned Liver

 260
Party Meatballs

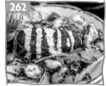 262
Gyro Skillet Sausages

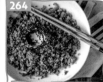 264
Protein Fried Rice

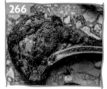 266
Pan-Seared Rib-Eye with Arugula

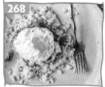 268
Lazy Moco

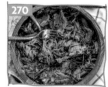 270
Slow Cooker Shawarma

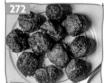 272
Sticky Pistou Meatballs

Pork

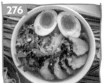
Pork Char Siu +
Ramen
276

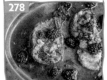
Berry Bliss
Slow Cooker Pork
278

Pork Sausage
280

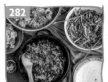
Crispy Kalua Pork +
Korean Vegetable
Salad
282

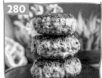
Cauliflower
Carbonara
284

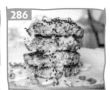
Scallion Pork
Patties with
Ginger Sauce
286

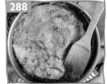
Cabbage + Sausage
Casserole
288

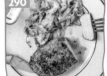
Braised Pork Chops
with Creamy
Green Beans
290

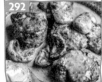
Spiced Pork
Tenderloin with
Rustic Mushroom
Sauce
292

Seafood + Fish

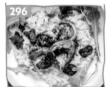
Shrimp + Grits
296

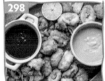
Calamari Two Ways
298

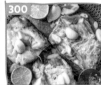
Pan-Seared Cod
300

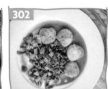
Seared Golden
Scallops with Wilted
Bacon Spinach
302

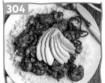
Camarones
Enchilados
304

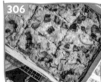
Salmon Zoodle
Casserole
306

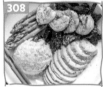
Deconstructed
Dragon Roll
308

Shrimp Linguine
310

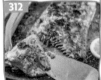
Toasted Coconut
Salmon
312

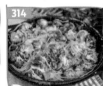
Little Lobster Mac
Skillet
314

Sides + Beverages

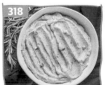
Creamy Cauliflower
Mash
318

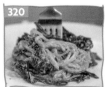
Creamy Kale
Noodles
320

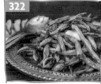
Crispy Bacon
Green Beans
322

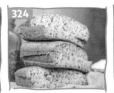
Nut-Free Keto
Bread
324

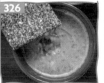
Everything Flaxseed
Meal Crackers
326

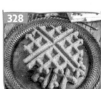
Savory Flax Waffles
328

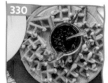
330
Mini Pumpkin Waffles with Blueberry Compote

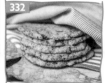
332
Street Taco Tortillas

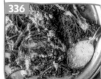
334
Loaded Roasted Carrots

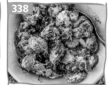
336
Spiced Broccolini with Cool Cilantro Sauce

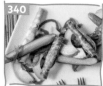
338
Curried Vegetable Salad

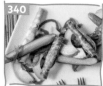
340
Half-Sour Pickled Salad

342
Creamy Cilantro Rice

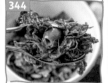
344
Tender Kale Salad

346
Crunchy Asian Salad

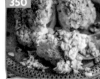
348
Spinach Salad

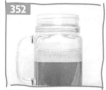
350
Garlicky Golden Cauliflower

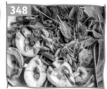
352
Butter Coffee

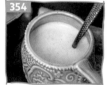
354
Golden Milk

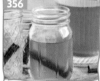
356
Korean Cinnamon Tea

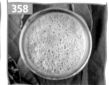
358
Coconut Butter Matcha Latte

Treats

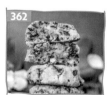
362
Chewy Chocolate Chip Cookies

364
Key Lime Pie Pots de Crème

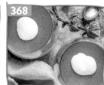
366
Coconut Citrus Tart

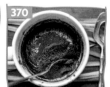
368
Cortado Panna Cotta

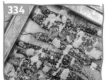
370
Chocolate Pudding Mug Cake

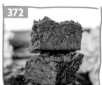
372
Flourless Brownies

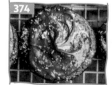
374
Dark Chocolate Muffins with Chocolate Ganache

376
Egg-Free Vanilla Spice Cookies

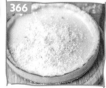
378
Super Seed Slice

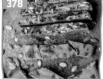
380
Coconut Caramel Slice

Allergen Index

RECIPE	PAGE	AIP	🥚	🥥	🌱
Cheesy Yellow Sauce	68	✓	✓	*	✓
Hard Cheese	70	✓	✓	*	✓
Toum	72	✓	✓	✓	✓
Pistou	74	*	✓	✓	*
Garlic Confit	76	✓	✓	✓	✓
Roasted Beet Marinara	78	*	✓	✓	✓
Chimichurri	80	✓	✓	✓	✓
Homemade Mayo	82			*	✓
Everything Bacon	84	*	✓	✓	*
Cauliflower Alfredo	86	*	✓	*	✓
Pickled Red Onions	88	✓	✓	✓	✓
Fiesta Guacamole	90	✓	✓	✓	✓
Pie Crust	92				✓
Ranch Dressing	94	*	✓		
Coconut Yogurt	96	✓	✓		✓
Tzatziki	98	*	✓		✓
Bone Broth	100	✓	✓	*	✓
Ginger Sauce	102	*	✓		*
Raspberry Vinaigrette	104	*	✓	✓	*
Green Goddess Dressing	106	*	✓		*
Greek Marinade + Dressing	108	*	✓	✓	✓
Croquetas de Jamón	112				✓
Deli Skewers	114	*	✓	*	*
Fried Hard-Boiled Eggs	116		✓		
Prosciutto Chips	118	*	✓	✓	✓
Zucchini Latkes	120				✓
Protein Porridge	122		*		
Smooth Chia Pudding	124		✓	*	
Ceviche	126	*	✓	✓	✓
Cold Soup Smoothie	128	✓	✓	✓	✓
Parfaits	130		✓		
Chocolate Shake	132	*	✓	✓	✓
Crispy Thin Flatbread	134				✓
Roasted Vegetable Soup	138	✓	✓		✓
Feel-Good Soup	140	*	✓		✓
"Corn" Chowder	142	*	✓		✓
Creamy Broccoli Soup	144	*	✓	✓	✓
Egg Drop Soup	146	*	*		✓
Thai Coconut Soup	148	✓	✓		✓
Pumpkin Chili	150	*	*	*	✓
Chicken + Dumpling Soup	152	*			✓
Salmon Salad Avocado Boats	154	*	*	✓	✓
Curried Crab Cake Salad	156		*	✓	*
Broiled Salmon Salad	158	*	✓	✓	*
Chicken Caesar Lettuce Cups	160	*	*	✓	*
Taco Salad	162	*	✓	✓	✓
Castaway Chicken Salad	164	*		✓	✓
Kailua Breakfast Bowl	170				✓
Mini Quiche Muffins	172				
Crispy Eggs + Cabbage	174			✓	✓
Eggs Benny	176				
Baked Scotch Eggs	178			✓	*
Brussels + Bacon Frittata	180			*	✓

* modification available

RECIPE	PAGE	AIP			
Egg Tart	182				✓
Smoky Shrimp Omelet	184			✓	✓
Egg Roll-ups	186			*	*
Persian Herb Frittata	188			✓	✓
Sheet Pan Dinner: Pad Thai	192	*	✓		*
Spinach Alfredo Chicken Bake	194	✓	✓	*	✓
Crispy Chicken Milanese with Hollandaise	196				✓
Orange Chicken Skewers	198	*	✓	✓	✓
Fricase de Pollo	200	*	✓	✓	✓
Cristina's Roast Chicken	202	*	✓		*
Collard Chicken Wraps	204	*	*	✓	✓
Chicken Kofta Kebabs	206	*	✓		*
Slow Cooker Arroz con Pollo	208	*	✓	✓	*
Prosciutto-Wrapped Chicken Tenders	210	*	*	✓	✓
Turkey Cheeseburgers with Crispy Rainbow Slaw	212	*	✓	*	✓
Vietnamese Crispy Chicken	214	*	✓		✓
Turkey Falafel	216	*	✓		*
Shredded Jerk Chicken	218		✓		✓
Chicken Katsu	220				✓
Sheet Pan Dinner: Chicken	222	*	✓		✓
Chicken Satay + Grilled Zucchini with Lemon Tahini Sauce	224	*	✓		*
Coconut-Braised Curried Chicken	226	*	✓	*	✓
Herbed Turkey Meatballs with Lemon Caper Sauce	228	*	*	*	✓
Chicken + Broccoli Bowls	230	*	✓	✓	✓
Savory Meat Pie	234		*		✓
Flank Steak Pinwheels	236	*	✓	*	✓
Multinational Beef + Rice	238	*	✓	✓	*
Vaca Frita	240	✓	✓	✓	✓
Stuffed Cabbage, Dolmas-Style	242	*	✓	✓	✓
Carne Molida	244	*	✓	✓	✓
Beef Carnitas	246	*	✓		✓
Spaghetti + Meatballs	248	*	✓	✓	*
Churrasco + Chimichurri	250	✓	✓	✓	✓
Suya Stir-Fry	252		✓		
Bacon-Wrapped Meatloaf	254	*	✓	✓	*
Braised Short Ribs	256	*	✓	✓	✓
Saucy Seasoned Liver	258	*	✓	✓	✓
Party Meatballs	260	*	*	✓	✓
Gyro Skillet Sausages	262	*	*		✓
Protein Fried Rice	264	*	✓		*
Pan-Seared Rib-Eye with Arugula	266	✓	✓	✓	✓
Lazy Moco	268	*	*		✓
Slow Cooker Shawarma	270		✓	✓	✓
Sticky Pistou Meatballs	272	*	✓	✓	*
Pork Char Siu + Ramen	276			*	*
Berry Bliss Slow Cooker Pork	278	*	✓	✓	✓
Pork Sausage	280	*	✓	✓	✓
Crispy Kalua Pork + Korean Vegetable Salad	282	*	✓		
Cauliflower Carbonara	284			*	✓
Scallion Pork Patties with Ginger Sauce	286	*	*		*
Cabbage + Sausage Casserole	288	*	✓	✓	✓
Braised Pork Chops with Creamy Green Beans	290	*	*		✓
Spiced Pork Tenderloin with Rustic Mushroom Sauce	292	*	*	*	✓

* modification available

RECIPE	PAGE	AIP	Egg-Free	Coconut-Free	Nut-Free
Shrimp + Grits	296	*	✓	*	✓
Calamari Two Ways	298	*	*		✓
Pan-Seared Cod	300	✓	✓	✓	✓
Seared Golden Scallops with Wilted Bacon Spinach	302	*	✓		✓
Camarones Enchilados	304	*	✓		✓
Salmon Zoodle Casserole	306	*	*		✓
Deconstructed Dragon Roll	308	*	✓	*	*
Shrimp Linguine	310	*	✓	*	✓
Toasted Coconut Salmon	312	✓	✓		
Little Lobster Mac Skillet	314	*	*	*	✓
Creamy Cauliflower Mash	318	*	*	*	✓
Creamy Kale Noodles	320	*	✓	*	✓
Crispy Bacon Green Beans	322		✓	✓	✓
Nut-Free Keto Bread	324				
Everything Flaxseed Meal Crackers	326		✓	✓	
Savory Flax Waffles	328				
Mini Pumpkin Waffles with Blueberry Compote	330				✓
Street Taco Tortillas	332		✓		
Loaded Roasted Carrots	334	*	✓	*	*
Spiced Broccolini with Cool Cilantro Sauce	336	*	*		✓
Curried Vegetable Salad	338			✓	✓
Half-Sour Pickled Salad	340	✓	✓	✓	✓
Creamy Cilantro Rice	342	*	*	*	✓
Tender Kale Salad	344	✓	✓	✓	✓
Crunchy Asian Salad	346	✓	✓		✓
Spinach Salad	348	*	✓	✓	*
Garlicky Golden Cauliflower	350	*	✓	✓	✓
Butter Coffee	352	*	✓	✓	✓
Golden Milk	354	*	✓	*	✓
Korean Cinnamon Tea	356	*	✓	✓	✓
Coconut Butter Matcha Latte	358	✓	✓		✓
Chewy Chocolate Chip Cookies	362				✓
Key Lime Pie Pots de Crème	364		✓		
Coconut Citrus Tart	366				✓
Cortado Panna Cotta	368		✓		✓
Chocolate Pudding Mug Cake	370				
Flourless Brownies	372			*	
Dark Chocolate Muffins with Chocolate Ganache	374			*	✓
Egg-Free Vanilla Spice Cookies	376		✓		
Super Seed Slice	378		✓		
Coconut Caramel Slice	380	*	✓		✓

* modification available

General Index